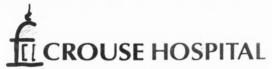

SPORTS MEDICINE CONDITIONS
RETURN TO PLAY:
RECOGNITION, TREATMENT, PLANNING

SPORTS MEDICINE CONDITIONS

RETURN TO PLAY:

RECOGNITION, TREATMENT, PLANNING

EDITORS

MARK D. MILLER, MD

S. Ward Casscells Professor of Orthopaedic Surgery
Head, Division of Sports Medicine
University of Virginia
Team Physician
James Madison University
Charlottesville, Virginia

A. BOBBY CHHABRA, MD

Charles J. Frankel Professor and Vice Chair
Department of Orthopaedic Surgery
Professor of Plastic Surgery
University of Virginia Health System
Charlottesville, Virginia

JEFF KONIN, PhD, ATC, PT, FACSM, FNATA

Department of Orthopaedic Surgery
University of Virginia Health System
Charlottesville, Virginia

DILAAWAR MISTRY, MD, MS, ATC

Primary Care Team Physician, Colorado Rockies
(Grand Junction)
Team Physician, USA Swimming
Western Orthopedics and Sports Medicine
Grand Junction, Colorado

ASSOCIATE EDITORS

JUSTIN W. GRIFFIN, MD

Resident Physician
Department of Orthopaedic Surgery
University of Virginia Health System
Charlottesville, Virginia

SIOBHAN M. STATUTA, MD, CAQSM

Director
Primary Care Sports Medicine Fellowship
Assistant Professor
Family Medicine and Physical Medicine & Rehabilitation
Team Physician, UVA Sports Medicine
University of Virginia Health System
Charlottesville, Virginia

SECTION EDITORS

BRIAN BUSCONI, MD

Associate Professor
Department of Orthopedics & Physical
Rehabilitation
Division of Sports Medicine
University of Massachusetts Medical School
Worcester, Massachusetts

A. BOBBY CHHABRA, MD

Charles J. Frankel Professor and Vice Chair
Department of Orthopaedic Surgery
Professor of Plastic Surgery
University of Virginia Health System
Charlottesville, Virginia

MARK D. MILLER, MD

S. Ward Casscells Professor of Orthopaedic Surgery
Head, Division of Sports Medicine
University of Virginia
Team Physician
James Madison University
Charlottesville, Virginia

DILAAWAR MISTRY, MD, MS, ATC

Primary Care Team Physician, Colorado Rockies
(Grand Junction)
Team Physician, USA Swimming
Western Orthopedics and Sports Medicine
Grand Junction, Colorado

JOSEPH S. PARK, MD

Assistant Professor
Division Head, Foot and Ankle Service
Department of Orthopaedic Surgery
University of Virginia Health System
Charlottesville, Virginia

FRANCIS H. SHEN, MD

Warren G. Stamp Professor of Orthopaedic
Surgery
Division Head, Spine Division
Director Spine Fellowship
Co-Director, Spine Center
University of Virginia Medical Center
Charlottesville, Virginia

 Wolters Kluwer | Lippincott Williams & Wilkins
Health

Philadelphia · Baltimore · New York · London
Buenos Aires · Hong Kong · Sydney · Tokyo

Acquisitions Editor: Brian Brown
Product Manager: David Murphy
Production Manager: David Saltzberg
Manufacturing Manager: Beth Welsh
Design Manager: Doug Smock
Production Service: Aptara, Inc.

Printed in China

Library of Congress Cataloging-in-Publication Data
Sports medicine conditions : return to play : recognition, treatment, planning / editors, Mark D. Miller, A. Bobby Chhabra, Jeff Konin, Dilaawar Mistry ; associate editors, Justin W. Griffin, Siobhan M. Statuta, Brian Busconi, A. Bobby Chhabra, Mark D. Miller, Dilaawar Mistry, Joseph S. Park, Francis H. Shen.
    p. ; cm.
  Includes bibliographical references and index.
  ISBN 978-1-4511-2103-2 (alk. paper)
  I. Miller, Mark D., editor. II. Chhabra, Anikar, editor. III. Konin, Jeff G., editor. IV. Mistry, Dilaawar J., editor. V. Griffin, Justin W., editor.
  [DNLM: 1. Athletic Injuries–diagnosis. 2. Athletic Injuries–rehabilitation. 3. Patient Care Planning. 4. Sports Medicine–methods. QT 261]
  RD97
  617.1′027–dc23   2013024675

To all athletes who are seeking a better understanding of their injury and their ability to Return to Play—and to all health care providers who are anxious to provide it.

—*Mark D. Miller*

To my loving family for their unwavering support. To Mark D. Miller for opening so many doors for me.

—*Bobby Chhabra*

To my wife Carter, for her loving endurance and pivotal insight. And to my mentor, Dr. Mark Miller, a true pioneer in Sports Medicine whose contagious creativity continues to teach me the sustained sense of wonder found in helping others Return to Play.

—*Justin W. Griffin*

To Mark D. Miller, for allowing me to be his wing man and teaching what dedication and commitment is all about.

—*Jeff Konin*

For my wife Kelly, whose endless patience is an indefinable inspiration and a gift.

—*Dilaawar Mistry*

Thank you to my amazing wife, Ann Marie, for her patience and guidance throughout the years. And to Isabelle and Stephen, who have learned that dad has to spend way too much time away from them to "fix bones." I am also eternally grateful to my parents, teachers, and mentors for their wisdom and encouragement. I am truly humbled to have been involved in this project.

—*Joseph S. Park*

To my daughter Mia who's vivid imagination and creativity always reminds me that the possibilities are endless.

—*Francis H. Shen*

To my father—Thomas, who instilled in me a passion for life-long learning. To my husband—Jason, children—Annabelle and Thomas, and mother—Martha for their endless love and support. Lastly, to Dr. Danny Mistry for his teaching, mentoring, and most importantly, friendship.

—*Siobhan M. Statuta*

CONTRIBUTORS

BRIAN BUSCONI, MD
Associate Professor
Department of Orthopedics & Physical
    Rehabilitation
Division of Sports Medicine
University of Massachusetts Medical School
Worcester, Massachusetts

A. BOBBY CHHABRA, MD
Charles J. Frankel Professor and Vice Chair
Department of Orthopaedic Surgery
Professor of Plastic Surgery
University of Virginia Health System
Charlottesville, Virginia

APRIL DUE, DO
Lieutenant United States Navy
Intern
Fort Belvoir Army Community Hospital
Fort Belvoir, Virginia

SCOTT A. EISENHUTH, MD
Captain, USAF
Chief of Orthopaedic Surgery
Keesler AFB
Bilouxi, Mississippi

JUSTIN W. GRIFFIN, MD
Resident Physician
Department of Orthopaedic Surgery
University of Virginia Health System
Charlottesville, Virginia

MARK D. MILLER, MD
S. Ward Casscells Professor of Orthopaedic
    Surgery
Head, Division of Sports Medicine
University of Virginia
Team Physician
James Madison University
Charlottesville, Virginia

JOSEPH S. PARK, MD
Assistant Professor
Division of Head, Foot and Ankle Service
Department of Orthopaedic Surgery
University of Virginia Health System
Charlottesville, Virginia

FRANCIS H. SHEN, MD
Warren G. Stamp Professor of Orthopaedic
    Surgery
Division Head, Spine Division
Director Spine Fellowship
Co-Director, Spine Center
University of Virginia Medical Center
Charlottesville, Virginia

**SIOBHAN M. STATUTA, MD,
CAQSM**
Director
Primary Care Sports Medicine Fellowship
Assistant Professor
Family Medicine and Physical Medicine &
    Rehabilitation
Team Physician, UVA Sports Medicine
University of Virginia Health System
Charlottesville, Virginia

JON VIVOLO, MS
Rocky Mountain Vista University
Parker, Colorado

DAVID B. WEISS, MD
Assistant Professor
Department of Orthopaedic Surgery
University of Virginia Health System
Charlottesville, Virginia

PREFACE

Several years ago, my colleague and friend, Dr. Jeff Konin, approached me about the concept of creating a stand-alone textbook that could be used by certified athletic trainers, physical therapist orthopedic health care professionals, and patients alike that addressed the most common musculoskeletal injuries and conditions in athletes. Because I firmly believe the adage that *a picture is worth a thousand words* (especially in our field), I pushed hard to include "composite figures" to illustrate each entity. Many years, two publishers, several illustrators and numerous editors later, we have finally succeeded! Each "chapter" stands alone but uses a common format:

- Surgical Indications and Goals
- Procedure and Technique
- Postsurgical Precautions and Rehabilitation
- Expected Outcomes
- Return to Play
- Selected References
- Relevant Figure(s)

Dr. Konin and I quickly realized that we could not complete this project on our own, so we brought in some very talented experts to help us out. It is impossible to acknowledge everyone involved, but I would be remiss if I did not highlight the following individuals (in alphabetical order):

- Dr. Bill Athans, medical student at USF at the time, who helped with the foot and ankle section.
- Dr. Brian Busconi, who we brought in late to assist with the Hip and Pelvis chapters.
- Dr. A. Bobby Chhabra who was responsible for much of the elbow/wrist/hand chapters. He was assisted by Dr. Scott A. Eisenhuth, one of our former star residents at UVA who is now at Keesler AFB in Bilouxi, Miss.
- Dr. Justin Griffin, one of our fine UVA residents with an interest in Sports Medicine. His role as an Associate Editor included manuscript and figure review and organization.
- Dr. Jeff Konin, who wrote all of the rehabilitation sections and contributed greatly to the development and production of the entire text.
- Dr. German Maralunda, a spine fellow at Florida Orthopaedic Institute who assisted with the spine chapters.

- Dr. Dilaawar (Danny) Mistry who was responsible for the Primary Care chapters.
- Dr. Joseph Park who assisted with many of the Foot and Ankle chapters. He was assisted by Dr. MaCalus Hogan, a UVA resident at the time, who has moved on to become a Foot and Ankle specialist at the University of Pittsburgh.
- Dr. Frank Shen who was responsible for the Spine chapters.
- Dr. Siobhan Statuta (also an Associate Editor) who worked directly with Dr. Mistry in completing the Primary Care chapter.
- Dr. David Weiss who assisted with many of the fracture figures and text throughout the book.

There were many, many people at Lippincott Williams & Wilkins/Wolters Kluwer Health and their consultants (most notably the firm responsible for most of the beautiful artwork included in this text, Synapse Studios) to thank. Some of these outstanding men and women, including Mr. Jack Haley, Ms. Elise Paxson, Mr. Mark Myktuik, and others, have moved on, but their assistance was invaluable. Hats off to Ruchira Gupta and Abhishan Sharma of Aptara and especially to Mr. Dave Murphy (Product Manager) who finally brought this book to publication.

This project became much larger than Dr. Konin and I first envisioned—and much better! Although I struggled with it at times, I am especially pleased with the Primary Care section that Drs. Mistry and Statuta developed. I must admit that those chapters have been very helpful for me.

The publisher has been very kind in giving me permission to use the wonderful illustrations in this book in many of my presentations and projects that I am lucky enough to be asked to participate in. I am especially looking forward to using this book in the orthopaedic clinic, athletic training room, and physical therapy centers—to educate my patients and athletes alike.

Mark D. Miller, MD
S. Ward Casscells Professor
Department of Orthopaedic Surgery
University of Virginia
Team Physician
James Madison University
Editor in Chief, Return to Play

CONTENTS

SPORTS MEDICINE CONDITIONS

RETURN TO PLAY:

RECOGNITION, TREATMENT, PLANNING

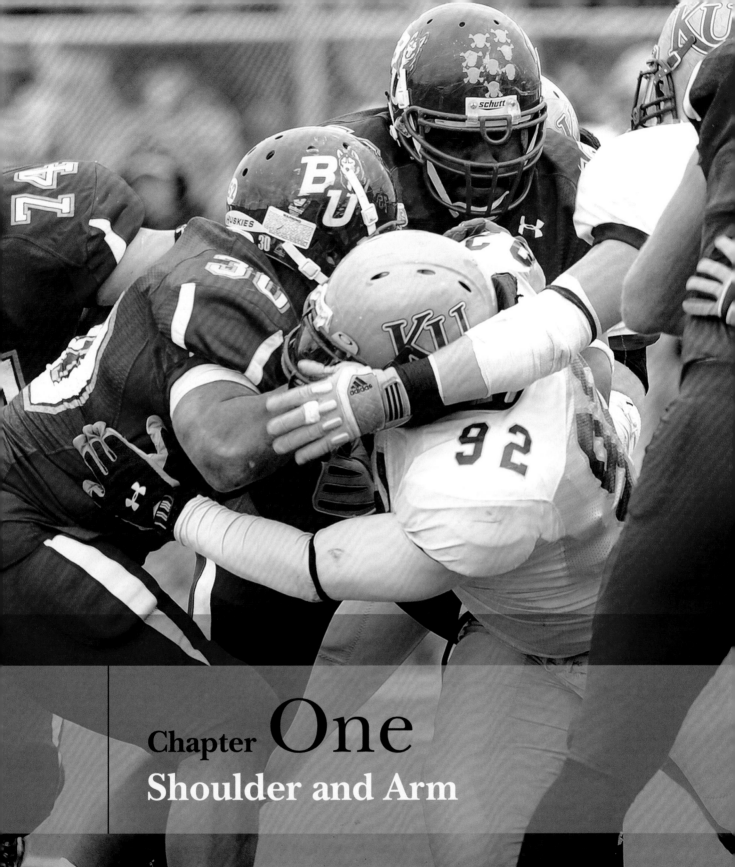

Chapter One
Shoulder and Arm

Shoulder Arthroscopy

Indications and Goals: Shoulder arthroscopy has probably had more advancements than anything in all of orthopaedic sports medicine in the last 10 years. Originally used only for diagnostic assistance, shoulder arthroscopy can be used to address a variety of injuries including instability, superior labral (SLAP) tears, and rotator cuff repair. The advantages of arthroscopy over open procedures include smaller incisions, less pain (allowing outpatient surgery), and quicker rehabilitation.

Procedures and Technique: There are two ways to perform shoulder arthroscopy, beach chair and lateral decubitus. For the beach chair technique, the patient is placed supine in a sitting position, and traction is typically not used. For the lateral decubitus technique, patients are placed on their side with the injured shoulder up and traction (typically 10 to 15 pounds) is used to distract the joint. The arthroscope is introduced from a posterior portal (2 cm distal and 2 cm medial to the posterolateral corner of the acromion) and probing/instrument insertion is done through an anterior superior portal (just anterior to the AC-joint). A variety of additional portals can be made depending upon the procedure. A systematic evaluation of the joint is carried out and all areas in the glenohumeral joint and subacromial space can be evaluated and treated. It is often very helpful to move the arthroscope to different portals (especially the anterior superior portal for glenohumeral visualization and lateral portal for subacromial/rotator cuff visualization). Instruments typically used in shoulder arthroscopy include various motorized shavers and burrs, handheld biters and graspers, and devices used to pass sutures through tissue.

Post-surgical Precautions/Rehabilitation: Depending upon the procedure done, patients are typically placed in a sling and encouraged to do elbow motion and pendulum exercises early. The type of rehabilitation involved following a shoulder arthroscopy depends upon whether or not the tissue was repaired or removed. If the procedure involves removing or debriding tissue without any repair, then acute rehabilitation can focus on pain relief and scar management at the portal sites. Range of motion can begin immediately, with supervision needed based upon the extent of the procedure performed and the confidence in the patient's/athlete's compliance. Strengthening exercise can begin within a few days. All exercises can use pain limitations as a guide for progression, but one should be careful not to be overly cautious and end up with adhesive capsulitis. Full active range of motion and functional strength should be restored within a few weeks. If the procedure involved a repair, then care should be taken to avoid placing too much stress on the repaired tissue until adequate and safe healing has occurred. More specific guidelines would depend upon which tissue was involved and the status of the tissue that is being repaired.

Expected Outcomes: The time frame for rehabilitation progression will depend upon the specific tissue that is repaired and the stability of the repair. Numerous procedures can be performed arthroscopically at the glenohumeral joint, thus outcomes will vary based upon the procedure.

Return to Play: This depends upon the procedure. In general, if the procedure does not involve soft tissue repair (e.g., debridement or acromioplasty), then the rehabilitation and return to play is relatively short. For most repairs (labrum, rotator cuff, etc.), return to play is often 4 to 6 months or more.

Recommended Readings

Carson WG. Arthroscopy of the shoulder: Anatomy and technique. *Orthop Rev.* 1992; 21(2):143–153.

Faber E, Kuiper JI, Burdorf A, Miedema HS, Verhaar JA. Treatment of impingement syndrome: A systematic review of the effects on functional limitations and return to work. *J Occup Rehabil.* 2006;16(1):7–25.

Lenters TR, Franta AK, Wolf FM, Leopold SS, Matsen FA 3rd. Arthroscopic compared with open repairs for recurrent anterior shoulder instability. A systematic review and meta-analysis of the literature. *J Bone Joint Surg Am.* 2007;89(2):244–254. Review.

Mazzocca AD, Cole BJ, Romeo AA. Shoulder: Patient positioning, portal placement, and normal arthroscopic anatomy. In: Miller MD, Cole BJ, eds. *Textbook of Arthroscopy.* Philadelphia, PA: Saunders; 2004.

Mohtadi NG, Bitar IJ, Sasyniuk TM, Hollinshead RM, Harper WP. Arthroscopic versus open repair for traumatic anterior shoulder instability: A meta-analysis. *Arthroscopy.* 2005;21(6):652–658.

Nho SJ, Shindle MK, Sherman SL, Freedman KB, Lyman S, MacGillivray JD. Systematic review of arthroscopic rotator cuff repair and mini-open rotator cuff repair. *J Bone Joint Surg Am.* 2007;89(suppl 3):127–136. Review.

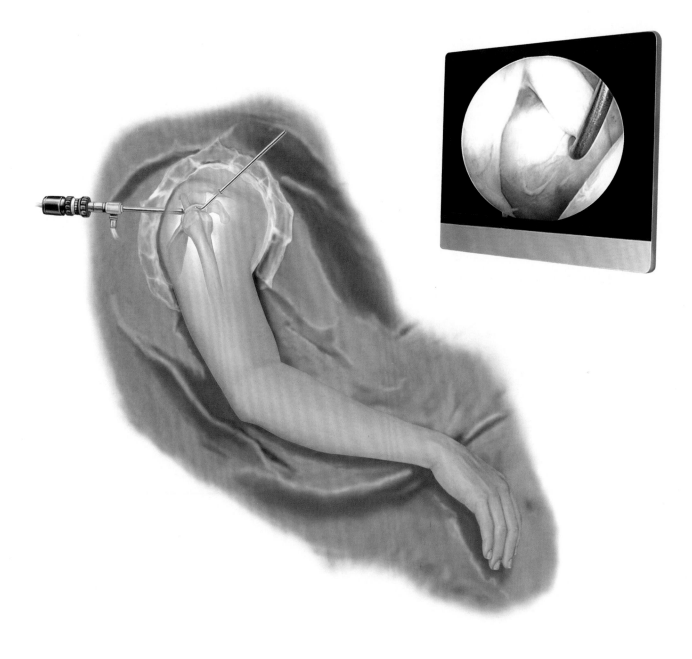

Figure 1. Shoulder Arthroscopy. Visualization through a standard posterior viewing portal with the patient in a beach chair position with arthroscopic instruments placed through and anterior superior portal.

Debridement/Loose Body Removal/ Synovectomy

Indications and Goals: This is merely an extension of shoulder arthroscopy, and is indicated for patients with symptomatic foreign or loose bodies in their glenohumeral joint or synovial disease.

Procedure and Technique: Motorized shavers and handheld instruments are used to remove pathologic synovium and loose bodies. For larger loose bodies, it is sometimes necessary to enlarge the portal. Another helpful trick is to bring the object up to the mouth of a large arthroscopic cannula and then pull it out with the cannula, which allows it to follow the path of the cannula. For posttraumatic loose bodies, it is important to do a thorough evaluation of the joint for a donor site and associated pathology.

Post-surgical Precautions/Rehabilitation: There are very little concerns related to postsurgical precautions following these types of procedures. Rehabilitation begins immediately for range of motion and strengthening exercises, guided by a person's pain tolerance. Return to participation and activity can occur relatively quickly and is often patient-limited.

Expected Outcomes: Outcomes related to arthroscopic debridement or removal of tissue should yield excellent results relatively quickly. Factors influencing the outcomes may include the age and prior activity level of the patient.

Return to Play: Since this procedure does not involve any structural tissue, return to play can be relatively quick—even within a week of the index procedure.

Recommended Readings

Lunn JV, Castellanos-Rosas J, Walch G. Arthroscopic synovectomy, removal of loose bodies and selective biceps tenodesis for synovial chondromatosis of the shoulder. *J Bone Joint Surg Br.* 2007;89(10):1329–1335.

Smith AM, Sperling JW, O'Driscoll SW, Cofield RH. Arthroscopic shoulder synovectomy in patients with rheumatoid arthritis. *Arthroscopy.* 2006;22(1):50–56.

Tokis AV, Andrikoula SI, Chouliaras VT, Vasiliadis HS, Georgoulis AD. Diagnosis and arthroscopic treatment of primary synovial chondromatosis of the shoulder. *Arthroscopy.* 2007;23(9):1023.e1–1023.e5.

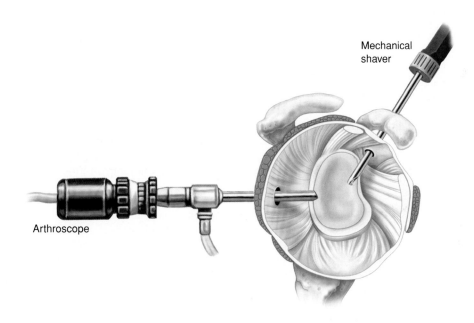

Mechanical
shaver

Arthroscope

Figure 2. Debridement of the Glenohumeral Joint Using an Arthroscopic Shaver

Acromioplasty

Indications and Goals: Three types of acromial shapes have been described on the basis of their appearance on lateral, or outlet, view—flat, curved, and hooked (I to III, respectively). Hooked acromions are thought to be more likely to result in rotator cuff tears, although this is somewhat controversial. The concept of outlet impingement—where the coracoacromial arch (acromion, coracoid, and coracoacromial ligament) causes pain and eventually rotator cuff tearing—has been challenged recently. Nevertheless, some patients do have subacromial impingement with positive exam findings (pain with passive forward flexion of approximately 120 to 150 degrees [Neer's sign] and pain with flexion to 90 degrees and internal rotation [Hawkins' sign]) and may benefit from acromioplasty. This typically also involves resection or recession of the coracoacromial ligament, although many surgeons attempt to preserve this ligament—especially with larger rotator cuff tears because it may prevent "escape" of the proximal humerus anterosuperiorly with massive tears. Surgical indications include pain refractory to cuff rehabilitation and subacromial injections with positive exam and imaging findings.

Procedure and Technique: Acromioplasty is most commonly performed arthroscopically. A shaver and burr is used to flatten the acromion (into a type I acromion). Most surgeons begin with the arthroscope in the posterior portal and, following arthroscopy of the glenohumeral joint, the scope is placed above the supraspinatus tendon into the subacromial space. A mechanical shaver, and sometimes ablater (electrocautery or radiofrequency device), is used to clear off the acromion and identify its borders. The acromioplasty proceeds from lateral to medial. The arthroscope is then moved to the lateral portal and the burr is placed in the posterior portal. Using the posterior acromion as a guide, the remaining acromion is flattened to allow a smooth undersurface (cutting-block technique).

Post-surgical Precautions/Rehabilitation: Since no muscle is taken down and nothing really needs to "heal," rehabilitation can progress quickly. Early motion is encouraged. Patients/athletes may find horizontal adduction to be painful during the first few weeks postoperatively, and general pain can be used as a guideline for progression. Strengthening exercises can begin as tolerated and full range of motion should be restored within 2 to 3 weeks.

Expected Outcomes: Though some general tenderness may remain in the area for months, full unrestricted range of motion and strength should be restored without complications.

Return to Play: As long as the deltoid origin is not affected, return to play can be within 2 to 3 weeks or as pain is tolerated and function restored to acceptable performance levels.

Recommended Readings

Barfield LC, Kuhn JE. Arthroscopic versus open acromioplasty: A systematic review. *Clin Orthop Relat Res*. 2007;455:64–71. Review.

Izquierdo R, Stanwood WG, Bigliani LU. Arthroscopic acromioplasty: History, rationale, and technique. *Instr Course Lect*. 2004;53: 13–20. Review.

Kesmezacar H, Babacan M, Erginer R, Oğüt T, Cansü E. The value of acromioplasty in the treatment of subacromial impingement syndrome. *Acta Orthop Traumatol Turc*. 2003;37(suppl 1):35–41. Review.

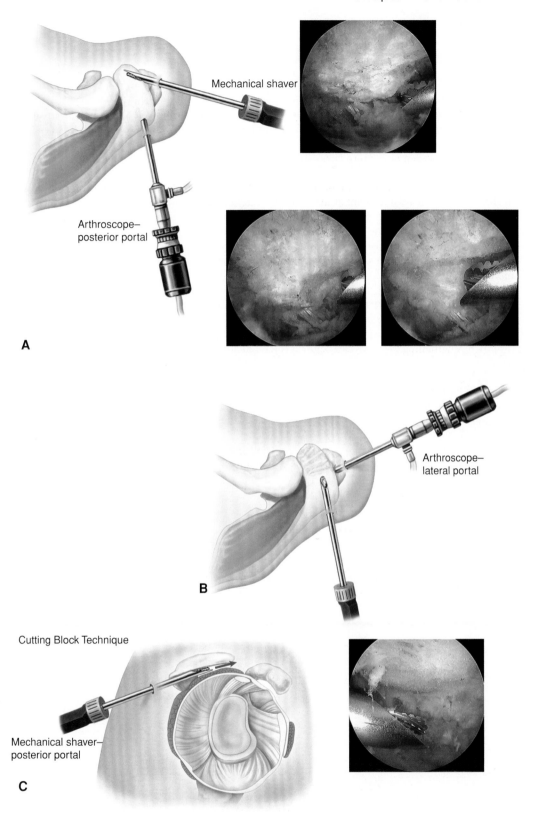

Mechanical shaver

Arthroscope—
posterior portal

A

Arthroscope—
lateral portal

B

Cutting Block Technique

Mechanical shaver-
posterior portal

C

Figure 3. Arthroscopic Acromioplasty (subacromial decompression). **A.** This procedure is performed using a posterior viewing portal in the subacromial space. A lateral portal for debridement of bursa and impinging subacromial spur is illustrated. **B.** Placement of the arthroscope through the lateral portal allows assessment of acromion for residual unresected bone **C.** Cutting block technique proceeds in a posterior to anterior and lateral to medial direction to flatten the acromion.

Distal Clavicle Resection

Indications and Goals: Distal clavicle resection is most commonly indicated in patients with acromioclavicular arthritis (sometimes following low-grade AC separations) and distal clavicle osteolysis (a stress phenomenon commonly seen in weight lifters). Patients typically have localized pain, pain with cross-chest adduction, and radiographic changes (best seen on a Zanca view—10-degree cephalic tilt with soft tissue technique).

Procedure and Technique: The procedure is most commonly performed arthroscopically. It is not uncommon to first perform at least a minimal acromioplasty to appreciate the landmarks for distal clavicle resection. A 70-degree scope can also be helpful to ensure complete resection (the posterior superior portion of the distal clavicle is sometimes missed). The superior acromioclavicular ligament fibers should be preserved to prevent anterior–posterior AC instability. After removing the capsule with a shaver and electrothermal device, the lateral 1 cm of distal clavicle is resected from a portal directly anterior or posterior to the AC-joint. All debris is removed prior to completion of the resection.

Post-surgical Precautions/Rehabilitation: Rehabilitation is similar to acromioplasty. In fact, these procedures are commonly done concurrently. Early motion is encouraged. Patients/athletes may find horizontal adduction to be painful during the first few weeks postoperatively, and general pain can be used as a guideline for progression. Strengthening exercises can begin as tolerated and full range of motion should be restored within 2 to 3 weeks.

Expected Outcomes: Full range of motion and normal restoration of strength should be expected within 1 to 2 months. Return to activities without restrictions should be expected, with the time frame dependent upon the activity requirement.

Return to Play: With appropriate rehabilitation, return to play can be as early as 4 weeks and typically up to 8 weeks, all dependent upon one's pain tolerance and ability to restore necessary strength and range of motion.

Recommended Readings

Bigliani LU, Nicholson GP, Flatow EL. Arthroscopic resection of the distal clavicle. *Orthop Clin North Am.* 1993;24(1):133–141. Review.

Hawkins BJ, Covey DC, Thiel BG. Distal clavicle osteolysis unrelated to trauma, overuse, or metabolic disease. *Clin Orthop Relat Res.* 2000;(370):208–211. Review.

Kharrazi FD, Busfield BT, Khorshad DS. Acromioclavicular joint reoperation after arthroscopic subacromial decompression with and without concomitant acromioclavicular surgery. *Arthroscopy.* 2007;23(8):804–808.

Rabalais RD, McCarty E. Surgical treatment of symptomatic acromioclavicular joint problems: A systematic review. *Clin Orthop Relat Res.* 2007;455:30–37. Review.

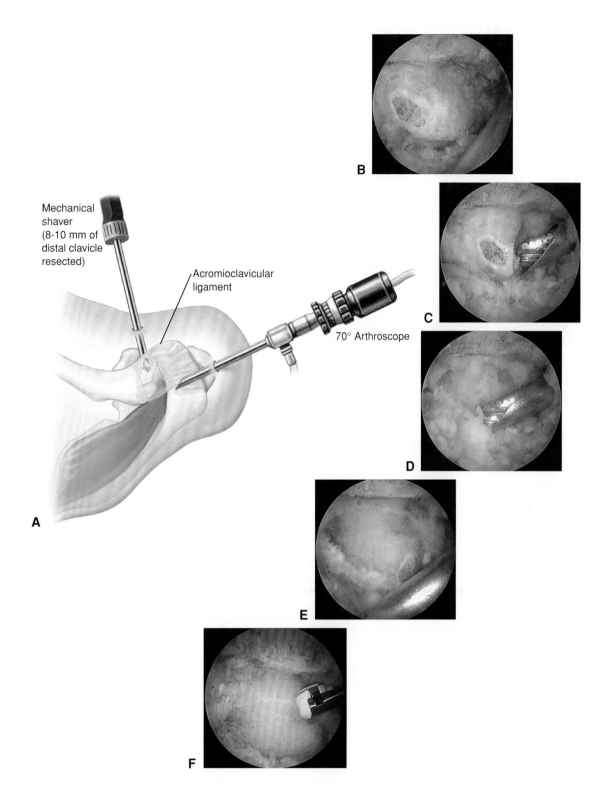

Figure 4. Distal Clavicle Resection. A. Arthroscopic distal clavicle resection using the arthroscopic burr from the anterior portal. The burr tip, which is 10–12 mm long, is used to measure the resection length (typically 8–10 mm) **B–F.** The clavicle if beveled progressively following exposure of the distal clavicle from an anteroinferior to posterosuperior direction. The clavicle in viewed end-on after completion.

Lysis of Adhesions/Manipulation Under Anesthesia

Indications and Goals: This procedure is indicated for adhesive capsulitis (frozen shoulder) that is refractory to rehabilitation and glenohumeral injection(s). Because the process can recur unless immediate postoperative motion is initiated, and the patient is the key to success, we prefer to make an oral "contract" with the patients preoperatively, emphasizing their important role in maintaining their motion.

Procedure and Technique: The patient is positioned in the beach chair position for shoulder arthroscopy. At this point, the arthroscope is detached and used to take preoperative photos of their shoulder motion (forward flexion, abduction, and external rotation). Arthroscopy is then carried out using a smaller sheath, and adhesions (particularly in the rotator interval between the biceps and the subscapularis tendons) are thoroughly removed. The shoulder is then manipulated and remaining adhesions can be felt as they break up. Range of motion pictures are repeated, documenting the improvement in motion and proving to the patients that motion was restored.

Post-surgical Precautions/Rehabilitation: It is critical that the patient maintain his/her motion! A postoperative block and adequate pain medications can be helpful in this process. Although the clinician can be helpful in this process, it is the patient's responsibility to perform passive range of motion exercises multiple times per day! Range of motion in all directions, and specifically accessory motion such as inferior glenohumeral glides, should begin immediately and preferably under supervision to facilitate improved outcomes and restored range of motion.

Expected Outcomes: Following a manipulation of this kind, the goal is to restore as much range of motion as possible. A reasonable functional goal can be determined at the time of manipulation under anesthesia and should be conveyed to the treating clinician. The most common complication is a recurrence of adhesions as a result of nonaggressive rehabilitation, noncompliance with rehabilitation, or rapid scarring from the trauma of the procedure.

Return to Play: This condition is not commonly seen with younger aged athletes. Return to play can be within 2 to 3 weeks, as long as the athlete maintains his/her motion that was restored during the procedure.

Recommended Readings

Castellarin G, Ricci M, Vedovi E, Vecchini E, Sembenini P, Marangon A, Vangelista A. Manipulation and arthroscopy under general anesthesia and early rehabilitative treatment for frozen shoulders. *Arch Phys Med Rehabil.* 2004;85(8):1236–1240.

Hand GC, Athanasou NA, Matthews T, Carr AJ. The pathology of frozen shoulder. *J Bone Joint Surg Br.* 2007;89(7):928–932.

Kivimäki J, Pohjolainen T, Malmivaara A, Kannisto M, Guillaume J, Seitsalo S, Nissinen M. Manipulation under anesthesia with home exercises versus home exercises alone in the treatment of frozen shoulder: A randomized, controlled trial with 125 patients. *J Shoulder Elbow Surg.* 2007;16(6):722–726. Epub 2007 Oct 10.

Loew M, Heichel TO, Lehner B. Intraarticular lesions in primary frozen shoulder after manipulation under general anesthesia. *J Shoulder Elbow Surg.* 2005;14(1):16–21.

Quraishi NA, Johnston P, Bayer J, Crowe M, Chakrabarti AJ. Thawing the frozen shoulder: A randomised trial comparing manipulation under anaesthesia with hydrodilatation. *J Bone Joint Surg Br.* 2007;89(9):1197–1200.

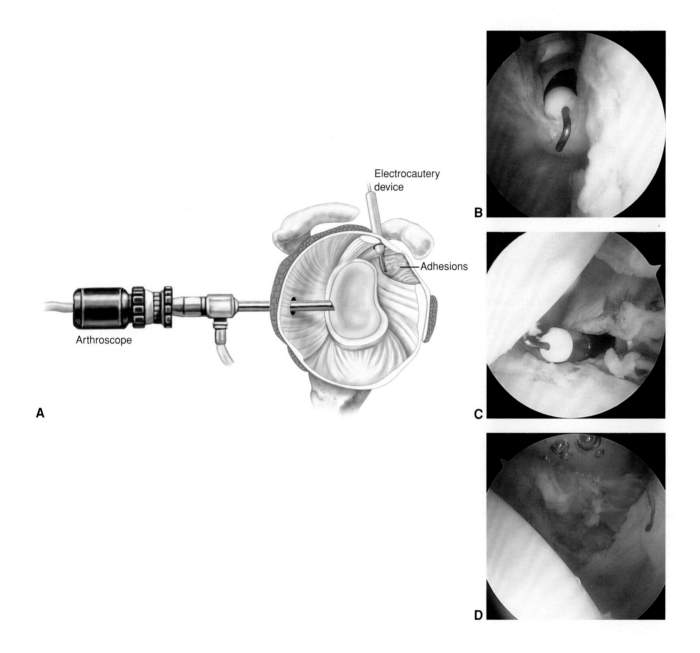

Figure 5. Lysis of Adhesions. A. Arthroscope introduced posteriorly with hook-tip electrocautery device through anterosuperior instrumentation portal. **B.** Electrocautery utilized through anterior portal to lyse adhesions. **C.** Thick scar tissue shown being released with arthroscopic bovie device. **D.** Post release image demonstrating increased space within glenohumeral joint.

Capsulotomy

Indications and Goals: This is an unusual but simple procedure that is often done in conjunction with other arthroscopic procedures in the shoulder. Throwing athletes that develop internal impingement with loss of internal rotation that do not respond to posterior capsular stretching (sleeper-stretches) and other therapy may have thickened posterior capsular tissues. Likewise, patients with long-standing glenohumeral arthritis may have capsular tightness.

Procedure and Technique: This procedure is simply a matter of identifying tight structures and releasing them. The tight capsule, which is most commonly found posteriorly, appears as thickened and shortened tissue. This capsule is divided, usually with electrocautery, from just posterior to the biceps tendon on the superior glenoid rim and continuing inferiorly. The rotator cuff is superficial to the capsule at this point, protecting them during the release as long as the dissection stays adjacent to the glenoid rim. Care should also be taken not to disrupt other normal structures, including the axillary nerve inferiorly.

Post-surgical Precautions/Rehabilitation: With the intent of this procedure to improve shoulder range of motion, supervised rehabilitation should begin immediately and include passive range of motion exercises, with the patient/athlete being encouraged to actively perform range of motion and muscle-strengthening exercises as soon as possible. Typically supervised physical therapy is recommended 5 days a week for the first 2 weeks and accompanied by a home exercise program. For the next 4 weeks, supervised sessions may be reduced to three times a week but the home program is continued daily.

Expected Outcomes: Similar to a manipulation under anesthesia, the goal of capsulotomy is to restore as much motion as possible. A reasonable functional goal can be determined at the time of manipulation under anesthesia and should be conveyed to the treating clinician. Complications primarily consist of a recurrence of adhesions as a result of nonaggressive rehabilitation, noncompliance with rehabilitation, or rapid scarring from the trauma of the procedure.

Return to Play: As long as the patient rehabilitates properly, return to play can be within 2 to 3 weeks or once pre-injury functional strength is restored for required performance levels.

Recommended Readings

Bach HG, Goldberg BA. Posterior capsular contracture of the shoulder. *J Am Acad Orthop Surg.* 2006;14(5):265–277. Review.

Bhatia DN, de Beer JF. The axillary pouch portal: A new posterior portal for visualization and instrumentation in the inferior glenohumeral recess. *Arthroscopy.* 2007;23(11):1241.e1–1241.e5. Epub 2007 Apr 6.

Ticker JB, Beim GM, Warner JP. Recognition and treatment of refractory posterior capsular contracture of the shoulder. *Arthroscopy.* 2000;16:27–34.

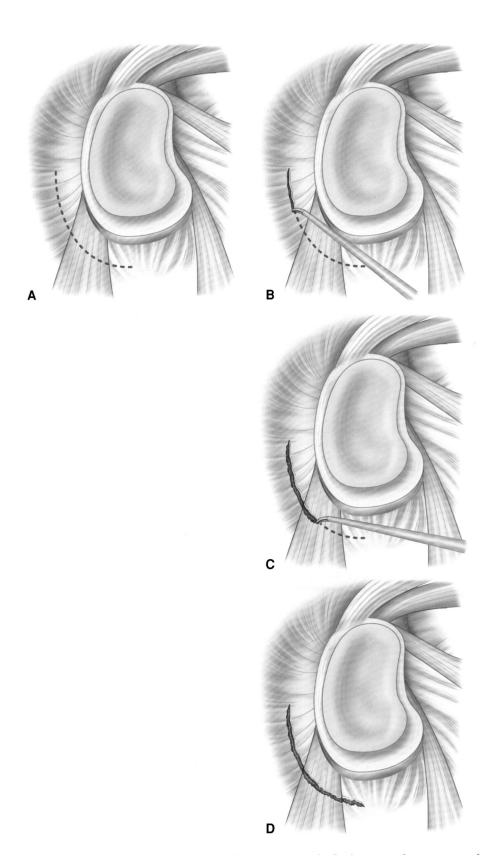

Figure 6. Posterior Capsulotomy. A. Location for a posteroinferior quadrant capsulotomy.
B–D. A hook-tip electrocautery device is used to perform full thickness capsulotomy
from 3–6 o'clock position.

Anterior Bankart Repair/Capsulorrhaphy

Indications and Goals: Traumatic anterior shoulder dislocations almost always result in a Bankart injury (avulsion of the anterior inferior labrum and inferior glenohumeral ligament/capsule from the glenoid). Recurrent atraumatic shoulder instability is usually a result of capsular patholaxity. Surgical indications include symptomatic recurrent instability that has failed rehabilitation (rotator cuff strengthening). Extended rehabilitation (for up to 6 months) has been proven to be beneficial for atraumatic instability, but has not been shown to reduce recurrence for traumatic anterior instability. Bracing has also not been shown to reduce recurrence rates, at least in the United States. In addition, recurrence for traumatic anterior instability is directly related to age—younger patients (18 to 20 years old) may have a recurrence rate of over 80%! This has led many surgeons to consider surgery even for traumatic first-time dislocators. Classic exam findings in anterior instability include a positive apprehension test (abduction and external rotation of the affected arm causes apprehension) and relocation text (a posteriorly directed force relieves this apprehension). The goal for shoulder stabilization procedures is to reduce the recurrence of instability.

Procedures and Techniques: Most anterior instability procedures are now done arthroscopically. The goal is to restore normal anatomy by repairing the Bankart lesion back to bone and to reduce capsular patholaxity (by shifting the Bankart repair laterally and superiorly on the glenoid and creating a bumper pad on the glenoid surface; and [sometimes] reducing capsular volume by plicating [using sutures to make "tucks" of tissue] the capsule of the glenohumeral joint [including the rotator interval [tissue between the subscapularis and biceps]]). A Bankart tear (if present) is mobilized (it often scars down onto the neck of the glenoid medially—an anterior labral periosteal sleeve avulsion [ALPSA]). The glenoid is then prepared (using a shaver or a burr to roughen up the bone and create a bleeding surface). Suture anchors (devices that have sutures imbedded in them that are fixed into bone and are often bioabsorbable) are then placed immediately off the articular surface, and the attached suture is passed through the torn tissue and tied using arthroscopic knots. Plication stitches are added based on the surgeon's assessment of associated capsular laxity (or for atraumatic instability, may be the only technique utilized). Thermal capsulorrhaphy (heat shrinkage) has been largely abandoned because of high recurrence and morbidity rates. Open procedures use similar techniques, but are done through a deltopectoral approach that usually involves dissecting the subscapularis tendon off of the underlying capsule.

Post-surgical Precautions/Rehabilitation: The patient is immobilized in a sling but encouraged to perform elbow motion and pendulum exercises several times a day. Passive range of motion is initiated but active motion is discouraged the first 4 to 6 weeks. External rotation is delayed until after the first 6 weeks and abduction-external rotation is discouraged the first 3 months. Closed kinetic chain exercises can begin for proprioception and strength at 6 weeks postoperatively. Return to contact sports is not allowed until 4 to 6 months postoperatively. With an open procedure, additional caution is placed on active and passive external rotation as well as active internal rotation to avoid a strong contraction of the subscapularis muscle and/or strain to the repair. Postoperative subscapularis tendon rupture (excessive external rotation and a positive "lift-off test") is a well-described but avoidable complication.

Expected Outcomes: The intent of the procedure is to restore joint stability. With restoration of the labrum and tightening of the capsule, this can be successfully accomplished in up to 90% of the cases. Failures are related to recurrent instability and bony defects.

Return to Play: With activities of daily living that do not require excessive forces to the glenohumeral joint, full return to activity is very reasonable within 4 to 6 months after surgery. For throwers who place added stress to the capsule, it may take up to 12 months or longer for a safe return to competition. Complications of recurrent instability have been reported 2 years after surgery suggesting long-term monitoring of patients.

Recommended Readings

Kartus C, Kartus J, Matis N, Forstner R, Resch H. Long-term independent evaluation after arthroscopic extra-articular Bankart repair with absorbable tacks. A clinical and radiographic study with a seven to ten-year follow-up. *J Bone Joint Surg Am.* 2007;89(7):1442–1448.

Mohtadi NG, Bitar IJ, Sasyniuk TM, Hollinshead RM, Harper WP. Arthroscopic versus open repair for traumatic anterior shoulder instability: A meta-analysis. *Arthroscopy.* 2005;21(6):652–658.

Rhee YG, Lim CT, Cho NS. Muscle strength after anterior shoulder stabilization: Arthroscopic versus open Bankart repair. *Am J Sports Med.* 2007;35(11):1859–1864. Epub 2007 Jul 30.

Thal R, Nofziger M, Bridges M, Kim JJ. Arthroscopic Bankart repair using Knotless or BioKnotless suture anchors: 2- to 7-year results. *Arthroscopy.* 2007;23(4):367–375.

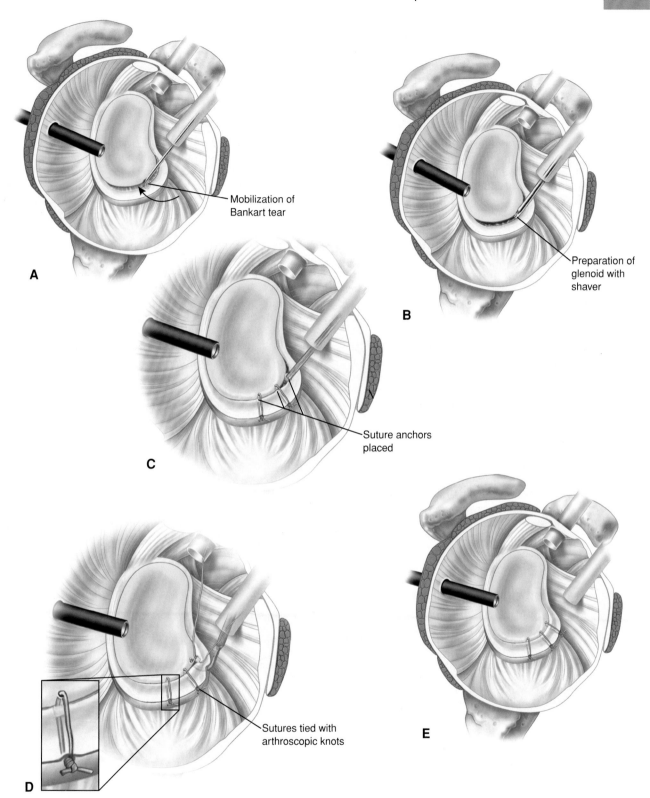

A. Mobilization of Bankart tear

B. Preparation of glenoid with shaver

C. Suture anchors placed

D. Sutures tied with arthroscopic knots

E.

Figure 7. Athroscopic Bankart Repair. A. Following identification of the lesion, an elevator is used to mobilize labral and capsular tissue off the glenoid. **B.** The glenoid is prepared with an arthroscopic shaver. **C.** Suture anchors are placed on the articular face of the glenoid. **D.** A shuttling instrument is passed through the capsule and then labrum and suture retrieved. Arthroscopic knots are tied away from the glenoid. **E.** The "bumper" effect is recreated preventing recurrent instability.

Posterior Bankart Repair/Capsulorrhaphy

Indications and Goals: Posterior instability is less common than anterior instability, but can be associated with certain sports/activities. Football interior linemen can develop posterior instability and labral tears from repetitive stress from blocking. Throwing athletes can also develop posterior laxity. Traumatic injuries are also responsible for some posterior instability, but, unlike traumatic anterior instability, these injuries have a more favorable prognosis with acute reduction and immobilization (in a neutral or externally rotated position). Classic exam findings for posterior instability include increased posterior translation with a load and shift test and a positive jerk test (passive abduction/adduction of the affected arm may reproduce the instability). Again, the goal of these procedures is to restore stability.

Procedures and Technique: Posterior shoulder procedures—both arthroscopic and open—are best performed with the patient in the lateral decubitus position. Standard portals are created and diagnostic arthroscopy is carried out. It is often helpful to switch the scope and instrumentation portals and to view the lesion from the anterior superior portal. An additional posterior (7 o'clock) portal is helpful for anchor placement and suture passage. The technique is similar to anterior Bankart repair and capsulorrhaphy. Open procedures are done through a deltoid-splitting approach with a posterior arthrotomy made in the infraspinatus/teres minor interval.

Post-surgical Precautions/Rehabilitation: Typically, the patient is placed in a neutral or external rotation brace for the first 4 to 6 weeks. Caution is emphasized to maintain this position early on to facilitate optimal healing of the repaired tissue. As one progresses, range of motion should be carefully increased, with no urgency to aggressively push the amount of internal rotation. Upon return to activity, bracing is not necessary and has not been shown to be effective in preventing against posterior shoulder dislocations. Passive forceful stretching into internal rotation and extension should be avoided for 3 months.

Expected Outcomes: The intent of the procedure is to restore joint stability. Again, with proper anatomic repair, success rates of approximately 90% can be expected.

Return to Play: With activities of daily living that do not require excessive forces to the glenohumeral joint, full return to activity is very reasonable within 6 months after surgery. This procedure is not performed as often as the anterior Bankart, yet precautions remain similar and expected outcomes should be similar. The posterior procedure is not as common as the anterior with throwing sport athletes, thus return to play may occur sooner in this case.

Recommended Readings

Ahmad CS, Wang VM, Sugalski MT, Levine WN, Bigliani LU. Biomechanics of shoulder capsulorrhaphy procedures. *J Shoulder Elbow Surg*. 2005;14(1 suppl S):12S–18S. Review.

Bottoni CR, Franks BR, Moore JH, DeBerardino TM, Taylor DC, Arciero RA. Operative stabilization of posterior shoulder instability. *Am J Sports Med*. 2005;33(7):996–1002.

Bradley JP, Baker CL III, Kline AJ, Armfield DR, Chhabra A. Arthroscopic capsulolabral reconstruction for posterior instability of the shoulder: A prospective study of 100 shoulders. *Am J Sports Med*. 2006;34(7):1061–1071.

Millett PJ, Clavert P, Hatch GF III, Warner JJ. Recurrent posterior shoulder instability. *J Am Acad Orthop Surg*. 2006;14(8):464–476.

Robinson CM, Aderinto J. Recurrent posterior shoulder instability. *J Bone Joint Surg Am*. 2005;87(4):883–892.

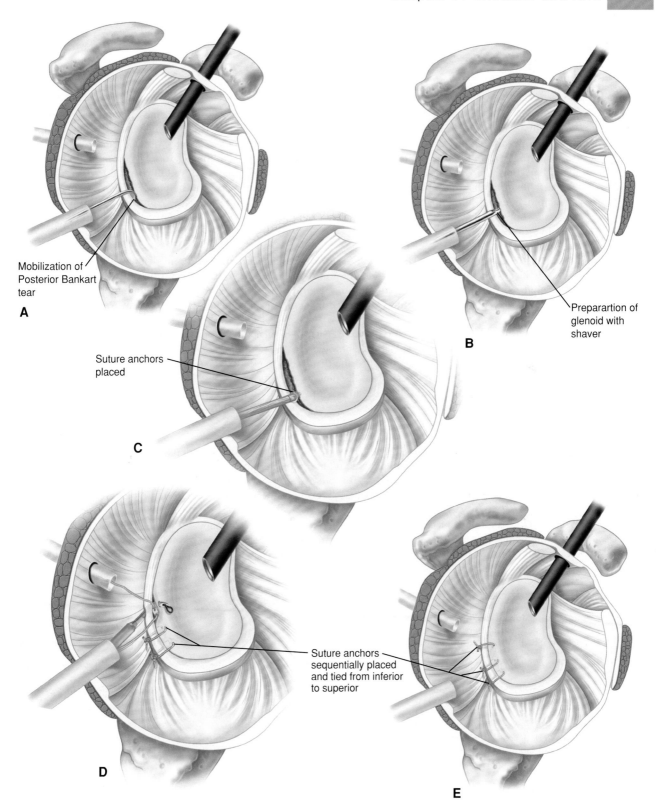

Figure 8. Posterior Labral Repair. A. Viewing from anterosuperior portal, the lesion is identified and an elevator is used to release labral and capsular tissue off the glenoid. **B.** The glenoid is prepared with an arthroscopic shaver. **C.** Suture anchors are placed on the articular surface of the glenoid from inferior to superior. **D.** A shuttling instrument is passed through the capsule and labrum and suture retrieved followed by arthroscopic knot tying. **E.** The "bumper" effect is recreated preventing recurrent posterior instability.

SLAP Repair

Indications and Goals: Superior labral anterior to posterior (SLAP) tears are most commonly a result of traction injury and are also common in throwers (peel back phenomenon). They have been classified based upon the involvement of the biceps anchor (most commonly disrupted with a type II injury, which has been further subclassified on the basis of whether the tear is anterior, posterior, or both). Although a variety of examinations have been described for diagnosing SLAP tears, bicipital groove tenderness and a positive O'Brien's test (pain with resisted forward flexion with a fully pronated forearm and an adducted arm) are most helpful. Often MR arthrography can be helpful in establishing the diagnosis. Indications for surgery include refractory pain and inability to throw (typically a loss of velocity) in a patient that has failed rehabilitation. The goal is to repair the tear and restore normal shoulder mechanics.

Procedure and Technique: Standard arthroscopic portals are used and diagnostic arthroscopy carried out. The biceps anchor is carefully examined for evidence of injury to the articular surface and to see if it is overly mobile. For posterior SLAP repairs, an accessory lateral or posterolateral (Port of Wilmington) portal is helpful. Suture anchor(s) are used and sutures are passed through the labrum and secured with arthroscopic knots.

Post-surgical Precautions/Rehabilitation: Similar to anterior Bankart repair, the patient is immobilized in a sling but encouraged to perform elbow motion and pendulum exercises several times a day. Passive ROM is initiated but active motion is discouraged the first 4 to 6 weeks. External rotation is delayed until after the first 6 weeks and abduction-external rotation is discouraged the first 3 months. Return to contact sports is not allowed until 4 to 6 months postoperatively. With an open procedure, additional caution is placed on active and passive external rotation as well as active internal rotation to avoid a strong contraction of the subscapularis muscle and/or strain to the repair.

Expected Outcomes: While the outcome is expected to be similar in all patients, those with goals of returning to overhead activity must remain patient and allow for adequate healing and a gradual progression to activity without compromising repaired tissue. Redislocation rate is reported to be low. However, excessive laxity upon return may be a result of aggressive rehabilitation. Complications of postsurgical neurologic symptoms are rare.

Return to Play: With successful rehabilitation, return to play in some sports can be within 4 to 6 months. Throwing athletes may take a year or longer to return to play given the stresses placed on the anterior shoulder and eccentric load on the long head of the biceps. Professional throwers may never completely return to their pre-injury level.

Recommended Readings

Burkhart SS, Morgan CD, Kibler WB. The disabled throwing shoulder: Spectrum of pathology. Part II: Evaluation and treatment of SLAP lesions in throwers. *Arthroscopy.* 2003;19(5):531–539. Review.

Ghalayini SR, Board TN, Srinivasan MS. Anatomic variations in the long head of biceps: Contribution to shoulder dysfunction. *Arthroscopy.* 2007;23(9):1012–1018. Review.

Jones GL, Galluch DB. Clinical assessment of superior glenoid labral lesions: A systematic review. *Clin Orthop Relat Res.* 2007;455:45–51. Review.

Nam EK, Snyder SJ. The diagnosis and treatment of superior labrum, anterior and posterior (SLAP) lesions. *Am J Sports Med.* 2003;31(5):798–810. Review.

Park HB, Lin SK, Yokota A, McFarland EG. Return to play for rotator cuff injuries and superior labrum anterior posterior (SLAP) lesions. *Clin Sports Med.* 2004;23(3):321–334, vii. Review.

Tennent TD, Beach WR, Meyers JF. A review of the special tests associated with shoulder examination. Part II: Laxity, instability, and superior labral anterior and posterior (SLAP) lesions. *Am J Sports Med.* 2003;31(2):301–307. Review.

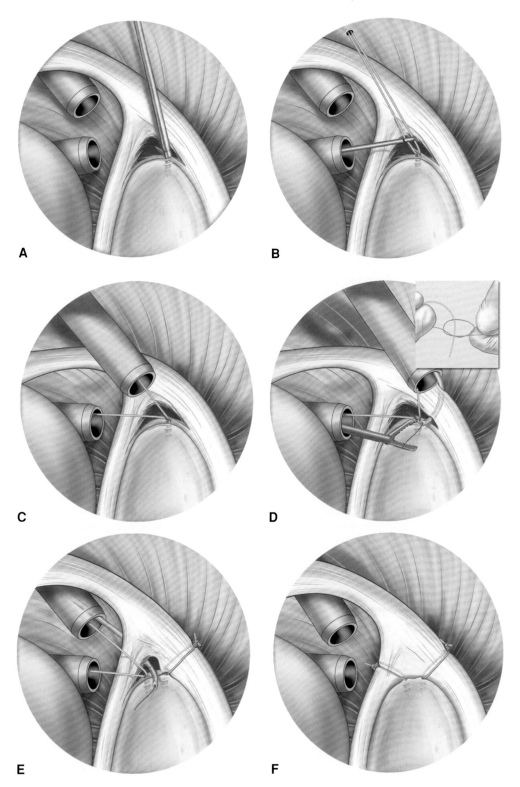

Figure 9. SLAP Repair. A. A Type II SLAP tear is visualized and a suture anchor placed on the superior glenoid face. **B.** The surgeon retrieves each limb of the suture into respective portals. **C.** Suture limbs are shown passing through each portal. **D.** Tissue penetrator is used to shuttle suture and a grasper is used to retrieve the monofilament. A knot is tied between the suture anchor suture and the monofilament to allow for passage. **E.** Another suture passer is used in the same manner. **F.** Athroscopic knots are tied for completion of superior labrum anterior-posterior repair.

Biceps Tenodesis

Indications and Goals: Pathology of the biceps tendon is increasingly recognized as a shoulder "pain generator." Biceps tendon pathology exists on a spectrum from tendinitis to tearing and rupture of the long head of the biceps tendon (1). The long head of the biceps brachii originates from the supraglenoid tubercle and superior aspect of the labrum traveling within the glenohumeral joint. The long head of the biceps is thought to contribute to humeral head stability and strength in overhead athletes though this is controversial (2).

Surgery is reserved for refractory cases. Indications for tenodesis include signs, symptoms, MRI, and arthroscopic findings consistent with biceps or superior labral pathology (3). Rotator cuff tears including subscapularis tears may need to be addressed concomitantly with biceps tendinopathy. Decision for tenodesis over tenotomy is largely based upon patient factors including age, sport, and body habitus. Other factors include surgeon arthroscopic experience and bone quality (3).

Procedures and Technique: Biceps tenodesis can be carried out either above or below the pectoralis tendon insertion on the humerus. In addition, tenodesis can be performed intraarticular as a soft tissue tenodesis at the proximal aspect of the bicipital groove or more distally at the superior border of the pectoralis tendon. Open techniques proceed subpectoral through a small anterior incision. The tendon is cut to leave the appropriate amount of tendon proximal to the musculotendinous junction and fixed in position.

Arthroscopic bony tenodesis with interference screws can also be performed (4). Standard arthroscopic portals are established for viewing and instrumentation, typically in the beach chair position. The biceps is examined during diagnostic arthroscopy, as is the labrum. This includes evaluation for subluxation. The biceps tendon is tagged and then released from its insertion on the labrum (Figure bony tenodesis with interference screw). The tendon is subsequently located within the subacromial space, bursectomy performed and the site for tenodesis prepared. Once the site for tenodesis is confirmed, a tunnel is drilled to the appropriate depth after sizing of the tendon. Various fixation methods are available.

Post-surgical Precautions/Rehabilitation: Postsurgical care often depends upon other pathology addressed at the time of tenodesis including rotator cuff injury. Sling immobilization is typical for 2 to 4 weeks following tenotomy and 4 to 6 weeks after tenodesis. Active elbow flexion is restricted for the first 6 weeks. True active strengthening is usually delayed for 8 to 12 weeks for patients undergoing tenodesis.

Expected Outcomes: When addressing isolated biceps pathology, both arthroscopic and open treatments appear to have good success in terms of pain relief. Minimal functional deficit is notable after either procedure. Biceps tenodesis, both arthroscopic and open techniques, may provide better cosmesis and maintains the length tension relationship of the biceps tendon and avoids the "popeye" deformity. Potential disadvantages are ongoing pain at the tenodesis site as well as attritional rupture at the tenodesis site (3–5). In addition, it takes significantly longer to recover following tenodesis compared to tenotomy.

Return to Play: Full return to play following biceps tenodesis can be expected around 3 months.

References

1. Murthi AM, Vosburgh CL, Neviaser TJ. The incidence of pathologic changes of the long head of the biceps tendon. *J Shoulder Elbow Surg*. 2000;9(5):382–385.
2. Warner JJ, McMahon PJ. The role of the long head of the biceps brachii in superior stability of the glenohumeral joint. *J Bone Joint Surg Am*. 1995;77(3):366–372.
3. Nho SJ, Strauss EJ, Lenart BA, Provencher MT, Mazzocca AD, Verma NN, Romeo AA. Long head of the biceps tendinopathy: Diagnosis and management. *J Am Acad Orthop Surg*. 2010;18(11):645–656.
4. Romeo AA, Mazzocca AD, Tauro JC. Arthroscopic biceps tenodesis. *Arthroscopy*. 2004;20(2):206–213.
5. Slabaugh MA, Frank RM, Van Thiel GS, Bell RM, Wang VM, Trenhaile S, Provencher MT, Romeo AA, Verma NN. Biceps tenodesis with interference screw fixation: A biomechanical comparison of screw length and diameter. *Arthroscopy*. 2011;27(2):161–166.

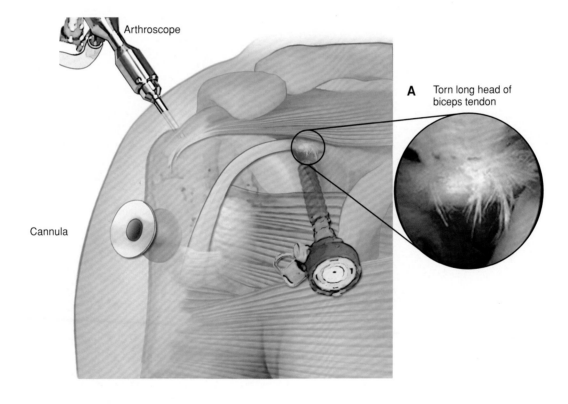

Figure 10. The damaged long head of the biceps tendon (**A**) is identified and the subdeltoid space developed. A more anterior lateral portal is established. (*continued*)

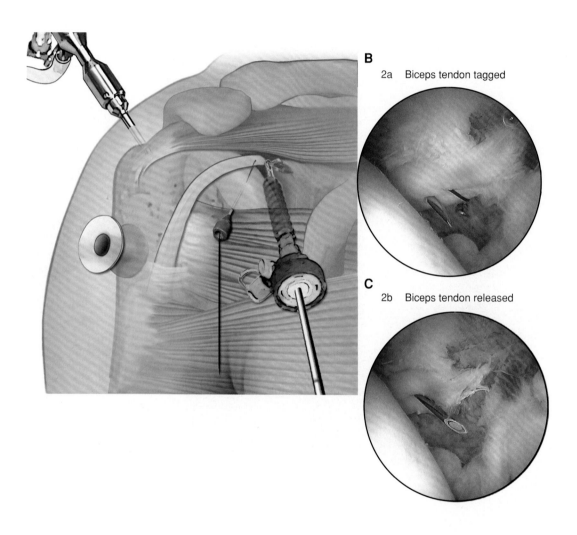

B

2a   Biceps tendon tagged

C

2b   Biceps tendon released

Figure 10. (*continued*) A tagging PDS suture is placed within the long head of the biceps (**B**) as well as a spinal needle to allow control of the tendon (**C**) and identification in the subdeltoid space. The tendon is release from it's insertion.

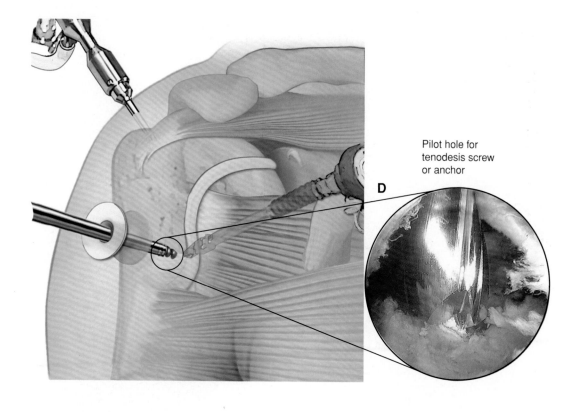

Pilot hole for
tenodesis screw
or anchor

D

Figure 10. (*continued*) A guidewire for the tenodesis screw is placed in the intertubercular groove
and drilled with an appropriate sized cannulated reamer (**D**). (*continued*)

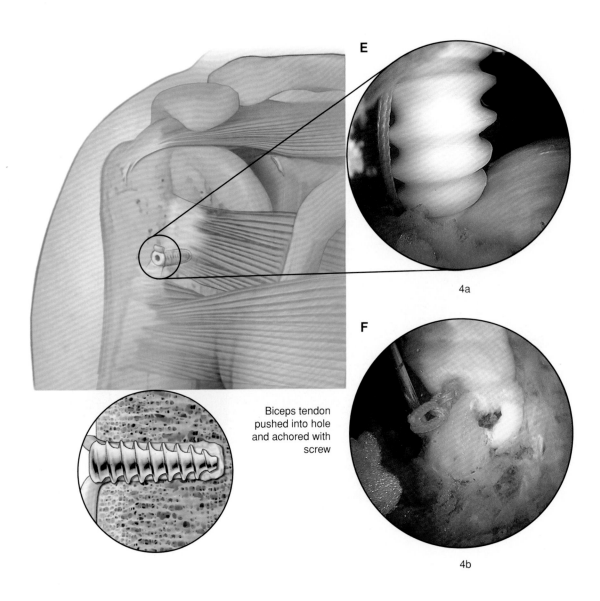

E

F

4a

4b

Biceps tendon
pushed into hole
and achored with
screw

Figure 10. (*continued*) The tenodesis screw is advanced to the appropriate depth within the tunnel (**E**) and secured by arthroscopically tying a suture on top of the interference screw (**F**).

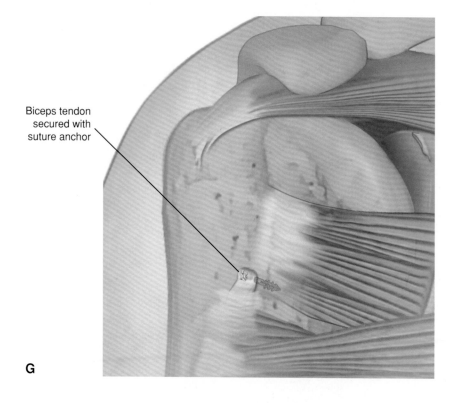

Biceps tendon
secured with
suture anchor

G

Figure 10. (*continued*) **G:** Completed tenodesis

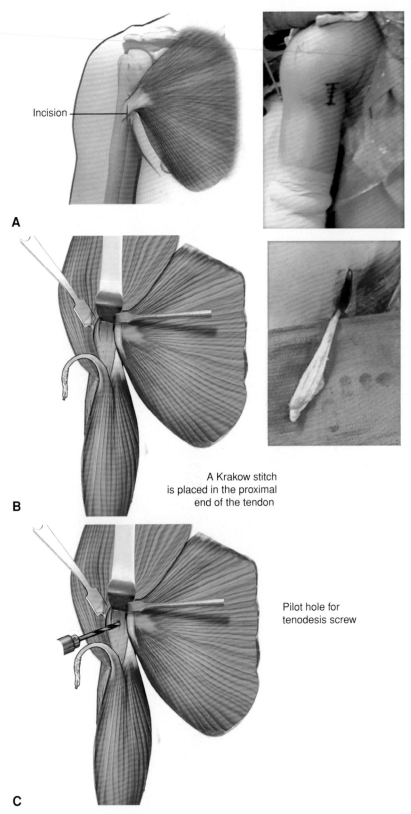

Incision

A

A Krakow stitch
is placed in the proximal
end of the tendon

B

Pilot hole for
tenodesis screw

C

Figure 11. A: Open subpectoral tenodesis is performed through a deltopectoral approach.
B: The tendon is released proximally and a running locking Krackow or whipstitch
is placed within the tendon. **C:** The pectoralis tendon is retracted superiorly and a
hole the size of the tendon is made in the subectoral region.

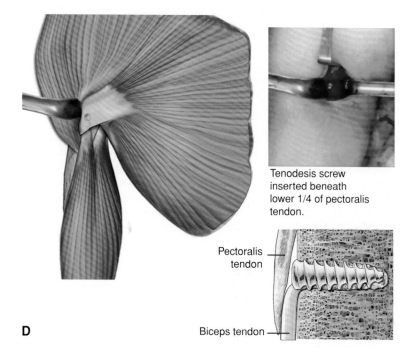

Tenodesis screw inserted beneath lower 1/4 of pectoralis tendon.

Pectoralis tendon

Biceps tendon

D

Figure 11. (*continued*) **D.** Completed open subpectoral biceps tenodesis

Rotator Cuff Repair

Indications and Goals: Rotator cuff tears, which typically involve the supraspinatus tendon, typically occur in older individuals. However, throwing athletes may develop cuff tears at a younger age and traumatic injuries can occur at any age. Atraumatic rotator cuff tears represent a continuum, beginning with mild fraying, or partial tears, progressing to full-thickness tears, continuing on to larger or even massive (>5 cm or two-tendon) tears, and, unfortunately, at the end of the spectrum are irreparable tears and rotator cuff arthropathy (proximal migration and arthrosis from long-standing cuff disease). Tears come in a variety of sizes and shapes; nevertheless, the goal is the same; to mobilize the tear and to attach it back to where it tore off—the greater tuberosity. In general, rotator cuff tears in younger, active individuals should be repaired as soon as they are recognized—especially if they are acute injuries—to avoid progression of the tear and enhance the surgeon's ability to repair it.

Procedure and Technique: Until recently, rotator cuff tears were treated with open (deltoid detaching) or mini-open (deltoid-splitting) approaches. Although this may still be appropriate for some larger tears, most surgeons now favor arthroscopic rotator cuff repair. Regardless of the approach—the goal is simple—mobilize and reattach the tendon to the tuberosity. This sometimes requires some tricks, including removing the bursal tissue (without making it bleed excessively), releasing adhesions above and below the cuff with blunt elevators, and sometimes releasing the connections between adjacent cuff tendons (interval slides). For "U"- or "L"-shaped tears, it is often helpful to place margin convergence (side-to-side) sutures prior to reattaching the tendon to the tuberosity. The tendon is repaired to bone using suture anchors in either a single- or double-row construct. Anchors are placed into the bone and their attached sutures are passed using passers and suture hooks from below up (antegrade) or top-down (retrograde) fashion using a mattress or simple stitch. They are tied over the tendon and can be further secured with another more laterally placed implant.

Post-surgical Precautions/Rehabilitation: Although patients recover much faster following arthroscopic rotator cuff repair, this is actually a double-edged sword. Regardless of how the repair is done (open, mini-open, or arthroscopic), the shoulder must be protected until the cuff can heal to the bone (at least 6 to 8 weeks). Passive motion is encouraged early; however, active and resisted motion and especially strengthening exercises must be delayed. Do not be fooled by a small incision when this procedure is performed arthroscopically; the same amount of surgery must be performed to repair the rotator cuff despite the size of the incision. As the tissue heals, the patient/athlete will want to "test" the shoulder, but it will likely take 6 months minimum to safely perform activities such as throwing and lifting.

Expected Outcomes: The evidence appears to be unclear regarding the relationship between demographic variables (duration of symptoms, timing of surgery, physical examination findings, and size of the tear) and treatment outcome.

Return to Play: Depending on the size of the tear, the quality of the tissue, the chronicity of the tear, and a variety of other factors, return to play may take 6 to 12 months. Professional throwing athletes rarely return to their pre-injury level.

Recommended Readings

Burns JP, Snyder SJ, Albritton M. Arthroscopic rotator cuff repair using triple-loaded anchors, suture shuttles, and suture savers. *J Am Acad Orthop Surg.* 2007;15(7):432–444. Review.

Cole BJ, ElAttrache NS, Anbari A. Arthroscopic rotator cuff repairs: An anatomic and biomechanical rationale for different suture-anchor repair configurations. *Arthroscopy.* 2007;23(6):662–669. Review.

Nho SJ, Shindle MK, Sherman SL, Freedman KB, Lyman S, MacGillivray JD. Systematic review of arthroscopic rotator cuff repair and mini-open rotator cuff repair. *J Bone Joint Surg Am.* 2007;89(suppl 3):127–136. Review.

Oh LS, Wolf BR, Hall MP, Levy BA, Marx RG. Indications for rotator cuff repair: A systematic review. *Clin Orthop Relat Res.* 2007;455:52–63. Review.

Reardon DJ, Maffulli N. Clinical evidence shows no difference between single- and double-row repair for rotator cuff tears. *Arthroscopy.* 2007;23(6):670–673. Review.

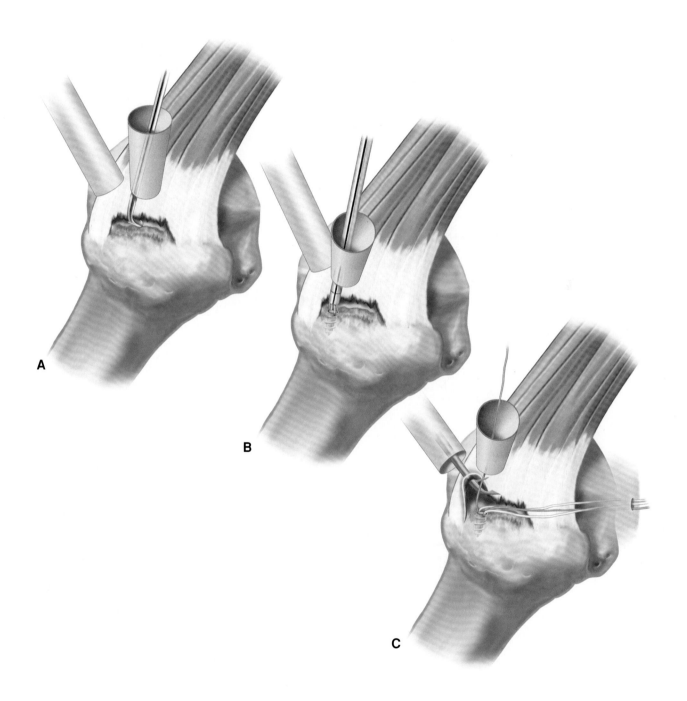

Figure 12. Arthroscopic Rotator Cuff Repair. A. Debridement of rotator cuff footprint. **B.** Screw-in anchors are placed at the footprint of the rotator cuff. **C–E.** Bridging horizontal mattress stitches are shuttled through the rotator cuff tendon medially. **G.** Athroscopic knots are used to bring the rotator cuff tissue to the footprint. **H.** A double row repair is created using two lateral anchors. (*continued*)

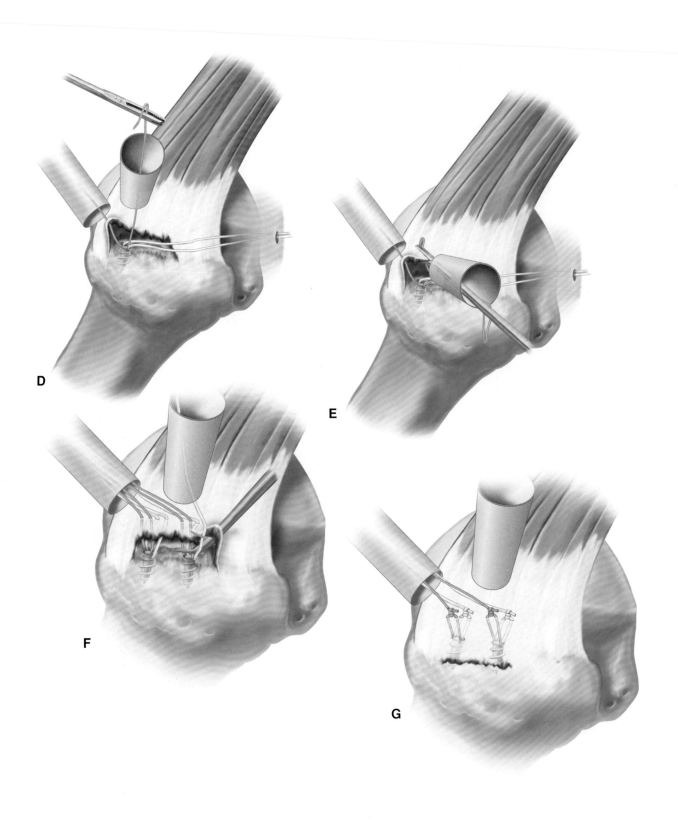

Figure 12. (*continued*)

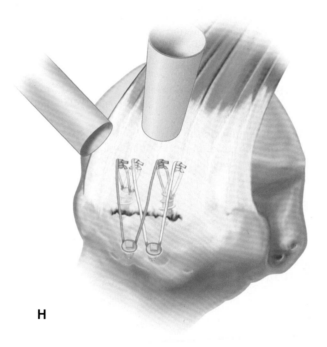

H

Figure 12. (*continued*)

Pectoralis Major Repair

Indications and Goals: Pectoralis major ruptures are relatively unusual, but can occur in weight lifters and other sports (football). The mechanism of injury usually involves a traction injury, and patients will have weak adduction and internal rotation. The loss of contour of the chest wall that occurs with pectoralis tears is referred to as "axillary webbing." Acute pectoralis major injury has never been reported in females! Repair is indicated in most active individuals, and late repair has also proven to be successful in many cases.

Procedure and Technique: The standard deltopectoral incision is extended distally and the ruptured muscle is identified, mobilized, and repaired to its normal insertion on the humerus. Suture anchor fixation has proven to be effective. Alternatively, sutures can be passed into a trough created at the pectoralis insertion.

Post-surgical Precautions/Rehabilitation: Primary rehabilitation is dependent upon the strength of the fixation. It is also important to know if the surgical tightening will result in a shortening of the muscle length, thus decreasing the amount of potentially available postoperative range of motion. Immediately postoperative, care should be taken to avoid external rotation and horizontal abduction. This will place tension on the repair. Cervical, elbow, and scapulothoracic range of motion can be performed immediately following surgery. Progression to shoulder elevation can be performed as tolerated. Return to exercises such as bench press and heavy weight lifting may take up to 6 months.

Expected Outcomes: Full strength is expected to return, with excellent functional ability as compared to pre-injury status. With a torn pectoralis muscle, surgical repair is oftentimes chosen versus conservative care.

Return to Play: Although the muscle will heal to bone within 6 to 12 weeks, return to play typically would be 4 to 6 months, and longer in a throwing athlete. Additional time is also required for those involved in activities that put heavy stresses on the anterior shoulder, such as weight lifting, wrestling, or tennis.

Recommended Readings

Anbari A, Kelly JD 4th, Moyer RA. Delayed repair of a ruptured pectoralis major muscle. A case report. *Am J Sports Med.* 2000;28(2): 254–256.

Kakwani RG, Matthews JJ, Kumar KM, Pimpalnerkar A, Mohtadi N. Rupture of the pectoralis major muscle: Surgical treatment in athletes. *Int Orthop.* 2007;31(2):159–163. Epub 2006 Jul 18.

Miller MD, Johnson DL, Fu FH, Thaete FL, Blanc RO. Rupture of the pectoralis major muscle in a collegiate football player. Use of magnetic resonance imaging in early diagnosis. *Am J Sports Med.* 1993;21(3):475–477.

Pavlik A, Csépai D, Berkes I. Surgical treatment of pectoralis major rupture in athletes. *Knee Surg Sports Traumatol Arthrosc.* 1998;6(2):129–133.

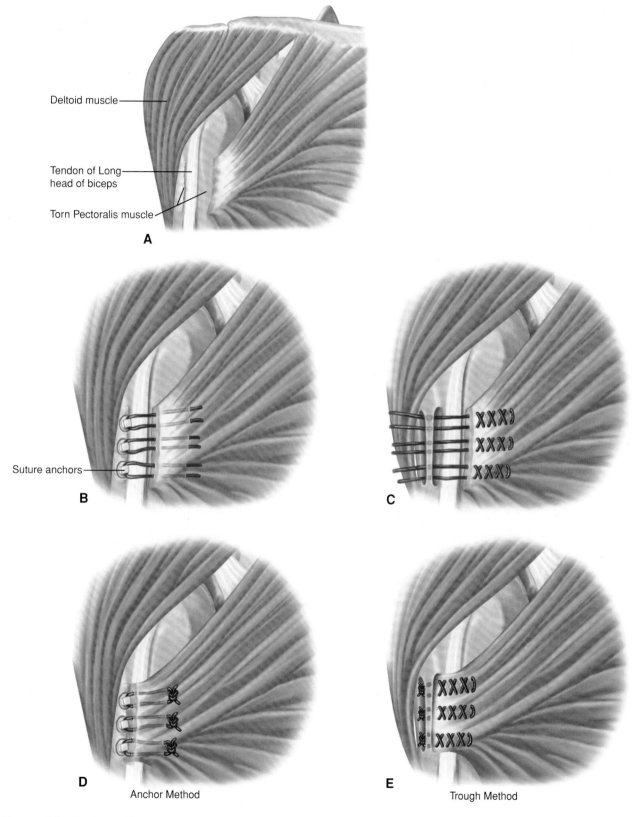

Deltoid muscle

Tendon of Long
head of biceps

Torn Pectoralis muscle

A

Suture anchors

B

C

D

Anchor Method

E

Trough Method

Figure 13. Pectoralis Major Repair. A. The torn pectoralis muscle is identified along with appropriate landmarks. **B,C.** Suture anchors placed lateral to the long head of biceps are tied to reapproximate the insertion. **D,E.** Bone tunnels can be used to create a through method for repair.

Subscapularis Tendon Repair

Indications and Goals: Subscapularis tendon ruptures are also rare, but can occur in association with traumatic anterior instability and degenerative conditions and, perhaps most commonly, following surgical closure of open glenohumeral procedures. Patients may recall an injury, or the tear may develop gradually. Exam findings include excessive external rotation (the subscapularis is a check-rein to external rotation beyond 70 to 90 degrees of rotation with the arm at the side) and a positive lift-off (patients unable to hold their hand off the small of their back) or belly-press (patients unable to symmetrically push their hand on their stomach) tests. MRI will confirm rupture of the tendon and medial biceps subluxation (no longer held by the tendon, so it can sublux medially). Operative treatment is usually indicated with the diagnosis being made.

Procedure and Technique: Although arthroscopic techniques have been described, most surgeons felt more comfortable with open repair of subscapularis tendon ruptures. A standard deltopectoral approach is made, the tendon is identified, and it is repaired anatomically, typically with suture anchors.

Post-surgical Precautions/Rehabilitation: The main precaution immediately postoperative is to avoid active internal rotation of the shoulder and passive and active external rotation of the shoulder for the first 4 weeks. These motions can gradually be addressed as tolerated using pain/discomfort as a guide.

Expected Outcomes: Studies report that arthroscopic repairs of an isolated subscapularis tear yield improvements with reduced pain, increased range of motion for forward flexion, external rotation, and internal rotation, as well as abduction strength. Though the structural integrity of the repair most often remains, cases have been reported involving partial re-ruptures.

Return to Play: Typically 4 to 6 months and longer in a throwing athlete. The quality of the repair will determine the ultimate success. Communication between the patient, clinicians, and surgeon is important to assess a safe timeline for return based upon the repair that was performed and the demands of the return to play.

Recommended Readings

Burkhart SS, Brady PC. Arthroscopic subscapularis repair: Surgical tips and pearls A to Z. *Arthroscopy.* 2006;22(9):1014–1027.

Flury MP, John M, Goldhahn J, Schwyzer HK, Simmen BR. Rupture of the subscapularis tendon (isolated or in combination with supraspinatus tear): When is a repair indicated? *J Shoulder Elbow Surg.* 2006;15(6):659–664. Epub 2006 Oct 19.

Ide J, Tokiyoshi A, Hirose J, Mizuta H. Arthroscopic repair of traumatic combined rotator cuff tears involving the subscapularis tendon. *J Bone Joint Surg Am.* 2007;89(11):2378–2388.

Lafosse L, Jost B, Reiland Y, Audebert S, Toussaint B, Gobezie R. Structural integrity and clinical outcomes after arthroscopic repair of isolated subscapularis tears. *J Bone Joint Surg Am.* 2007;89(6):1184–1193.

Maier D, Jaeger M, Suedkamp NP, Koestler W. Stabilization of the long head of the biceps tendon in the context of early repair of traumatic subscapularis tendon tears. *J Bone Joint Surg Am.* 2007;89(8):1763–1769.

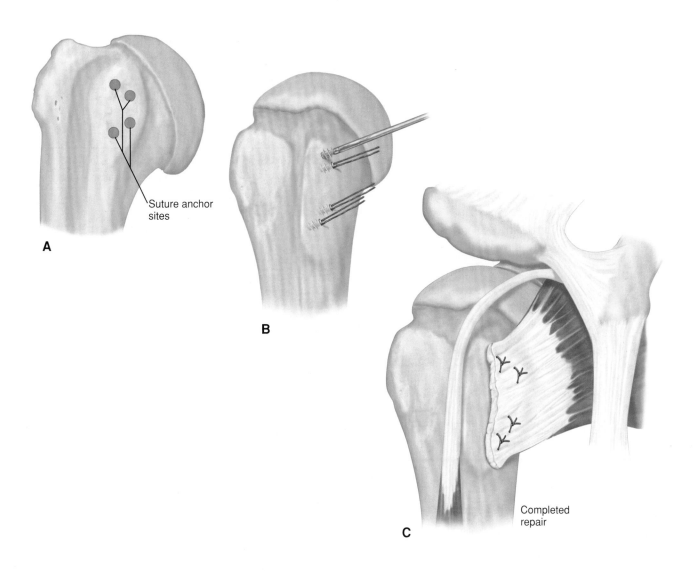

A

Suture anchor sites

B

C

Completed repair

Figure 14. Subscapularis Tendon Repair. A. Insertion site of the subscapularis is identified medial to the bicipital groove. **B.** Suture anchors are placed at the insertion site into the lesser tuberosity. **C.** Subscapularis tendon is mobilized and repaired to reapproximate the tendon insertion.

Release of Neurovascular Entrapment

Indications and Goals: There are a variety of nerve entrapment syndromes in and around the shoulder. Some of these syndromes extend beyond the boundaries of conventional "sports medicine." However, a brief description of them follows. For all of these syndromes, symptoms (numbness, weakness, paresthesias, etc.) follow the distribution of the entrapped nerve. Imaging is sometimes difficult and electrodiagnostic (EMG, NCS) studies are often helpful in making the diagnosis. Surgical release of the offending structure(s), either via arthroscopic or open procedures, is designed to relieve symptoms (although it may often take months to return). Vascular entrapment may be more difficult to identify, but ischemic pain may occur and vascular studies (both invasive and noninvasive) may help establish the diagnosis.

Procedure and Technique: The following are the common shoulder neurovascular entrapments and their treatments:

Nerve/Artery	Location of Entrapment	Treatment
Suprascapular nerve	Suprascapular notch (SS and IS)	Release transverse scapular ligament
	Spinoglenoid notch (IS only)	Decompress cyst and repair labrum
Thoracic outlet syndrome	Brachial plexus/subclavian A/V	First rib resection
Quadrilateral space syndrome	Axillary N/circumflex scap A	Release teres M
Axillary/subclavian		Remove clot/aneurysm
Thrombosis/aneurysm		

Post-surgical Precautions/Rehabilitation: Rehabilitation following the release of an entrapped neurovascular structure is relatively simplistic. Since no tissue was directly repaired, there are no precautions with extreme range of motion gains during the early postoperative days. In some cases, individuals may complain of minimal symptoms postoperatively that mimic preoperative symptoms, oftentimes related to the acute inflammation surrounding the surgical region. The individual will become asymptomatic once the inflammation is reduced. Scar management should be addressed early on to reduce the sensitivity to the area.

Expected Outcomes: Outcomes will vary based upon the procedure performed. Ultimately, an accurate diagnosis followed by a successful release will result in a reduction of neurovascular symptoms. Symptoms that remain within a few months postoperative should be re-assessed for diagnostic accuracy.

Return to Play: If symptoms resolve, the athlete should expect to return to play in 3 to 4 months. A gradual return should pay careful attention to any reoccurrence of symptoms.

Recommended Readings

Aval SM, Durand P Jr, Shankwiler JA. Neurovascular injuries to the athlete's shoulder: Part II. *J Am Acad Orthop Surg.* 2007;15(5): 281–289. Review.

Gosk J, Urban M, Rutowski R. Entrapment of the suprascapular nerve: Anatomy, etiology, diagnosis, treatment. *Orthop Traumatol Rehabil.* 2007;9(1):68–74. Review.

Hosseini H, Agneskirchner JD, Tröger M, Lobenhoffer P. Arthroscopic release of the superior transverse ligament and SLAP refixation in a case of suprascapular nerve entrapment. *Arthroscopy.* 2007;23(10):1134.e1–1134.e4. Epub 2007 Apr 19.

Lafosse L, Tomasi A, Corbett S, Baier G, Willems K, Gobezie R. Arthroscopic release of suprascapular nerve entrapment at the suprascapular notch: Technique and preliminary results. *Arthroscopy.* 2007;23(1):34–42.

Reeser JC. Diagnosis and management of vascular injuries in the shoulder girdle of the overhead athlete. *Curr Sports Med Rep.* 2007;6(5):322–327.

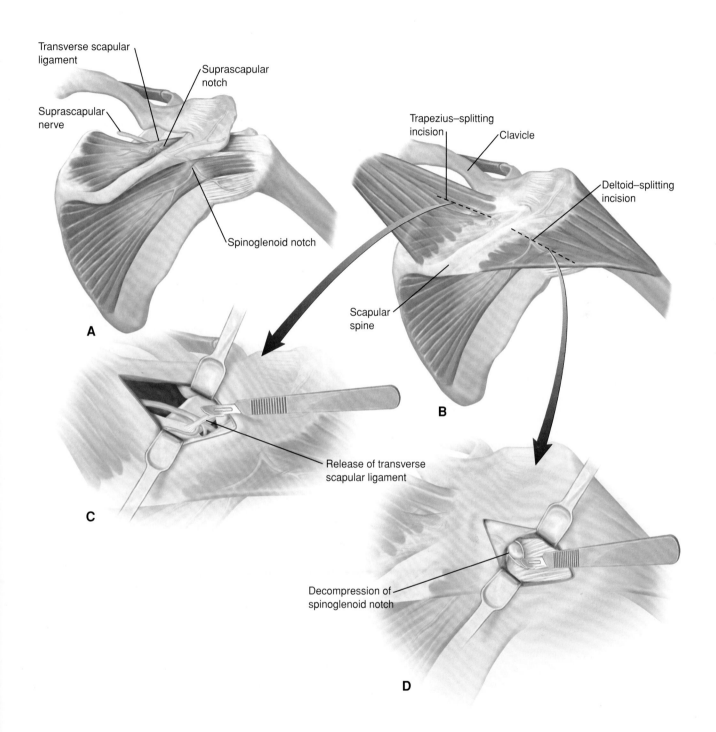

Figure 15. Suprascapular Nerve Release. A. Suprascapular nerve entrapment can occur within the suprascapular notch or from constriction at the pictured spinoglenoid notch. **B.** Open release through a trapezius or deltoid splitting incision allows access to release the transverse scapular ligament at the suprascapular notch **C,** or decompression of the spinoglenoid notch **D.**

Coracoclavicular Ligament Repair/ Reconstruction

Indications and Goals: Most acromioclavicular separations are low grade and do not require operative intervention. More significant separations (greater than 100% displacement [grade V] or posterior displacement of the clavicle [grade IV]) and occasionally chronic lower grade separations that continue to be symptomatic require surgery. The goal is to restore the normal relationship between the coracoid and the clavicle by mobilizing and reducing the joint and then placing some type of fixation between the two bones.

Procedure and Technique: A 5 cm (2 in.) saber incision is made over the distal clavicle and the end of the clavicle is stripped of all soft tissue. While a variety of options have been described (suture constructs, screws, soft tissue) we prefer to use a free tendon (autologous hamstring or allograft tibialis anterior) to pass under the coracoid and fix into the clavicle for chronic injuries (acute injuries typically do not require grafts). The joint is reduced and the tendon is passed through drill holes in the clavicle. Small bioabsorbable interference screws are used to secure the tendon. Most of the time, we prefer to preserve the distal clavicle; however, in chronic cases, the distal clavicle can be resected and the coracoacromial ligament is transferred into the resected end (Weaver–Dunn procedure).

Post-surgical Precautions/Rehabilitation: Since the glenohumeral joint is not violated, stiffness is rarely a problem and prolonged immobilization is appropriate following this procedure. Rare exception would be with an elderly patient, whereby disuse may lead to joint stiffness. However, this type of injury and subsequent surgical procedure are more likely to be seen with a younger population. Protective healing may take up to 8 weeks accompanied by a gradual increase of range of motion. Care should be taken early on to avoid any downward forces to the lateral upper arm region as this would place stress on the repair.

Expected Outcomes: With postoperative compliancy, outcomes are very positive for joint stabilization and return to activity without range of motion restrictions.

Return to Play: With anatomic restoration of the AC joint, return to play is possible at 3 to 4 months postoperatively.

Recommended Readings

Jin CZ, Kim HK, Min BH. Surgical treatment for distal clavicle fracture associated with coracoclavicular ligament rupture using a cannulated screw fixation technique. *J Trauma*. 2006;60(6):1358–1361.

Lee SJ, Nicholas SJ, Akizuki KH, McHugh MP, Kremenic IJ, Ben-Avi S. Reconstruction of the coracoclavicular ligaments with tendon grafts: A comparative biomechanical study. *Am J Sports Med*. 2003;31(5):648–655.

Mazzocca AD, Arciero RA, Bicos J. Evaluation and treatment of acromioclavicular joint injuries. *Am J Sports Med*. 2007;35(2): 316–329. Review.

Wellmann M, Zantop T, Weimann A, Raschke MJ, Petersen W. Biomechanical evaluation of minimally invasive repairs for complete acromioclavicular joint dislocation. *Am J Sports Med*. 2007;35(6):955–961. Epub 2007 Feb 22.

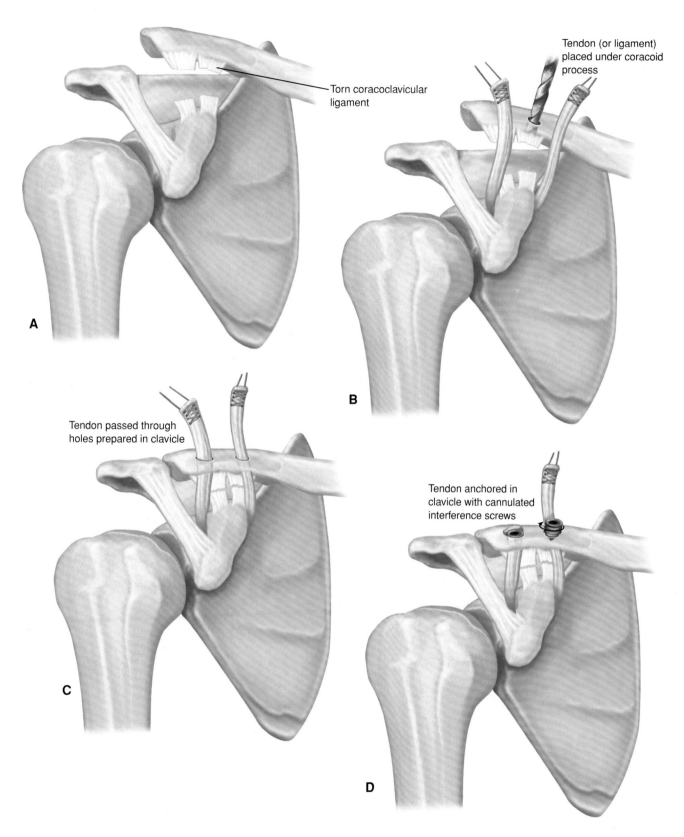

Torn coracoclavicular ligament

Tendon (or ligament) placed under coracoid process

Tendon passed through holes prepared in clavicle

Tendon anchored in clavicle with cannulated interference screws

A

B

C

D

Figure 16. Ligament Reconstruction. A. Complete disruption of the CC ligaments. Acromioclavicular ligament reconstruction: **B.** Graft is looped around the coracoid base with bone tunnel drilled through the clavicle. **C.** The graft is placed through the drill holes and the clavicle reduced. **D.** The graft is fixed in position using interference screw(s).

Sternoclavicular Procedures

Indications and Goals: Sternoclavicular dislocations are rare, but if they are significantly displaced, they may need surgical treatment. Chronic injuries may also occasionally need reduction and fixation. Most surgeons have a healthy respect for the major neurovascular structures that lie beneath the sternoclavicular joint, so surgical decision making is usually on the conservative side.

Procedure and Technique: Closed reduction through indirect traction or with the use of a sterile towel clip in the operating room may be successful for symptomatic (difficulty breathing or swallowing) posterior dislocations. Reduction of anterior dislocations is usually not successful because of recurrent instability, but is less of a problem. Rarely, the medial clavicle can be resected and a graft can be used to reconstruct the joint in chronic refractory cases. Extreme caution is used to protect the posterior structures.

Post-surgical Precautions/Rehabilitation: Activity and rehabilitation focuses on early protection of the sternoclavicular joint. While bracing is not necessary, limited shoulder elevation, abduction, and adduction should be encouraged for the first 2 weeks and only utilized as needed. This will facilitate localized scarring of the tissue without leading to postoperative recurrent instability. Mobilization to surrounding joints can be performed passively under supervision initially, and can progress to independent active exercises as tolerated. Activity that involves potential contact such as with team sports should be delayed for a minimum of 6 weeks, and consideration should be given to using a protective padding device to reduce forces that may be applied to the sternoclavicular joint, especially with a previously posteriorly directed instability.

Expected Outcomes: Functional outcomes approximately 2 years postoperatively are reported as excellent for children and adolescents, absent any respiratory or neurovascular complications. Stabilization appears to be accomplished relatively often with adult patients.

Return to Play: With anatomic reconstruction, return to play may be within 3 to 4 months.

Recommended Readings

Battaglia TC, Pannunzio ME, Chhabra AB, Degnan GG. Interposition arthroplasty with bone-tendon allograft: A technique for treatment of the unstable sternoclavicular joint. *J Orthop Trauma.* 2005;19(2):124–129.

Brinker MR, Bartz RL, Reardon PR, Reardon MJ. A method for open reduction and internal fixation of the unstable posterior sternoclavicular joint dislocation. *J Orthop Trauma.* 1997;11(5):378–381.

Thomas DP, Williams PR, Hoddinott HC. A 'safe' surgical technique for stabilisation of the sternoclavicular joint: A cadaveric and clinical study. *Ann R Coll Surg Engl.* 2000;82(6):432–435.

Tubbs RS, Loukas M, Slappey JB, McEvoy WC, Linganna S, Shoja MM, Oakes WJ. Surgical and clinical anatomy of the interclavicular ligament. *Surg Radiol Anat.* 2007;29(5):357–360. Epub 2007 Jun 12.

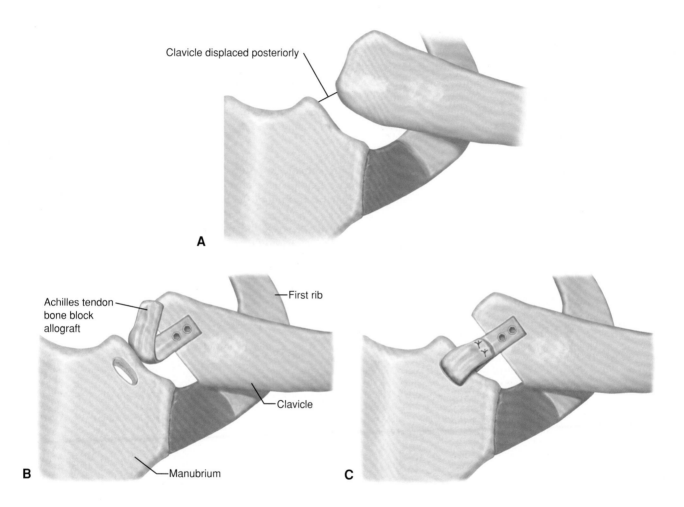

Figure 17. Sternoclavicular Reconstruction. A. Viewing from superior, posterior sternoclavicular dissociation is shown. **B.** Allograft reconstruction is attached to the medial clavicle and **(C)** fixed after passing through the sternum.

Articular Cartilage Procedures

Indications and Goals: Although it is less commonly encountered in the shoulder than the knee, focal full-thickness cartilage loss can occur, often as a result of trauma. Pain, mechanical catching, and other symptoms may necessitate consideration of operative intervention.

Procedure and Technique: Shoulder arthroscopy is carried out in either the beach chair or the lateral decubitus position. The base and edges of the lesion are smoothed out with a shaver or a curette (small spoon-like instrument). The lesion is then treated with microfracture (small holes are made into the bone to allow marrow cells to escape and fill the defect with a clot that will later mature into healing fibrocartilage) or other techniques. Larger defects in the humeral head can be filled with allograft cartilage or specially developed implants.

Post-surgical Precautions/Rehabilitation: A procedure that involves articular cartilage within the shoulder complex requires early protection against joint compressive forces. Closed kinetic chain activities should be avoided, and instead an emphasis should be placed on local joint distraction and adjacent joint mobilization. Range of motion can begin immediately following surgery, with minimal to no added resistance applied to exercises for the first 4 weeks since these can require an increase in muscle contractile forces which in turn will increase joint compressive forces.

Expected Outcomes: There appears to be good clinical results found when treating full-thickness osteochondral lesions of the glenohumeral joint. However, studies suggest that the development of osteoarthritis and the progression of preexisting osteoarthritic changes may be technique dependent.

Return to Play: This is totally dependent upon the size of the lesion and the extent of surgery. For small- to medium-sized focal lesions treated with microfracture, return to play can be within 3 to 4 months. Larger defects may delay return to play for 6 months or longer.

Recommended Readings

Gold GE, Reeder SB, Beaulieu CF. Advanced MR imaging of the shoulder: Dedicated cartilage techniques. *Magn Reson Imaging Clin N Am.* 2004;12(1):143–159, vii. Review.

Hamada J, Tamai K, Koguchi Y, Ono W, Saotome K. Case report: A rare condition of secondary synovial osteochondromatosis of the shoulder joint in a young female patient. *J Shoulder Elbow Surg.* 2005;14(6):653–656.

Kim SH, Noh KC, Park JS, Ryu BD, Oh I. Loss of chondrolabral containment of the glenohumeral joint in atraumatic posteroinferior multidirectional instability. *J Bone Joint Surg Am.* 2005;87(1):92–98.

Scheibel M, Bartl C, Magosch P, Lichtenberg S, Habermeyer P. Osteochondral autologous transplantation for the treatment of full-thickness articular cartilage defects of the shoulder. *J Bone Joint Surg Br.* 2004;86(7):991–997.

Thomas DP, Williams PR, Hoddinott HC. A 'safe' surgical technique for stabilisation of the sternoclavicular joint: A cadaveric and clinical study. *Ann R Coll Surg Engl.* 2000;82(6):432–435.

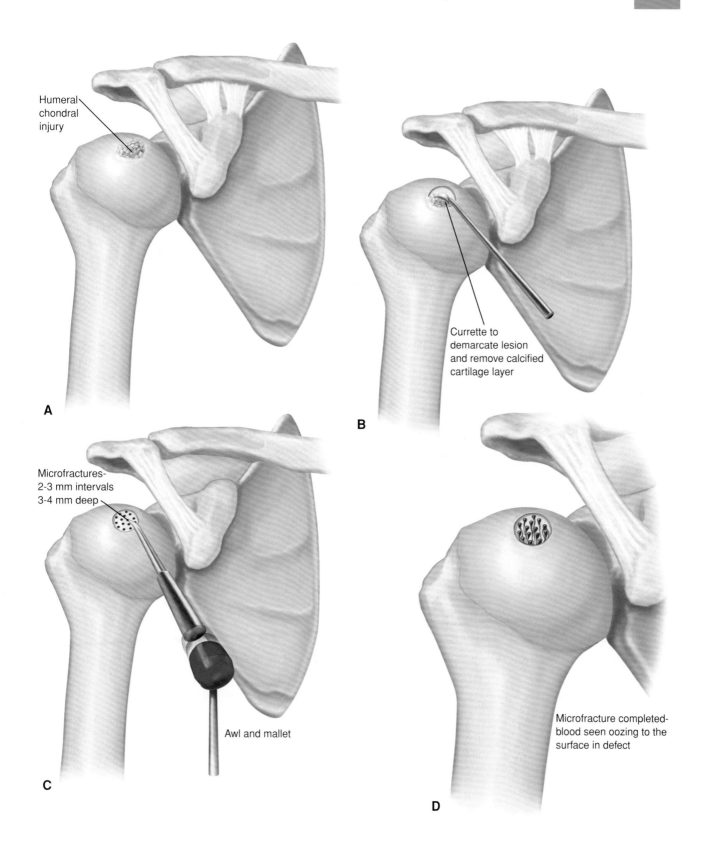

Figure 18. Microfracture/Osteochondral Autologous Transplantation. A. High grade chondral injury to humeral head surface shown. **B.** A curette is utilized to debride overlying calcified cartilage layer. **C.** A microfracture awl is used to make 3–4 mm deep holes. **D.** Bleeding bony bed at completion of procedure.

Shoulder Arthroplasty

Indications and Goals: Shoulder degenerative joint disease (thinning and loss of the articular cartilage) can be a result of repetitive trauma and overuse. When the cartilage loss is diffuse, then resurfacing of the joint may be the only surgical option. Obviously, this is not appropriate for younger, active individuals and represents a salvage option for patients with refractory pain and loss of motion.

Procedure and Technique: There are three basic options for shoulder arthroplasty: Placing a small implant that resurfaces the head only (Copeland-type prosthesis), placing a stem into the bony canal with an attached head (hemiarthroplasty), or adding a glenoid implant to resurface the socket with high-grade plastic (polyethylene) (total shoulder arthroplasty). All three procedures are done through a deltopectoral approach. The head-resurfacing implant involves reaming the head and placing a metal cover over it. The other implants require preparation of the canal with various reamers and rasps and then placing a size-matched implant into the canal with or without bone cement. A metal head is fixed onto the implant at the completion of the case. If a total shoulder arthroplasty is planned, the glenoid is prepared and the implant is cemented into place prior to inserting the head on the humeral implant. For younger patients with isolated humeral-sided arthrosis, humeral arthroplasty with soft tissue glenoid resurfacing may be a consideration.

Post-surgical Precautions/Rehabilitation: Immediately postoperative, the patient will be in a hospital stay may be 1 to 3 days. Motion exercises such as pendulums and Codman's can begin on day 1, with limitations on external rotation movements possibly up to 6 weeks as specified by the surgeon and the prosthetic design used. Exercises should be performed with supervision, but can be done active or active assisted if able. A focus should be on pain management to allow for pain-free range of motion exercises to be performed regularly. Around 6 weeks postoperatively, gradual resistive exercises can be implemented for the shoulder girdle. In addition, proprioceptive exercises can be added at this time to improve the functional use of the shoulder. Some form of cardiovascular exercise should accompany the rehabilitation procedure given the typical age of a patient undergoing this type of a procedure and the activity limitations following the surgery. Driving is not advised until a minimum of 6 weeks postoperatively. Ultimately, weight-lifting restrictions of about 10 pounds should be considered even after full recovery.

Expected Outcomes: It is important to note that the rate of postoperative rehabilitation progression will weigh primarily on four factors: surgeon preference, prosthetic devise used, type of procedure performed, and status of repaired tissue. Expected outcomes should focus more on decreased pain and increased function as commonly accepted goals.

Return to Play: Unlikely in a competitive athlete. Recreational athletes may return to some activities, but often in moderation after 6 to 12 months.

Recommended Readings

Bohsali KI, Wirth MA, Rockwood CA Jr. Complications of total shoulder arthroplasty. *J Bone Joint Surg Am.* 2006;88(10):2279–2292. Review.

Bryant D, Litchfield R, Sandow M, Gartsman GM, Guyatt G, Kirkley A. A comparison of pain, strength, range of motion, and functional outcomes after hemiarthroplasty and total shoulder arthroplasty in patients with osteoarthritis of the shoulder. A systematic review and meta-analysis. *J Bone Joint Surg Am.* 2005;87(9):1947–1956. Review.

Ho JY, Miller SL. Allografts in the treatment of athletic injuries of the shoulder. *Sports Med Arthrosc.* 2007;15(3):149–157. Review.

Matsen FA 3rd, Bicknell RT, Lippitt SB. Shoulder arthroplasty: The socket perspective. *J Shoulder Elbow Surg.* 2007;16(5 suppl): S241–S247. Epub 2007 Apr 19. Review.

Pennington WT, Bartz BA. Arthroscopic glenoid resurfacing with meniscal allograft: A minimally invasive alternative for treating glenohumeral arthritis. *Arthroscopy.* 2005;21(12):1517–1520.

Radnay CS, Setter KJ, Chambers L, Levine WN, Bigliani LU, Ahmad CS. Total shoulder replacement compared with humeral head replacement for the treatment of primary glenohumeral osteoarthritis: A systematic review. *J Shoulder Elbow Surg.* 2007;16(4):396–402. Epub 2007 Jun 20. Review.

Wilcox RB, Arslanian LE, Millett P. Rehabilitation following total shoulder arthroplasty. *J Orthop Sports Phys Ther.* 2005;35(12): 821–836. Review.

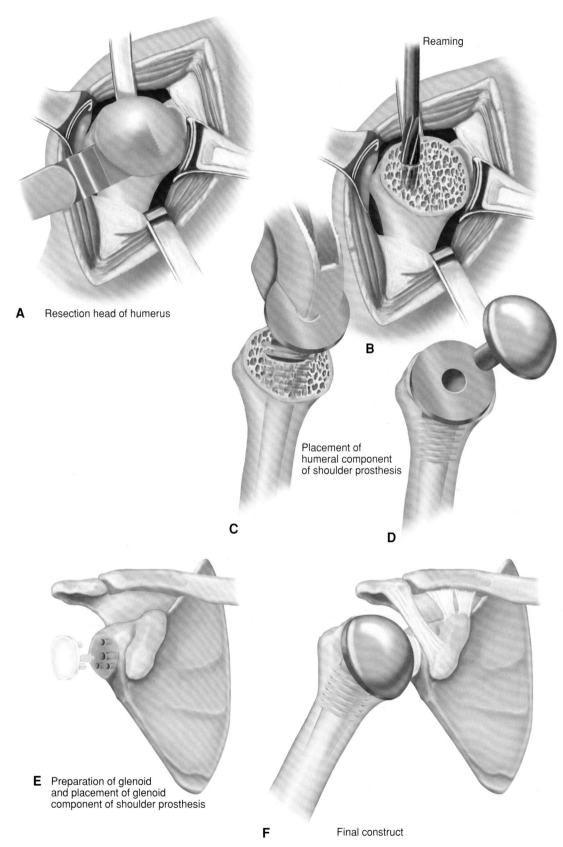

Figure 19. Shoulder Arthroplasty Technique. A. The exposed humeral head is resected to allow for placement of humeral stem. **B.** Reaming is performed to prepare the humeral shaft for stem insertion. **C,D.** The humeral component is inserted. **E,F.** The glenoid is reamed and glenoid component fixed.

ORIF Clavicle Fractures

Indications and Goals: The indications for clavicle open reduction and internal fixation (ORIF) have evolved, and surgical reduction and fixation is now recommended for significantly displaced (more than 2 cm) fractures and some distal clavicle fractures. Open fractures, neurovascular injury (or impending injury), and certain other fractures may require ORIF. Reduction and fixation with bone grafting is also indicated for chronic, symptomatic nonunions of the clavicle.

Procedure and Technique: Traditionally, plates and screws are used for clavicular fixation. More recently, intramedullary fixation has become popular. A direct approach to the fracture allows the ends to be mobilized and prepared, and then the fracture is reduced and fixed with the implant of choice. Vertical or oblique limited incisions can reduce iatrogenic injury to supraclavicular nerve branches.

Post-surgical Precautions/Rehabilitation: Prolonged immobilization is necessary to ensure that these fractures heal, possibly taking up to 12 weeks before satisfactory results. The patient will be required to wear a shoulder sling for approximately 6 weeks postoperatively, allowing for reduced gravitation loads to be placed on the clavicle. In the interim, a focus on scapulothoracic, glenohumeral, and elbow range of motion can be accomplished. Loss of motion is typically not a problem because the glenohumeral joint is not violated. Resistive exercises for the shoulder can begin lightly at week 2 and be guided for progression using discomfort as a measure of limits. There is no rush to regain strength; emphasis should be placed on the healing clavicle. Full activity that places stress on the clavicle should be reserved for a minimum of 6 months.

Expected Outcomes: Overall, the procedure has minor risks and complications, with good outcomes associated with proper hardware alignment and insertion.

Return to Play: After complete healing and rehabilitation, 6 months is a safe time frame to use as a guide for return to competition. The area may still be sensitive to contact, and any symptoms that return should be taken seriously and may warrant an x-ray to assure continued healing is taking place without unwanted stresses.

Recommended Readings

Denard PJ, Koval KJ, Cantu RV, Weinstein JN. Management of midshaft clavicle fractures in adults. *Am J Orthop*. 2005;34(11):527–536.

Jeray KJ. Acute midshaft clavicle fracture. *J Am Acad Orthop Surg*. 2007;15(4):239–248.

Kettler M, Schieker M, Braunstein V, König M, Mutschler W. Flexible intramedullary nailing for stabilization of displaced midshaft clavicle fractures: Technique and results in 87 patients. *Acta Orthop*. 2007;78(3):424–429.

Meier C, Grueninger P, Platz A. Elastic stable intramedullary nailing for midclavicular fractures in athletes: Indications, technical pitfalls, and early results. *Acta Orthop Belg*. 2006;72(3):269–275.

Mueller M, Burger C, Florczyk A, Striepends N, Rangger C. Elastic stable intramedullary nailing of midclavicular fractures in adults: 32 patients followed for 1–5 years. *Acta Orthop*. 2007;78(3):421–423.

Zlowodzki M, Zelle BA, Cole PA, Jeray K, McKee MD. Evidence based orthopaedic trauma working group. *J Orthop Trauma*. 2005;19(7):504–507.

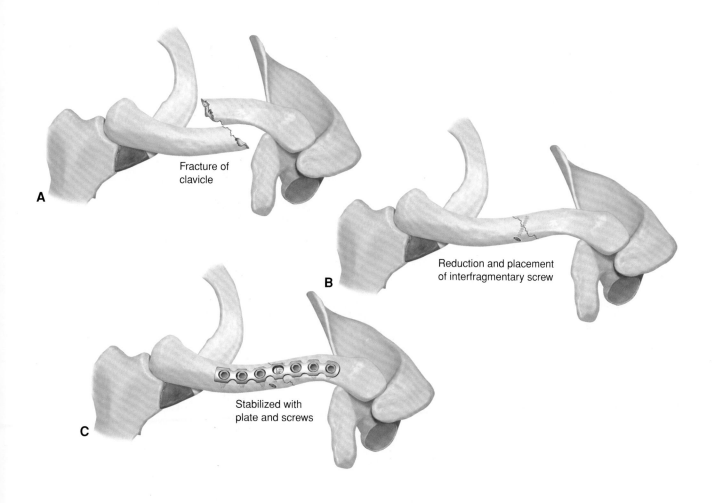

Fracture of
clavicle

A

Reduction and placement
of interfragmentary screw

B

Stabilized with
plate and screws

C

Figure 20. Open Reduction, Internal Fixation of Clavicle Fracture (A). B. A lag screw is placed perpendicular to the fracture line. **C.** Superior plate placed for stabilization.

ORIF Proximal Humerus Fractures

Indications and Goals: Proximal humerus fractures are relatively rare in the athletic population, and most of these injuries can be treated nonoperatively. These fractures are more common in the elderly population, especially in post-menopausal women. Open reduction and internal fixation is preferred over hemiarthroplasty whenever possible, but especially in the younger, more active patient.

Procedure and Technique: This procedure is typically done in a beach chair position with the use of x-ray (fluoroscopy). A deltopectoral incision is made and the fracture is reduced. Although a variety of implants are available, newer locking plates have made this operation much more successful. The plates are secured on the lateral side of the proximal humerus after reduction.

Post-surgical Precautions/Rehabilitation: A patient can expect to have at most an overnight hospital stay, and early supervised rehabilitation should be encouraged for educational purposes. Early joint range of motion for both the shoulder and the elbow region should be encouraged. Heavy resistance should be avoided for at least 3 to 4 months, allowing for a complete healing of the humerus. Strengthening activities can be implemented approximately during week 2 postoperatively and can be gradually increased as tolerated. Emphasis should be placed on restoring functional task abilities and avoiding secondary range of motion limitations that can occur from overly cautious immobilization and decreased activity.

Expected Outcomes: Fractures to the head or neck may take slightly longer to heal versus those to the shaft of the humerus. Postoperative risks of avascular necrosis and nonunions may exist in older populations.

Return to Play: Depends upon the extent of the fracture and whether anatomic restoration is possible. In the best circumstances, 4 to 6 months may be possible. Return to play may also be determined by the health status of the bone and the general age of the patient.

Recommended Readings

Hodgson S. Proximal humerus fracture rehabilitation. *Clin Orthop Relat Res*. 2006;442:131–138.

Kocher MS, Waters PM, Micheli LJ. Upper extremity injuries in the pediatric athlete. *Sports Med*. 2000;30(2):117–135.

Sperling JW, Cuomo F, Hill JD, Hertel R, Chuinard C, Boileau P. The difficult proximal humerus fracture: Tips and techniques to avoid complications and improve results. *Instr Course Lect*. 2007;56:45–57.

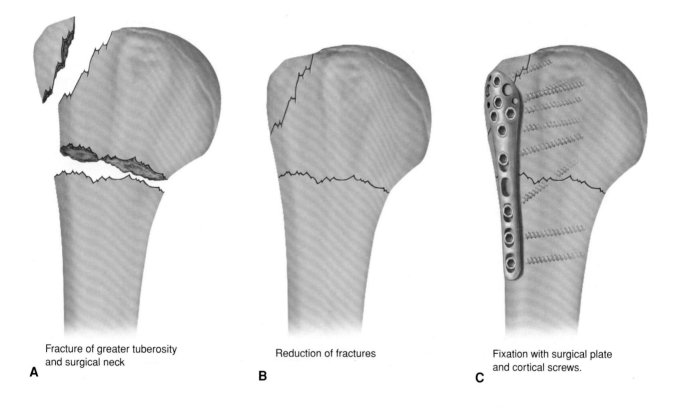

Fracture of greater tuberosity
and surgical neck

A

Reduction of fractures

B

Fixation with surgical plate
and cortical screws.

C

Figure 21. Open Reduction, Internal Fixation of Proximal Humerus Fracture. A. Proximal
humerus fracture shown with displacement of the greater tuberosity and surgical
neck. **B,C.** Open reduction and internal fixation with plate shand screws.

ORIF Humeral Shaft Fractures

Indications and Goals: Most humeral shaft fractures can be treated nonoperatively with a brace. Open fractures, certain fractures with neurovascular injuries, and fractures in multitrauma victims may require ORIF. Humeral shaft fractures can be characterized as simple (spiral, oblique, or transverse) or complex (comminution). The goal of the procedure is to restore the length and alignment of the humerus.

Procedure and Technique: An incision is made centered on the fracture and reduction is accomplished. Typically, an anterior (extended deltopectoral) incision is used. A large broad plate is selected and secured to the side of the bone with screws. It is critical to protect the radial nerve which spirals around the back of the humerus during fixation (especially if cerclage wires are used). Another alternative is to place an intramedullary (IM) nail down the shaft of the humerus to secure the fracture. The problem with IM devices is that they can cause rotator cuff problems.

Post-surgical Precautions/Rehabilitation: A patient can expect to have at most an overnight hospital stay, and early supervised rehabilitation should be encouraged for educational purposes. As the healing component is within the long shaft of the bone, early joint range of motion for both the shoulder and the elbow region should be encouraged. Heavy resistance should be avoided for at least 3 to 4 months, allowing for a complete healing of the humerus. Strengthening activities can be implemented approximately during week 2 postoperatively and can be gradually increased as tolerated. Emphasis should be placed on restoring functional task abilities and avoiding secondary range of motion limitations that can occur from overly cautious immobilization and decreased activity.

Expected Outcomes: Fractures to the shaft may heal in less time versus those of the neck or head of the humerus. Outcomes may be correlated with the severity of the fracture, anatomical reduction results, and positioning of the hardware. Though minimally reported, one should be cautious for vascular complications.

Return to Play: With anatomic restoration and complete healing, return to play can be within 4 to 6 months. The age of the patient and the health status of the bone may alter this timeline.

Recommended Readings

Changulani M, Jain UK, Keswani T. Comparison of the use of the humerus intramedullary nail and dynamic compression plate for the management of diaphyseal fractures of the humerus. A randomised controlled study. *Int Orthop.* 2007;31(3):391–395. Epub 2006 Aug 10.

Hierholzer C, Sama D, Toro JB, Peterson M, Helfet DL. Plate fixation of ununited humeral shaft fractures: Effect of type of bone graft on healing. *J Bone Joint Surg Am.* 2006;88(7):1442–1447.

Rubel IF, Kloen P, Campbell D, Schwartz M, Liew A, Myers E, Helfet DL. Open reduction and internal fixation of humeral nonunions: A biomechanical and clinical study. *J Bone Joint Surg Am.* 2002;84-A(8):1315–1322.

Zhiquan A, Bingfang Z, Yeming W, Chi Z, Peiyan H. Minimally invasive plating osteosynthesis (MIPO) of middle and distal third humeral shaft fractures. *J Orthop Trauma.* 2007;21(9):628–633.

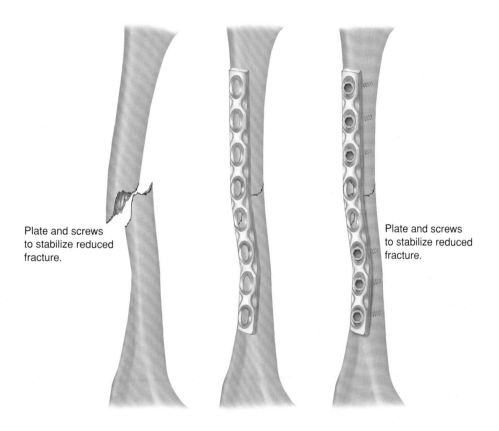

Plate and screws
to stabilize reduced
fracture.

Plate and screws
to stabilize reduced
fracture.

Figure 22. Open Reduction and Internal Fixation of Humeral Shaft Fracture with Plate and Screw Construct

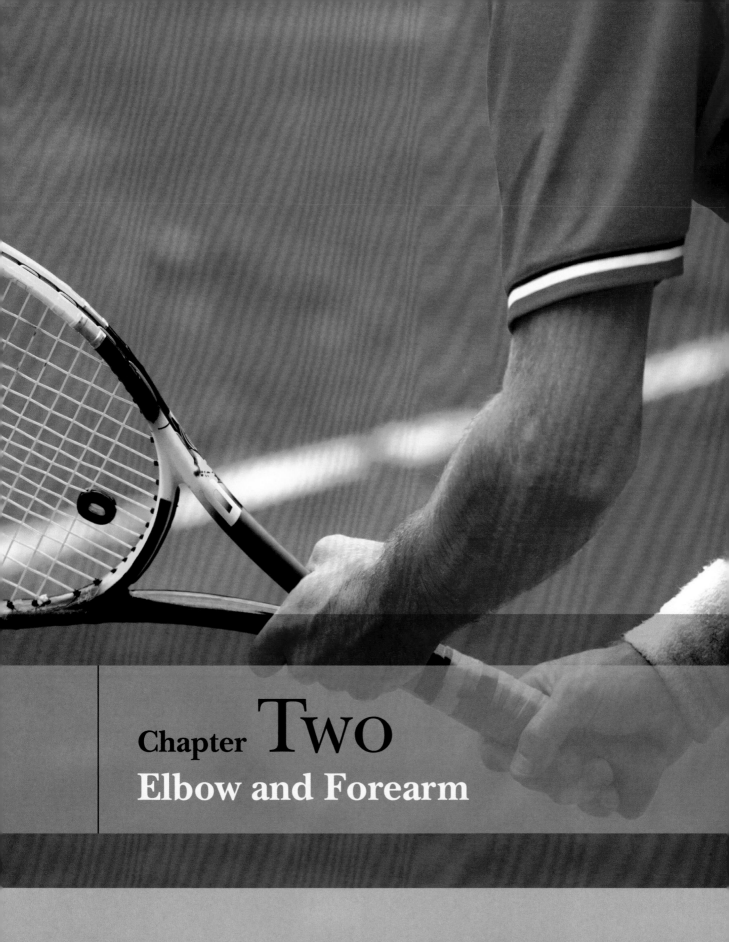

Chapter TWO
Elbow and Forearm

Elbow Arthroscopy

Indications and Goals: Elbow arthroscopy is a valuable treatment modality in a variety of pathologic conditions, including loose body removal, synovectomy, osteophyte debridement, treatment of osteochondral injuries (usually of the capitellum), evaluation of joint stability, and even radial head excision and extensor carpi radialis brevis (ECRB) release for tennis elbow.

Procedure and Technique: On the basis of the surgeon's preference, the patient can be placed in the lateral decubitus, prone, or supine position. There are seven portals that have been most commonly described for elbow arthroscopy and that can be further divided into anterior and posterior portals. Anterior portals are the proximal medial portal, the anterolateral portal, and the proximal lateral portal. The posterior portals consist of the midlateral (soft spot) portal, the posterior lateral portal, the transtriceps portal, and the accessory lateral portal. Anterior portals must be made with the elbow in flexion in order to reduce the risk of injury to the neurovascular structures.

Anterior Portals: The proximal medial portal is usually the first portal created as it provides visualization of the entire anterior compartment. It is located 2 cm proximal to the medial epicondyle and anterior to the intermuscular septum. The septum protects the ulnar nerve while the trochar is advanced into the central portion of the elbow against the anterior margin of the humerus. Any history of a subluxating or previously transposed ulnar nerve must be obtained as these conditions place the ulnar nerve at risk and require exposure and protection of the nerve under direct visualization. This portal provides the best access to the radial head and capitellum.

The proximal lateral portal is 2 cm proximal to the lateral epicondyle of the humerus and lies on the anterior margin of the humerus. It is considered the safest of all anterior portals. This portal can access the distal humerus, trochlear ridges, and coronoid process.

The anterolateral portal is located 2 cm distal and 1 cm anterior to the lateral epicondyle. It is less commonly used as it puts the radial nerve at risk. If used, it is safest to create this portal with an inside-out technique to reduce the risk of injury to the radial nerve. This portal can access the distal humerus, trochlear ridges, coronoid process, and radial head.

Posterior Portals: The midlateral or soft spot portal is located at the center of a triangle bordered by the olecranon, the lateral epicondyle, and the radial head. It is used initially for insufflation (approximately 20 mL) before arthroscopy and for visualization and instrumentation of the inferior radiocapitellar joint and the proximal radioulnar joint.

The posterolateral portal is created at the level of the tip of the olecranon and just lateral to the border of the triceps. The posterior lateral portal is the main viewing portal for the posterior compartment of the elbow.

The transtriceps portal is created 3 cm proximal to the tip of the olecranon and is used for visualization and instrumentation of the tip of the olecranon, the humeral fossa, and the humeral trochlea.

The accessory or adjacent lateral portal is made in the area of the soft spot portal and is used for visualization and instrumentation of the radiocapitellar joint, in particular for osseous and chondral procedures related to osteochondritis dissecans of the joint.

Post-surgical Precautions/Rehabilitation: Rehabilitation following an elbow arthroscopy that does not involve tissue repair can be relatively progressive. Performed as an outpatient procedure, an individual can utilize a compression wrap to reduce postoperative swelling. Range of motion exercises can be begun immediately as needed to restore normal movement. Splints and immobilization braces are usually not needed. Scar management and pain control can be addressed from the onset, and a return to participation and/or activity can occur on an individual basis as one feels comfortable. If the original condition was the result of a repetitive stress injury, then education regarding appropriate biomechanics ergonomics may need to occur to prevent against a recurrence.

Expected Outcomes: If diligent attention is paid to anatomic detail, arthroscopy of the elbow is safe and effective, with success rates for various procedures around 90%. An overall complication rate of 12.6% has been reported, but this can be minimized by limiting joint distension by limiting fluid pressure, placing portals with the elbow flexed at 90 degrees, recognizing that the radial nerve is at greatest risk at the anterior lateral portal, and avoiding posterior medial and direct anterior portals.

Return to Play: Depends upon the procedure. Procedures that do not affect the structural integrity of the joint may allow return within weeks and more extensive procedures months. Throwing athletes who have more extensive procedures including ligament reconstruction may require several months before the athlete can return to play.

Recommended Readings

Brownlow HC, O'Connor-Read LM, Perko M. Arthroscopic treatment of osteochondritis dissecans of the capitellum. *Knee Surg Sports Traumatol Arthrosc.* 2006;14(2):198–202. Epub 2005 Apr 26.

Coleman SH, Altchek DW. Arthroscopy and the thrower's elbow. In: Green DP, et al., eds. *Green's Operative Hand Surgery.* 5th ed. Philadelphia, PA: Elsevier; 2005:959–972.

Elbow arthroscopy: Surgical techniques and rehabilitation. *J Hand Ther.* 2006;19(2):228–236. Review.

Kelly EW, Morrey BF, O'Driscoll SW. Complications of elbow arthroscopy. *J Bone Joint Surg Am.* 2001;83-A(1):25–34.

McGinty JB, et al., eds. The elbow. In: *Operative Arthroscopy.* 3rd ed. Baltimore: Lippincott Williams and Wilkins; 2003:661–717.

O'Holleran JD, Altchek DW. Elbow arthroscopy: Treatment of the thrower's elbow. *Instr Course Lect.* 2006;55:95–107. Review. Brach P, Goitz RJ.

Savoie FH 3rd. Guidelines to becoming an expert elbow arthroscopist. *Arthroscopy.* 2007;23(11):1237–1240.

Steinmann SP. Elbow arthroscopy: Where are we now?*Arthroscopy.* 2007;23(11):1231–1236. Review.

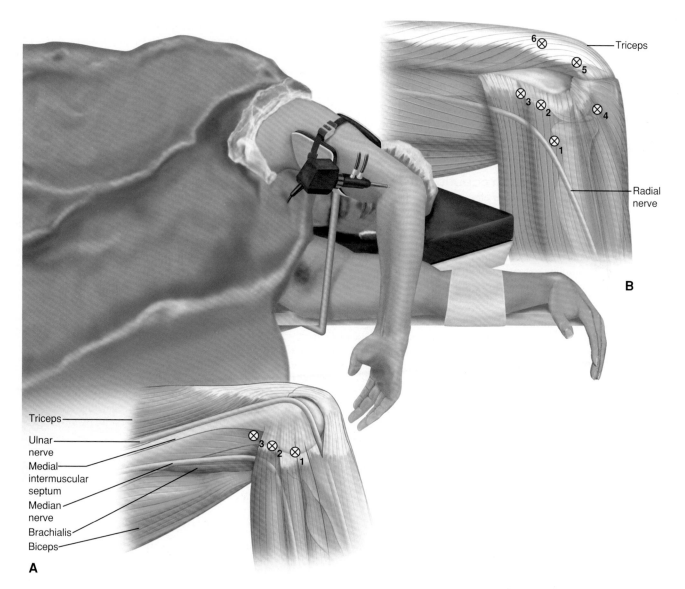

Figure 23. Elbow Arthroscopy Portals: A. Anatomy of medial arthroscopic portal sites *1)* standard anteromedial; *2)* midanteromedial; *3)* proximal anteromedial. **B.** *1)* distal anterolateral; *2)* mid-anterolateral; *3)* proximal anterolateral; *4)* direct posterolateral; *5)* posterolateral; and *6)* posterior central.

Elbow Articular Cartilage Surgery

Indications and Goals: Articular cartilage problems in the elbow include osteochondritis dissecans (OCD), which typically involves the capitellum in younger patients, traumatic chondral injuries, and arthrosis.

OCD of the capitellum occurs primarily in adolescent throwing athletes or upper extremity weight-bearing athletes such as gymnasts as a result of repetitive compressive microtrauma, resulting in injury to the subchondral blood supply, osteonecrosis, and loose body formation. Surgical options after a failed period of rest include removal of loose bodies, debridement and chondroplasty, microfracture, or fragment fixation.

More recently, a technique for osteochondral mosaicplasty using autograft transplantation from the knee has been described. It is indicated for large capitellar lesions that comprise greater than 50% of the capitellar surface area. These lesions typically involve the lateral aspect of the capitellum and result in the loss of the lateral buttress to the radial head.

Procedure and Technique: Typically, arthroscopy is carried out and the problem is characterized. Most commonly, the technique used involves loose body removal and abrasion chondroplasty or microfracture. The midlateral, anterolateral, and proximal medial portals are used. Visualization from the proximal medial portal with instruments that enter from the lateral portals allows good access to fragments. Following removal of the fragment(s), the resulting defect is microfractured with a 45-degree awl.

If mosaicplasty is chosen, an open technique using a Kocher approach between the anconeus and extensor carpi ulnaris muscles is performed. The lateral collateral ligament is preserved and the forearm is pronated to protect the posterior interosseous nerve. The defect is drilled and appropriately sized osteochondral plugs are transplanted from the ipsilateral knee using an osteochondral transplant system.

Post-surgical Precautions/Rehabilitation: Rehabilitation following elbow articular cartilage surgery is very similar to an elbow arthroscopy with the addition of tissue that has been intentionally insulted to enhance a bleeding response for healing. Performed as an outpatient procedure, an individual can utilize a compression wrap to reduce postoperative swelling. Range of motion exercises can be begun immediately for the elbow, as well as the shoulder and wrist as needed to restore normal movement. Splints and immobilization braces are not typically necessary. However, depending upon which bone was microfractured, there may be a 2-week period of limited complete extension in an attempt to reduce bone-to-bone compression at the elbow. Scar management and pain control can be addressed from the onset, and a return to participation and/or activity can occur on an individual basis as one feels comfortable.

For mosaicplasty procedures, the patient's elbow is immobilized at 90 degrees with the forearm in neutral rotation for 3 weeks, after which active and passive range of motion exercises are initiated. Strengthening exercises are commenced in the third postoperative month.

Expected Outcomes: In general, patients with loose bodies causing mechanical symptoms will have the most significant improvement in symptoms after elbow arthroscopy and loose body removal. Complications are generally minimal. If the original condition was the result of a repetitive stress injury, then education regarding appropriate biomechanics and ergonomics may need to occur to prevent against a recurrence. Early results of mosaicplasty procedures are promising, but longer term follow-up is needed.

Return to Play: Depends upon the size of the lesion and the procedure. In the best circumstances, 6 to 8 months may be required.

Recommended Readings

Brownlow HC, O'Connor-Read LM, Perko M. Arthroscopic treatment of osteochondritis dissecans of the capitellum. *Knee Surg Sports Traumatol Arthrosc.* 2006;14(2):198–202.

Davis JT, Idjadi JA, Siskosky MJ, ElAttrache NS. Dual direct lateral portals for treatment of osteochondritis dissecans of the capitellum: An anatomic study. *Arthroscopy.* 2007;23(7):723–728.

Iwasaki N, Kato H, Ishikawa J, Saitoh S, Minami A. Autologous osteochondral mosaicplasty for capitellar osteochondritis dissecans in teenaged patients. *Am J Sports Med.* 2006;34(8):1233–1239. Epub 2006 Mar 27.

Rahusen FT, Brinkman JM, Eygendaal D. Results of arthroscopic debridement for osteochondritis dissecans of the elbow. *Br J Sports Med.* 2006;40(12):966–969. Epub 2006 Sep 15.

Takahara M, Mura N, Sasaki J, Harada M, Ogino T. Classification, treatment, and outcome of osteochondritis dissecans of the humeral capitellum. *J Bone Joint Surg Am.* 2007;89(6):1205–1214.

Wahegaonkar AL, Doi K, Hattori Y, Addosooki A. Technique of osteochondral autograft transplantation mosaicplasty for capitellar osteochondritis dissecans. *J Hand Surg [Am].* 2007;32(9):1454–1461.

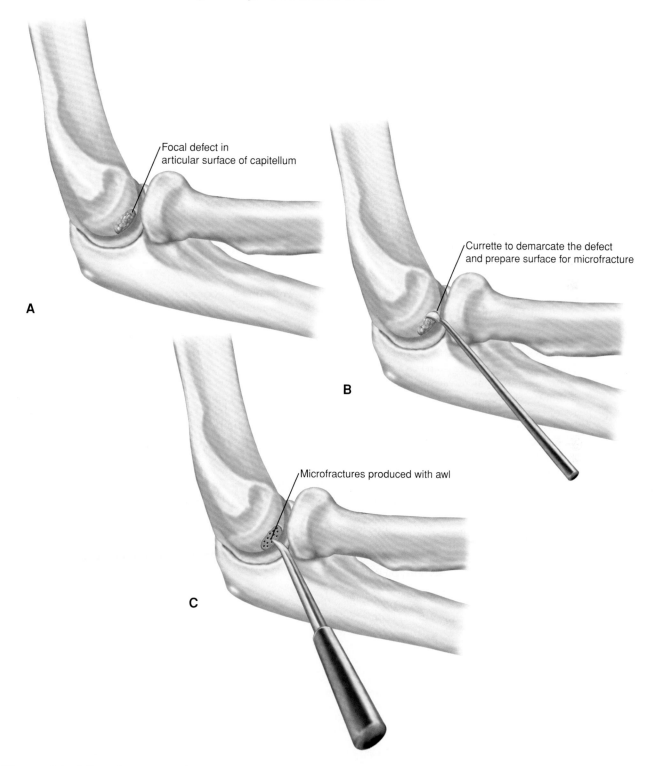

Figure 24. Microfracture of Osteochondritis Dessicans (OCD) Lesion of the Capitellum. A. Defect is identified on articular surface of the capitellum. **B.** A curette is utilized to debride calcified cartilage layer and define borders of the lesion. **C.** Small perforations are made using the awl.

Elbow Ulnar (Medial) Collateral Ligament Reconstruction (Tommy John Procedure)

Indications and Goals: This procedure is usually indicated for torn or stretched elbow ulnar (medial) collateral ligaments in throwing athletes. The goal is to allow the athlete to return to play.

Procedure and Technique: The patient is positioned supine on the operating table with the arm extended on a hand table. A 10 cm posteromedial longitudinal incision, centered on the joint line, is made and the ulnar nerve is exposed. Typically, the nerve is mobilized and transposed subcutaneously. The flexor-pronator tendon is split between its anterior and middle thirds and the medial epicondyle and coronoid process are exposed. The palmaris longus tendon is harvested through a transverse incision at the wrist and a whip-stitch is placed at both ends. Converging drill holes (typically 3.2 mm) are made in the coronoid process and diverging drill holes are made in the medial epicondyle. The tendon is weaved through the tunnels in a figure-of-eight fashion and sutured to itself. Alternatively, the docking technique can be used. With this technique, the ulnar tunnels are made as described above and the humeral tunnels are designed so that the free ends of the tendon are pulled into (docked) the tunnels and are secured by tying the free ends over a bony bridge on the medial epicondyle. Small bioabsorbable interference screws can also be used on one or both sides of these reconstructions.

Post-surgical Precautions/Rehabilitation: Following surgery, a long arm splint in 90 degrees of flexion at the elbow is worn. During the first 2 to 3 weeks, elbow range of motion is encouraged between 30 and 120 degrees of flexion, while shoulder and wrist motions are maintained. Both supervised and independent range of motion exercises should be performed daily, with pronation and supination being added as tolerated. Light grip strengthening activities can be performed using putty or other rehabilitation devices, with wrist flexor and forearm pronation strengthening exercises added between weeks 3 and 4. The brace can be adjusted to increase 10 degrees of extension movement each week past week 3, and complete range of motion at the elbow should be achieved within 6 weeks. Most of the exercises should be performed with the protection of the brace, though it can be removed several times daily for controlled, gentle range of motion exercises only. The brace can typically be discontinued if complete range of motion is achieved by the sixth postoperative week. While resistive exercise demand is increased over the first 3 to 4 months, forces that place a valgus stress on the elbow should be avoided during this time. Functional elbow braces may be worn when returning to an activity, job, or sport depending upon the feasibility. For throwers, a gradual increase in return to throwing must be supervised for compliance. This should be closely guided by the surgeon and may include an incremental increase in technique and objects utilized to throw with. For example, lighter objects that place less stress on the elbow may be used initially, progressing to a baseball or football.

Expected Outcomes: Average time to return to pre-injury status with throwers is approximately 1 year. While many have successful outcomes, others may experience ulnar nerve neurapraxia symptoms. If the goal of the individual is not to return to an activity that requires continued stress to the medial aspect of the elbow, then conservative care may be adequate for functional needs.

Return to Play: Six months to a year. In fact, the best results are often the following year. Competitive athletes may never return to their pre-injury status.

Recommended Readings

Armstrong AD, Dunning CE, Ferreira LM, Faber KJ, Johnson JA, King GJ. A biomechanical comparison of four reconstruction techniques for the medial collateral ligament-deficient elbow. *J Shoulder Elbow Surg*. 2005;14(2):207–215.

Dodson CC, Thomas A, Dines JS, Nho SJ, Williams RJ 3rd, Altchek DW. Medial ulnar collateral ligament reconstruction of the elbow in throwing athletes. *Am J Sports Med*. 2006;34(12):1926–1932. Epub 2006 Aug 10.

Gibson BW, Webner D, Huffman GR, Sennett BJ. Ulnar collateral ligament reconstruction in major league baseball pitchers. *Am J Sports Med*. 2007;35(4):575–581. Epub 2007 Jan 31.

Jobe FW, Stark H, Lombardo SJ. Reconstruction of the ulnar collateral ligament in athletes. *J Bone Joint Surg Am*. 1986;68(8): 1158–1163.

Koh JL, Schafer MF, Keuter G, Hsu JE. Ulnar collateral ligament reconstruction in elite throwing athletes. *Arthroscopy*. 2006;22(11): 1187–1191.

McAdams TR, Lee AT, Centeno J, Giori NJ, Lindsey DP. Two ulnar collateral ligament reconstruction methods: The docking technique versus bioabsorbable interference screw fixation—a biomechanical evaluation with cyclic loading. *J Shoulder Elbow Surg.* 2007;16(2):224–228. Epub 2007 Jan 24.

Paletta GA Jr, Wright RW. The modified docking procedure for elbow ulnar collateral ligament reconstruction: 2-year follow-up in elite throwers. *Am J Sports Med.* 2006;34(10):1594–1598. Epub 2006 Jul 10.

Purcell DB, Matava MJ, Wright RW. Ulnar collateral ligament reconstruction: A systematic review. *Clin Orthop Relat Res.* 2007;455:72–77.

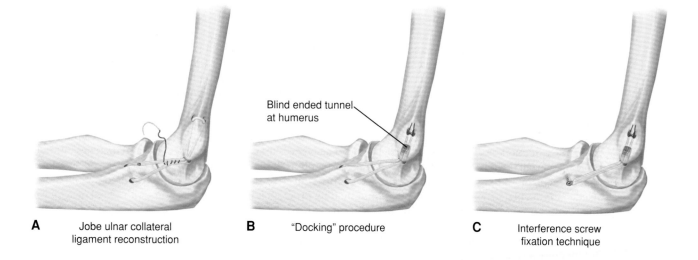

A   Jobe ulnar collateral ligament reconstruction

B   "Docking" procedure

C   Interference screw fixation technique

Blind ended tunnel at humerus

Figure 25. Types of Ulnar Collateral Ligament Reconstruction. A. Traditional UCL reconstruction with graft woven through drilled holes and sutured. **B.** Docking procedure. **C.** Interference screw fixation technique.

Lateral Elbow Collateral Ligament Reconstruction

Indications and Goals: Lateral-sided injuries are less common than medial collateral ligament injuries and often follow elbow instability (dislocations). The recurrent instability and the posterolateral rotatory instability (PLRI) are most likely caused by failure of the lateral complex to heal in its anatomic position on the lateral epicondyle following nonoperative treatment of an elbow dislocation. Patients with PLRI may describe recurrent elbow dislocations with normal daily activities, such as pushing on armrests while rising from a chair. This instability can be recreated by the lateral pivot shift test by starting with the elbow in supination and extension and slowly flexing the elbow while applying a slight valgus force and axial load, and is best performed with examination under anesthesia. Arthroscopy may be used as an adjunct to further assess the degree of instability, evaluate for osteochondral injury to the trochlea and radial head, and debride the joint. Reconstruction of the lateral ulnar collateral ligament may need to be carried out in isolation or in conjunction with surgical repair of other injuries, including the "terrible triad" injury of the elbow (elbow dislocation, radial head fracture, and coronoid fracture), transolecranon fracture-dislocations, and the posterior Monteggia lesion. The goal of reconstruction is early mobilization within a stable arc of motion.

Procedure and Technique: The Kocher approach utilizing the interval between the anconeus and extensor carpi ulnaris muscles is performed with the forearm in pronation to protect the posterior interosseous nerve. The lateral epicondylar origin of the Lateral Collateral Ligament is exposed by incising the capsule transversely, proximal to the annular ligament. If adequate ligamentous tissue is present, primary repair can be performed to reconstitute elbow stability. If adequate tissue is not present, a ligamentous graft such as palmaris longus is harvested and utilized for reconstruction. Two converging 3.2 mm drill holes are drilled in the supinator tubercle 1 cm apart and a suture is passed through them. Isometry is checked by holding the suture ends over the lateral epicondyle and flexing and extending the elbow. Diverging drill holes in the lateral epicondyle are created, originating from the isometric point. The palmaris graft is weaved through the drill holes and sutured to itself.

Post-surgical Precautions/Rehabilitation: Postoperatively, the arm is immobilized in full pronation with the elbow in 90 degrees of flexion for the first week to 10 days. This is replaced with a hinged brace and a 30-degree extension block is set for the first 4 weeks. The brace is then unlocked for 2 weeks and then discontinued at 6 weeks. From the onset, shoulder and wrist range of motion should be maintained with exercises. Scar and pain management should be addressed to reduce sensitivity concerns. Elbow loading in extension and supination is avoided for the first 3 months. A graduated strengthening program is initiated at that point with a goal of achieving full extensor power by 6 to 9 months and unrestricted activity at 12 months.

Expected Outcomes: Results from this procedure generally demonstrate good outcomes. If there is no degenerative arthritis and the radial head is intact, then approximately 90% of patients have a satisfactory outcome. Less reliable results have been reported with synthetic or triceps grafts. Considerable care is required to prevent fracture of the bony bridges with the reconstruction. Recovery time is typically 1 year for activities that place stress on the reconstructed ligament, and possible residual scarring may be found.

Return to Play: Six months to a year or more. Competitive athletes may never return to their pre-injury status.

Recommended Readings

King GJ, Dunning CE, Zarzour ZD, Patterson SD, Johnson JA. Single-strand reconstruction of the lateral ulnar collateral ligament restores varus and posterolateral rotatory stability of the elbow. *J Shoulder Elbow Surg.* 2002;11(1):60–64.

Lehman RC. Lateral elbow reconstruction using a new fixation technique. *Arthroscopy.* 2005;21(4):503–505.

Mehta JA, Bain GI. Posterolateral rotatory instability of the elbow. *J Am Acad Orthop Surg.* 2004;12(6):405–415.

Sotereanos DG, Darlis NA, Wright TW, Goitz RJ, King GJ. Unstable fracture-dislocations of the elbow. *Instr Course Lect.* 2007;56: 369–376.

Yadao MA, Savoie FH 3rd, Field LD. Posterolateral rotatory instability of the elbow. *Instr Course Lect.* 2004;53:607–614.

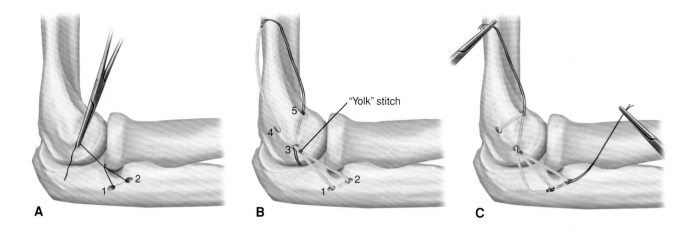

A   **B**   **C**

Figure 26. Lateral Collateral Ligament Reconstruction. A. Two drill holes for the graft insertion are made in the ulna. **B.** A suture is passed through the two holes, tied to itself and used to determine isometric point. **C.** Graft is passed through the Y-shaped tunnel and back through the isometric point, tensioned and fixed.

Distal Biceps Tendon Rupture

Indications and Goals: Distal biceps ruptures typically occur in the dominant extremity of men between the fourth and sixth decades of life as a result of an unexpected excessive extension force applied to an arm flexed to 90 degrees. The tendon typically avulses from the radial tuberosity in an area of preexisting tendon degeneration. Patients may note a sudden "pop", pain, and decreased strength of flexion and supination.

Procedure and Technique: The biceps tendon is anatomically reattached to its distal insertion on the radial tuberosity. This can be done through a one- or two-incision approach. A laterally based "L" incision or a transverse incision in the flexion crease is made. If a second incision is used, it is localized by putting the arm in maximum supination and placing a Kelly clamp in the first incision and passing it through the radioulnar interval and through the posterior muscles. Classically, the tendon is pulled into a trough and secured with sutures. If the second incision is made, the forearm is pronated to expose the radial tuberosity. The tuberosity is burred to accept the tendon end which is sutured through drill holes. Suture anchors, small bioabsorbable interference screws, endobuttons, and a variety of other devices have also been used. The surgeon must be careful to protect important neurovascular structures in the area (brachial artery, lateral antebrachial cutaneous nerve, and posterior interosseous nerve). Excessive dissection in the radioulnar interval can lead to heterotopic ossification.

Symptomatic partial ruptures that do not respond to conservative measures such as physical therapy are best treated by releasing the remaining portion of the biceps tendon from the tuberosity, debriding the frayed tendon end, and anatomically reattaching the tendon to the radial tuberosity as if there were a complete rupture. Chronic ruptures may have significant tendon retraction and shortening, especially if the bicipital aponeurosis is also ruptured. This may require autogenous tendon graft, such as the semitendinosus, to complete the reconstruction.

Post-surgical Precautions/Rehabilitation: Following a brief period of immobilization of 7 to 10 days with the elbow flexed at 90 degrees and the forearm in supination, active extension and passive flexion is initiated. The patient should avoid active supination and passive/active pronation for the first 4 to 6 weeks. A hinged flexion-assist splint with a 30-degree extension block is used to protect the repair until 8 weeks postoperatively. In addition, no lifting involving the biceps brachii muscle (elbow flexion, shoulder flexion) should occur. Exercises for range of motion of the shoulder and wrist flexion can be performed from the onset, while wrist extension should be avoided to reduce the stress on the repair. Scar and pain management can be addressed immediately postoperatively. Heavy lifting should be avoided for 9 to 12 months following repair.

Expected Outcomes: Results at this time appear to be excellent clinically and functionally, with significant improvement in flexion and supination strength over nonoperative management, nearing 95% of strength compared to the uninjured side. Strength assessed via isokinetics and range of motion is restored within 1 year of surgery. A slight deficit in the amount of pronation may be found in some occasions. Heterotopic bone formation of the radial tuberosity has been noted on radiographs at 2 months postoperatively with excellent anatomical structural status. Older reports of radial nerve neurapraxia with the single incision technique have been lessened with the advent of suture anchors and biotenodesis screws.

Return to Play: Athletes may return nine to twelve months following repair based upon the type of resistance required of the arm with the sport participation.

Recommended Readings

Hartman MW, Merten SM, Steinmann SP. Mini-open 2-incision technique for repair of distal biceps tendon ruptures. *J Shoulder Elbow Surg.* 2007;16(5):616–620. Epub 2007 May 9.

Henry J, Feinblatt J, Kaeding CC, Latshaw J, Litsky A, Sibel R, Stephens JA, Jones GL. Biomechanical analysis of distal biceps tendon repair methods. *Am J Sports Med.* 2007;35(11):1950–1954. Epub 2007 Jul 30.

Kettler M, Lunger J, Kuhn V, Mutschler W, Tingart MJ. Failure strengths in distal biceps tendon repair. *Am J Sports Med.* 2007;35(9): 1544–1548. Epub 2007 Mar 29.

Kettler M, Tingart MJ, Lunger J, Kuhn V. Reattachment of the distal tendon of biceps: Factors affecting the failure strength of the repair. *J Bone Joint Surg Br.* 2008;90(1):103–106.

Khan AD, Penna S, Yin Q, Sinopidis C, Brownson P, Frostick SP. Repair of distal biceps tendon ruptures using suture anchors through a single anterior incision. *Arthroscopy.* 2008;24(1):39–45. Epub 2007 Nov 28.

Klein DM, Ghany N, Urban W, Caruso SA. Distal biceps tendon repair: Anchor versus transosseous suture fixation. *Am J Orthop.* 2007;36(1):34–37.

Ramsey M. Distal biceps tendon injuries: Diagnosis and management. *J Am Acad Orthop Surg.* 1999;7:199–207.

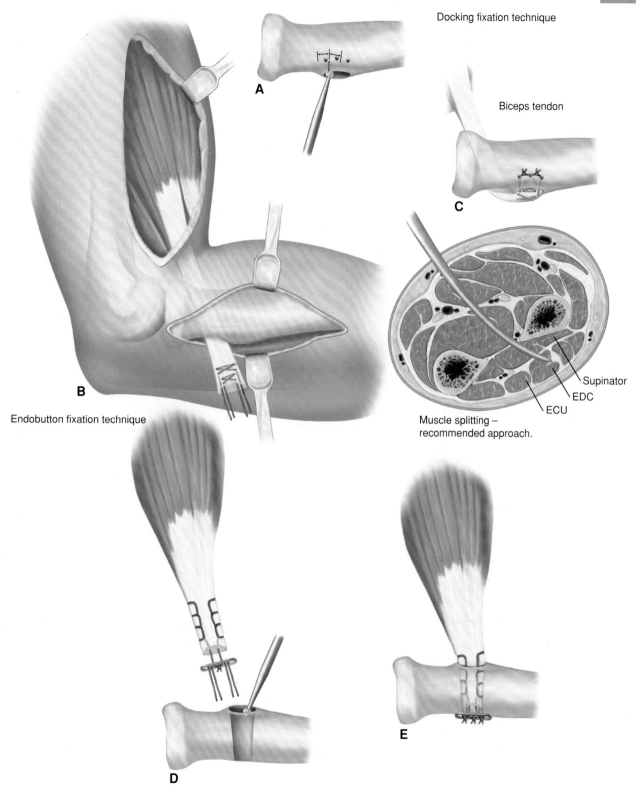

Docking fixation technique

A.

Biceps tendon

C.

B.

Endobutton fixation technique

Supinator
EDC
ECU

Muscle splitting –
recommended approach.

D.

E.

Figure 27. Distal Biceps Repair Two Incision Technique. A. Docking site is created at the bicipital tuberosity with a burr with drill holes placed next to the cavity. **B.** An anterior incision is made to locate the distal tendon stump and facilitate passage. **C.** The biceps tendon is advanced into the docking site and fixed through drill holes adjacent to the site and tied over bone with suture. **Endobutton fixation technique. D.** Distal biceps tendon pulled into the proximal hole as the endobutton is advanced. **E.** The Endobutton is flipped to prevent pullout of the tendon.

Cubital Tunnel Decompression/Ulnar Nerve Transposition

Indications and Goals: Cubital tunnel and ulnar nerve entrapment is the second most common nerve entrapment syndrome of the upper extremity (behind carpal tunnel syndrome) that causes pain, tingling, numbness, and even weakness in the elbow, forearm, and hand. The classic complaint includes numbness and tingling in the ring and small fingers and medial forearm pain, especially at night, and is exacerbated by elbow flexion. Ulnar motor neuropathy can present with a Wartenberg's sign (spontaneous abduction of the small finger with finger extension caused by weakness of the third palmar interosseous and unopposed extensor digiti minimi) early, followed by Froment's sign (weak thumb adduction with compensatory Flexor Pollicus Longus flexion during pinch), and finally clawing of the ulnar digits with long-standing compression.

Potential sites of compression of the ulnar nerve along its course through the elbow include the arcade of Struthers (extension of the coracobrachialis fascia 8 cm proximal to the medial epicondyle), the medial intermuscular septum (between the biceps and triceps), the cubital tunnel (arcuate ligament of Osborn), the humeral and ulnar heads of the flexor carpi ulnaris, the proximal flexor digitorum profundus arch, and the anconeus epitrochlearis. Surgical decompression should be considered in patients that fail nonoperative measures including bracing, injections, or therapy, or those with progressive motor or sensory deficits.

Procedure and Technique: The patient can be placed supine with the arm extended on a hand table and the shoulder abducted and externally rotated. Alternatively, the arm can be placed across the chest. A 10 cm incision is placed medial to the posterior midline of the elbow, just off the olecranon. The nerve is identified proximal to the arcuate ligament and posterior to the medial intermuscular septum. The nerve is dissected from proximal to distal. All sites of compression must be eliminated. It is commonly compressed at the fascial arcade between the two heads of the Flexor Carpi Ulnaris. The nerve can be transposed either subcutaneously or submuscularly. Subcutaneous transposition is typically done by creating a fascial sling from the superficial surface of the flexor–pronator mass. Submuscular transposition is accomplished by elevating the flexor–pronator mass off the medial epicondyle, carefully protecting the MCL, moving the nerve adjacent to the median nerve, and then reapproximating the flexor–pronator mass.

Post-surgical Precautions/Rehabilitation: This is performed as an outpatient procedure. Early motion is important and perhaps the most critical element. Active and passive joint movement, as well as gentle nerve gliding, will facilitate an optimal healing response with functional range of motion and decreased pain. There is no formal repair performed, but there is a fascial sling that was created which will take 6 to 8 weeks to heal. As such, aggressive resistive exercises should be avoided for this time frame. Resistive exercises can begin with surgeon approval primarily based upon tissue status.

Expected Outcomes: Patients who present early, typically have excellent relief of symptoms. Late presentation with progressive motor or sensory deficits decreases the likelihood of full recovery and good clinical outcome. Patients may have persistent symptoms due to incomplete decompression or perineural scarring. Injury to the posterior branch of the medial antebrachial cutaneous nerve can lead to hyperesthesia, hyperalgesia in the forearm, and a painful surgical scar. Subluxation of the ulnar nerve may occur with simple decompression alone. Injury to the medial collateral ligament of the elbow may occur as a complication of a submuscular transposition procedure. For individuals involved in high-level upper extremity activities, such as a throwing sport or a job that requires lifting, a slightly extended rehabilitation period may be required.

Return to Play: In the best circumstances, a full unrestricted return to activity for most can occur within 3 to 4 months.

Recommended Readings

Baek GH, Kwon BC, Chung MS. Comparative study between minimal medial epicondylectomy and anterior subcutaneous transposition of the ulnar nerve for cubital tunnel syndrome. *J Shoulder Elbow Surg.* 2006;15(5):609–613.

Catalano LW 3rd, Barron OA. Anterior subcutaneous transposition of the ulnar nerve. *Hand Clin.* 2007;23(3):339–344, vi. Review.

Elhassan B, Steinmann SP. Entrapment neuropathy of the ulnar nerve. *J Am Acad Orthop Surg.* 2007;15(11):672–681.

Henry M. Modified intramuscular transposition of the ulnar nerve. *J Hand Surg [Am].* 2006;31(9):1535–1542. Review.

Isaković E, Delić J, Bajtarević A, Davis GA, Bulluss KJ. Submuscular transposition of the ulnar nerve: Review of safety, efficacy and correlation with neurophysiological outcome. *J Clin Neurosci.* 2005;12(5):524–528.

Ruchelsman DE, Lee SK, Posner MA. Failed surgery for ulnar nerve compression at the elbow. *Hand Clin.* 2007;23(3):359–371, vi–vii.

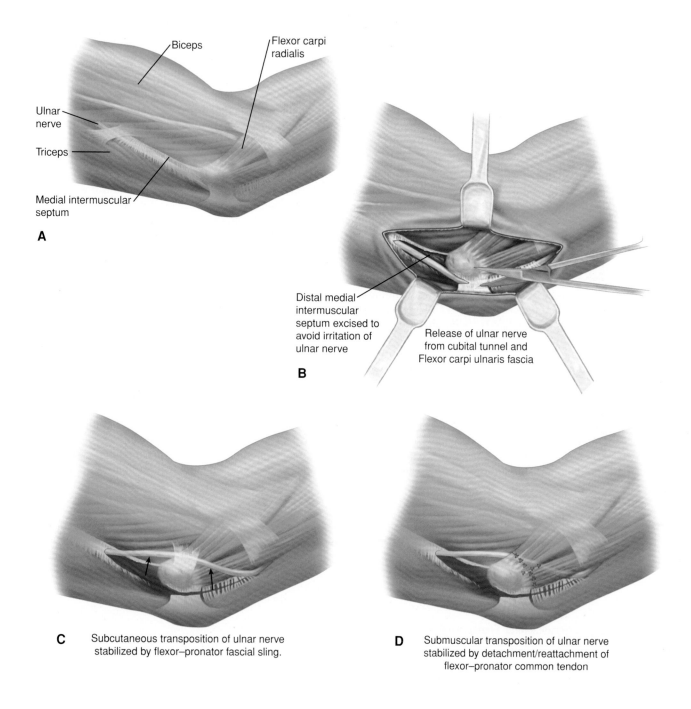

Figure 28. **A.** Relevant anatomy for ulnar nerve transposition. **B.** Standard incision centered over medial epicondyle with release of compressive structures. **C.** Subcutaneous transposition demonstrating nerve lying anterior to medial epicondyle with fascial sling. **D.** Submuscular transposition below flexor pronator mass.

Radial Tunnel/PIN Release

Indications and Goals: Posterior interosseous nerve (PIN) syndrome is a compression neuropathy that includes weakness of all or some of the muscles innervated by this nerve (supinator, extensor digitorum communis (EDC), extensor carpi ulnaris, extensor digiti minimi, abductor pollicis longus, extensor pollicis brevis, extensor pollicis longus, and extensor indicis proprius). Patients will have radial deviation upon wrist extension as the extensor carpi radialis longus (ECRL) and the extensor carpi radialis brevis (ECRB) are innervated by the radial nerve proper.

Radial tunnel syndrome presents with pain from the lateral elbow to the radial forearm without motor or sensory deficit. Patients typically have tenderness to palpation over the supinator arch (mobile wad), pain with resisted supination or passive forearm pronation, and pain distal to lateral epicondyle. They will have relief of symptoms and a wrist drop after injection of anesthetic into the radial tunnel. A significant number of patients will have concomitant lateral epicondylitis.

Sites of compression of the PIN are the same in both syndromes and include the fascial band anterior to the radiocapitellar joint, the recurrent leash of Henry (radial recurrent vessels), the leading edge of the ECRB, the arcade of Frohse at the proximal edge of the supinator muscle (most common), and the distal edge of the supinator muscle. Surgical release of all compression points is indicated if there is no improvement in 1 to 3 months with conservative measures such as splinting, therapy, nonsteroidal anti-inflammatory medications, and activity modification.

Procedure and Technique: Three different approaches have been described: brachioradialis (BR) splitting, BR–ECRL interval, and posterior (Thompson) approach in the EDC–ECRB interval. The Thompson approach can be combined with the BR–ECRL approach proximally. A lateral incision is made and the fascial septum between the EDC and the ECRB is identified. An incision is made along the ulnar border of this septum. The supinator is dissected and the plane between the supinator and the ECRB is developed and the PIN is visualized as it enters the arcade of Frohse. Release of the fascia on the deep surface of the ECRB improves exposure. Proximal release is accomplished by exploring the BR–ECRL interval.

Post-surgical Precautions/Rehabilitation: This is performed as an outpatient procedure and, like with any isolated release, there is typically no tissue repair involved. Therefore, the immediate postoperative care focuses on pain control, scar management, control of localized inflammation, and gentle and gradual range of motion. A bandage wrap may be worn initially to protect the surgical area, and perhaps to add some minimal compression if swelling persists. Patients can begin early range of motion exercises to promote nerve gliding and prevent adhesions and can be taught an independent home exercise program as soon as possible.

Expected Outcomes: Surgical decompression of the PIN for the PIN syndrome typically gives excellent relief of symptoms. Decompression for radial tunnel syndrome, however, gives less predictable results. Satisfaction rates are between 60% and 70% because of residual pain. Worker's compensation and litigation patients have even worse results. Potential complications include paresthesias or paralysis in the PIN distribution.

Return to Play: Return to work or mild activity can occur relatively quickly, using functional ability and postoperative symptoms as a guide. Full recovery should take no longer than 2 to 3 months on average.

Recommended Readings

Kim DH, Murovic JA, Kim YY, Kline DG. Surgical treatment and outcomes in 45 cases of posterior interosseous nerve entrapments and injuries. *J Neurosurg.* 2006;104(5):766–777.

Markiewitz A, Merryman J. Radial nerve compression in the upper extremity. *J Am Soc Surg Hand.* 2005;5(2):87–99.

Stanley J. Radial tunnel syndrome: A surgeon's perspective. *J Hand Ther.* 2006;19(2):180–184. Review.

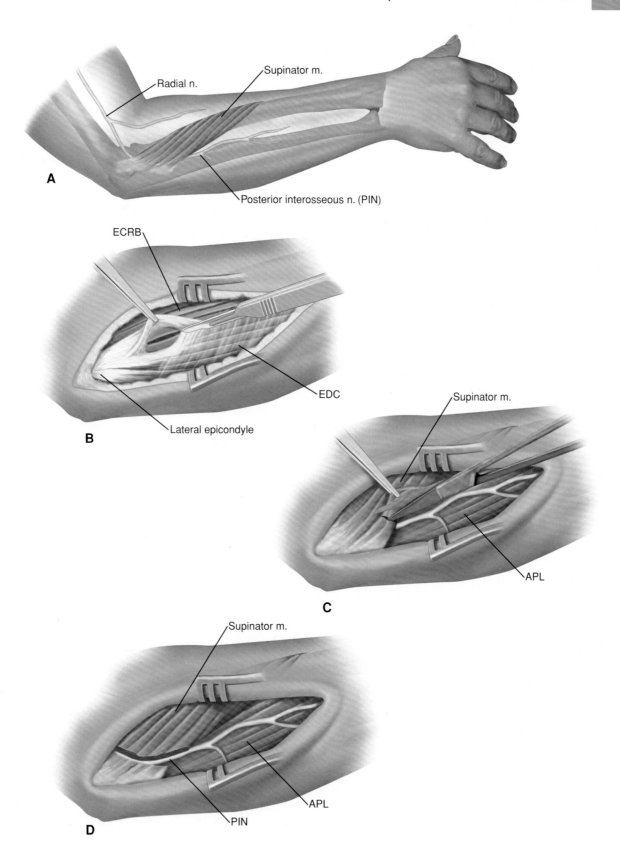

Figure 29. Radial Tunnel Entrapment Sites. A. Radial nerve divides into the PIN and superficial radial sensory nerve distal to the lateral epicondyle. **B.** The interval between EDC and ECRB in developed. The leading edge of ECRB fascia is released. **C.** Compressive supinator fibers overlying the PIN are released. **D.** Course of the PIN following release.

Lateral and Medial Epicondylitis Debridement/Repair

Indications and Goals: This condition, associated with overuse, is a tendinosis of the common extensor (lateral) or common flexor (medial) origin. The extensor carpi radialis brevis (ECRB) is the tendon primarily affected laterally and the pronator teres and flexor carpi radialis (FCR) are primarily affected medially. Patients present with tenderness just distal to the affected epicondyle. Lateral epicondylitis will show weakness in wrist extension and grip strength, and medial epicondylitis is aggravated by resisted pronation and wrist flexion. Lateral epicondylitis is much more common than medial, but medial epicondylitis has a high incidence of concomitant cubital tunnel syndrome. Conservative measures include rest, nonsteroidal anti-inflammatory drugs, physical therapy, bracing, cortisone, blood, and botulinum toxin injections, but surgical treatment is indicated in recalcitrant disease.

Procedure and Technique: The patient is placed supine on the operating table with the arm on a hand table. For lateral epicondylitis, a 7 cm longitudinal incision is made just posterior to the lateral epicondyle. The ECRB is identified and incised in line with its fibers. Degenerative tissue within the ECRB, which often has a gray hue, is identified and debrided. The underlying epicondyle is decorticated and the remaining tendon is then reattached. For medial epicondylitis, a 7 cm oblique incision is made just anterior to the medial epicondyle. The common flexor–pronator tendon is incised and intratendinous degenerative tissue is excised and the tendon is reattached. Arthroscopic techniques have also been described.

Post-surgical Precautions/Rehabilitation: Splint immobilization is often used for 10 days following open release and extensor origin repair. Range of motion exercises are then commenced, and strengthening is started after 6 weeks. Postoperative splinting protocols are continued until strength is regained. It should be kept in mind that the condition that warrants this surgical procedure is often brought on by repetitive overuse.

Expected Outcomes: It is important to educate the patient about proper ergonomics and biomechanics to avoid an injury recurrence. Surgical intervention typically gives excellent results, but some patients may have mild intermittent recurrence of symptoms with activity. Potential complications include residual strength deficit, iatrogenic posterolateral rotatory instability from excessive debridement and damage to the lateral collateral ligament, and persistent postoperative pain or neuroma formation from injury to the posterior cutaneous nerve of the forearm (a cutaneous branch of the radial nerve crosses 1.5 cm anterior to the lateral epicondyle on the brachioradialis fascia).

Return to Play: Patients should gradually return to activities, including sports (e.g., golf, tennis), no earlier than 6 weeks postoperatively utilizing a gradual progression.

Recommended Readings

Calfee RP, Patel A, Dasilva MF, Akelman E. Management of lateral epicondylitis: Current concepts. *J Am Acad Orthop Surg*. 2008; 16(1):19–29.

Cummins CA. Lateral epicondylitis: In vivo assessment of arthroscopic debridement and correlation with patient outcomes. *Am J Sports Med*. 2006;34(9):1486–1491. Epub 2006 May 9.

Dunn JH, Kim JJ, Davis L, Nirschl RP. Ten- to 14-year follow-up of the Nirschl surgical technique for lateral epicondylitis. *Am J Sports Med*. 2008;36:261–266.

Gabel GT, Morrey BF. Operative treatment of medical epicondylitis. Influence of concomitant ulnar neuropathy at the elbow. *J Bone Joint Surg Am*. 1995;77(7):1065–1069.

Jobe FW, Ciccotti MG. Lateral and medial epicondylitis of the elbow. *J Am Acad Orthop Surg*. 1994;2(1):1–8.

Smith AM, Castle JA, Ruch DS. Arthroscopic resection of the common extensor origin: Anatomic considerations. *J Shoulder Elbow Surg*. 2003;12(4):375–379.

Thornton SJ, Rogers JR, Prickett WD, Dunn WR, Allen AA, Hannafin JA. Treatment of recalcitrant lateral epicondylitis with suture anchor repair. *Am J Sports Med*. 2005;33(10):1558–1564.

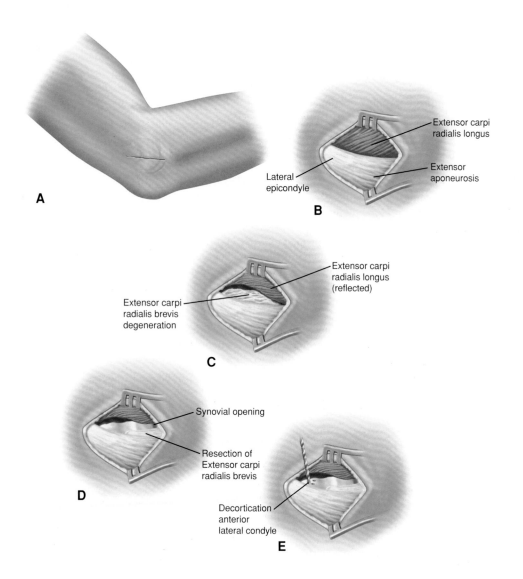

Figure 30. Open Treatment of Lateral Epicondylitis. A. Incision is made over the lateral epicondyle. **B.** The extensor aponeurosis is identified and ECRL is elevated off ECRB. **C.** Degenerative ECRB enthesopathy is identified. **D.** Sharp resection of degenerative ECRB. **E.** Anterior lateral epicondyle is decorticated.

Releases for Loss of Motion

Indications and Goals: Elbow loss of motion can be the result of a variety of factors including prolonged immobilization, fracture, dislocation, burns, head injury, cerebral palsy, and arthritis. Functional range of motion is 30 to 130 degrees, so this should be the minimal goal following releases. Surgical release is indicated for patients failing an extended trial of conservative therapy, including injections, range of motion and stretching therapy, and static splinting.

Procedure and Technique: Anterior capsular excision is facilitated by developing the plane between the brachialis and capsule and then by excising the capsule. In difficult cases, the Lateral Collateral Ligament can be released. The brachialis and triceps muscles may need to be elevated from the humeral shaft near the joint with an elevator to improve terminal flexion and extension.

Arthroscopic releases can avoid some of the complications associated with open procedures, including soft tissue trauma from open dissection and postoperative scarring of the capsule and anterior structures that may add to the risk of contracture recurrence, and increased time before physical therapy may be initiated due to surgical pain and scarring. The arthroscopic approach should only be attempted by experienced elbow arthroscopists, owing to the high risk of nerve or vascular injury. Anterior debridement and anterior capsular excision is carried out through the midlateral, proximal medial, and anterolateral portals. Posterior debridement of osteophytes and synovitis, ulnohumeral arthroplasty, and loose body removal can be accomplished through posterolateral and transtriceps portals.

Post-surgical Precautions/Rehabilitation: This is done as an outpatient procedure, and it is critical that immediate supervised rehabilitation be implemented starting on the day of surgery. Though somewhat uncomfortable at times, passive physiologic range of motion and joint accessory mobilization needs to occur early and often. There is no tissue repair with this technique, and therefore aggressive mobilization can be guided by pain tolerance and healing timelines to prevent a recurring limited functional range of motion.

Expected Outcomes: Outcomes for this procedure are similar to that of a release of adhesion at the glenohumeral joint. Progressive rehabilitation to facilitate joint mobilization will prevent a recurrence of tissue adhesion. Patient compliance is critical for a successful outcome.

Return to Play: As long as motion is maintained and with proper rehabilitation, return to play can be as early as 4 to 6 weeks or sooner if range of motion is restored.

Recommended Readings

Ball CM, Meunier M, Galatz LM, Calfee R, Yamaguchi K. Arthroscopic treatment of post-traumatic elbow contracture. *J Shoulder Elbow Surg.* 2002;11(6):624–629.

Gates HS 3rd, Sullivan FL, Urbaniak JR. Anterior capsulotomy and continuous passive motion in the treatment of post-traumatic flexion contracture of the elbow. A prospective study. *J Bone Joint Surg Am.* 1992;74(8):1229–1234.

Lindenhovius AL, Linzel DS, Doornberg JN, Ring DC, Jupiter JB. Comparison of elbow contracture release in elbows with and without heterotopic ossification restricting motion. *J Shoulder Elbow Surg.* 2007;16(5):621–625. Epub 2007 Jul 23.

Ring D, Adey L, Zurakowski D, Jupiter JB. Elbow capsulectomy for posttraumatic elbow stiffness. *J Hand Surg [Am].* 2006;31(8):1264–1271.

Ring D, Jupiter JB. Operative release of complete ankylosis of the elbow due to heterotopic bone in patients without severe injury of the central nervous system. *J Bone Joint Surg Am.* 2003;85-A(5):849–857.

Savoie FH. Arthroscopic management of the stiff elbow. In: McGinty JB, et al., eds. *Operative Arthroscopy.* 3rd ed. Baltimore: Lippincott Williams and Wilkins; 2003;708–717.

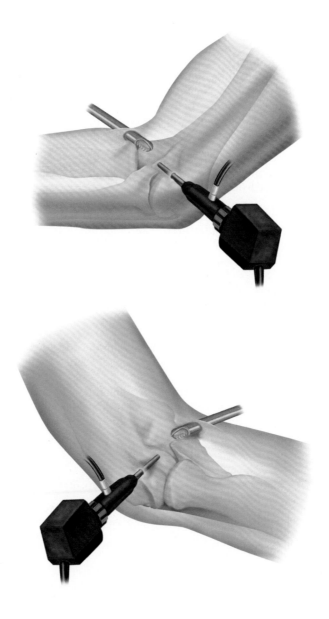

Figure 31. Arthroscopic Elbow Contracture Release.

Valgus Extension Overload Debridement

Indications and Goals: This condition occurs in overhead throwing athletes and involves repetitive abutment of the olecranon into the olecranon fossa combined with valgus torques, resulting in impaction and shear along the posteromedial olecranon. Patients may complain of insidious and progressive motion loss, crepitus, and tenderness at the posteromedial olecranon. Medial ligamentous laxity may exacerbate this condition. Posteromedial olecranon osteophytes and loose bodies may be identified on radiographs, computed tomography, or MRI.

Procedure and Technique: Although debridement is often done arthroscopically, the open technique is sometimes required, particularly with anterior and posterior osteophytes. The patient is placed supine with the arm across the chest. For posterior osteophytes, a triceps-splitting approach is used. Alternatively, a lateral Kocher approach can be used for access to both the anterior and posterior osteophytes. The anconeus–Extensor Carpi Ulnaris interval is used to access the joint anteriorly; the LCL is preserved and the extensor origin is subperiosteally reflected off the humerus for exposure. Posterior osteophytes are removed with a transverse and oblique osteotomy. The olecranon and coranoid fossas are debrided with a burr.

The Outerbridge–Kashiwagi procedure can be performed in elbow osteoarthritis through a midline posterior incision with a triceps split. A hole is trephined through the olecranon fossa to allow access to the anterior part of the elbow joint. Osteophytes are removed from the olecranon and coronoid process, and loose bodies are also removed from the joint.

Post-surgical Precautions/Rehabilitation: This procedure is performed on an outpatient basis. No tissue is repaired, so mobilization can occur immediately. The patient will experience some soreness from the osteotomy, which will subside over time. Emphasis should be on regaining full range of motion now that all bony obstructions have been removed. Scar and pain management are addressed as needed, and progressive resistive exercises can be initiated immediately postoperatively. This injury is usually the result of a repetitive type activity leading up to the osteophyte formation, so a gradual return to activity is required, as this is likely one's occupation or highly participative recreational hobby.

Expected Outcomes: Standard arthroscopic debridement for this condition has yielded good results thus far and has less operative morbidity than open procedures.

Return to Play: Gradual return to play can begin within 3 to 4 weeks. Moderation may delay recurrence. It is not uncommon for some residual soreness to be present from burring of the bone may last beyond the return to participation timeline.

Recommended Readings

Ahmad CS, ElAttrache NS. Valgus extension overload syndrome and stress injury of the olecranon. *Clin Sports Med.* 2004;23(4): 665–676, x. Review.

Chen FS, Rokito AS, Jobe FW. Medial elbow problems in the overhead-throwing athlete. *J Am Acad Orthop Surg.* 2001;9(2):99–113.

Forster MC, Clark DI, Lunn PG. Elbow osteoarthritis: Prognostic indicators in ulnohumeral debridement—the Outerbridge–Kashiwagi procedure. *J Shoulder Elbow Surg.* 2001;10(6):557–560.

Valkering KP, van der Hoeven H, Pijnenburg BC. Posterolateral elbow impingement in professional boxers. *Am J Sports Med.* 2008;36:328–332.

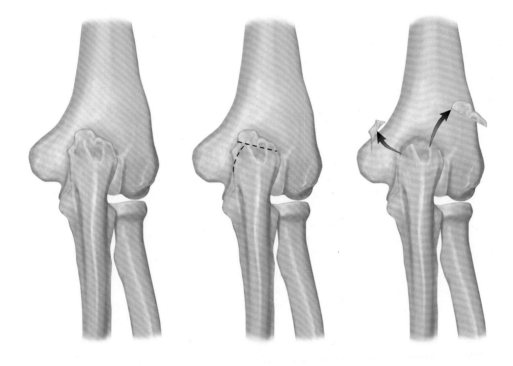

Figure 32. Posterior Osteophyte Debridement for Valgus Extension Overload.

ORIF Elbow Fractures

Indications and Goals: Displaced intraarticular fractures of the elbow should be fixed as anatomically as possible to allow congruent range of motion. There are a variety of elbow fractures, including distal humeral, olecranon, and radial head fractures.

Procedure and Technique: Distal humeral fractures may be addressed with a variety of approaches, including the triceps-sparing Bryan–Morrey approach, a triceps-splitting approach, or an olecranon osteotomy. The olecranon osteotomy provides the best visualization of the articular surface and may be necessary in highly comminuted intraarticular fractures, but this must be weighed against the potential complications of osteotomy nonunion and symptomatic hardware. Anatomic reduction of the articular surface (the "spool") is the primary goal of open reduction internal fixation (ORIF), followed by attachment of the spool back to the medial and lateral columns of the distal humerus. Headless compression screws may need to be used in highly comminuted intraarticular fractures. Anatomic locking plate technology has allowed for repair of fractures previously viewed as too comminuted or with too poor bone stock to attempt repair. However, in the elderly population, ORIF of comminuted distal humeral intraarticular fractures can result in failure of fixation, increased immobilization time with resultant stiffness, posttraumatic arthritis, and heterotopic ossification. Primary total elbow arthroplasty may be a better choice in these situations.

Radial head fractures are significant injuries, as the radiocapitellar joint bears 60% of the forearm axial load in full extension. These fractures are repaired if the patient has a mechanical block to motion. Extraosseous hardware is placed within a 100-degree "safe zone" centered laterally with the forearm in neutral rotation to avoid hardware impingement in the proximal radioulnar joint. Buried intraosseous hardware, such as headless compression screws, may be placed anywhere. Excision of small radial head fracture fragments (<25% of the articular surface) is an option, but even these small fragments may be critical to elbow stability. If the radial head is extensively comminuted (Mason 3-type injuries), then radial head replacement may be a better option. The surgeon should be prepared for radial head replacement in any planned ORIF procedure. Radial head fractures may also be associated with an Essex-Lopresti injury, medial collateral ligament rupture, terrible triad injury (elbow dislocation, radial head fracture, and coronoid fracture), or Monteggia proximal ulna fracture–dislocations. In Essex-Lopresti lesions, or acute longitudinal radioulnar dissociation (ALRUD), the distal radioulnar joint, interosseous membrane, and radial head are all injured. In these situations, it is critical to retain or replace the radial head to prevent proximal migration of the radius and resultant ulnocarpal impaction at the wrist.

In coronoid fractures, often associated with the terrible triad injury, even small fragments can lead to instability. Small fragments can be repaired with sutures passed through drill holes in the olecranon, and larger fragments can be repaired with new anatomic plates or screw fixation through a flexor carpi ulnaris–splitting medial approach. A hinged external fixator may be required if there is persistent instability despite surgically addressing all injured structures.

Displaced olecranon fractures can be repaired with K-wires or a screw in a tension-band technique or with a contoured reconstruction or anatomic locking plate construct. It is important not to decrease the arc of curvature of the olecranon, especially in comminuted fractures, as it will prevent the trochlea from seating fully and may cause postoperative instability.

Post-surgical Precautions/Rehabilitation: The amount of fixation required and the anatomical location of the fixation will determine the primary phase of immobilization and estimated length of time for healing. A hinged elbow brace is used postoperatively with range of motion restrictions also determined by the surgical procedure. Early mobilization to the shoulder and wrist can be initiated immediately, with elbow and forearm range of motion to be determined by the surgeon. Isometric exercises can be performed for the elbow musculature to prevent local atrophy following early immobilization periods.

Expected Outcomes: Range of motion improvements of the elbow can be achieved with fracture site union and successful elbow joint arthrolysis and soft-tissue releases when required. Chronic elevated joint stresses may ultimately lead to the development of elbow pain and osteoarthritis.

Return to Play: Totally dependent upon the extent of fracture and restoration of normal anatomy. In the best circumstances, return to participation will be 4 to 6 months postoperatively.

Recommended Readings

Bryan RS, Morrey BF. Extensive posterior exposure of the elbow: A triceps-sparing approach. *Clin Orth Rel Res.* 1982;166:188–192.

Helfet DL, Kloen P, Anand N, Rosen HS. ORIF of delayed unions and nonunions of distal humeral fractures. Surgical technique. *J Bone Joint Surg Am.* 2004;86-A(suppl 1):18–29.

McCarty LP, Ring D, Jupiter JB. Management of distal humerus fractures. *Am J Orthop.* 2005;34(9):430–438. Review.

Moed BR, Ede DE, Brown TD. Fractures of the olecranon: An in vitro study of elbow joint stresses after tension-band wire fixation versus proximal fracture fragment excision. *J Trauma.* 2002;53(6):1088–1093.

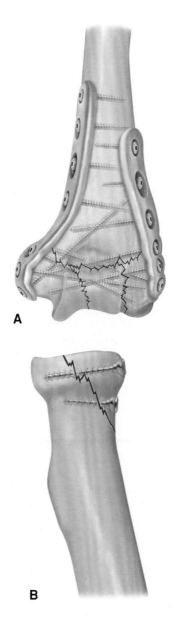

A

B

Figure 33. Open Reduction Internal Fixation (ORIF) of Elbow Fractures. A, ORIF of a distal humerus fracture using two parallel medial and lateral plates. **B,** Radial head ORIF.

ORIF Forearm Fractures

Indications and Goals: Forearm fractures are common, and most often need operative intervention to restore normal function to the upper extremity. The goals of surgery are to achieve anatomic reduction with restoration of length and restoration of the radial bow and to achieve rigid fixation to allow early range of motion. Restoration of the radial bow with the apex radial and dorsal is the key to regaining full forearm rotation, so intraoperative reduction must be scrutinized prior to final fixation.

Procedure and Technique: The radius can be exposed through the anterior (Henry) approach or the posterior (Thompson) approach based on the fracture location and the surgeon preference. The anterior Henry approach is a safe and commonly used approach for most diaphyseal fractures of the radius. A longitudinal incision is made in a line just lateral to the biceps tendon proximally down to the radial styloid distally. Proximally, the internervous plane is between the brachioradialis (radial nerve) and the pronator teres (median nerve). Distally, the internervous plane is between the brachioradialis and flexor carpi radialis (median nerve). The superficial branch of the radial nerve and the radial artery are deep to the brachioradialis must be identified and protected. Usually the nerve is taken laterally with the brachioradialis and the artery is taken medially after contributions to the brachioradialis are ligated. The forearm must be kept fully supinated with this approach to move the posterior interosseous nerve (PIN) away from the field. If this approach is used for proximal third radial fractures, the supinator muscle must be elevated subperiosteally to protect the PIN. The PIN may come into direct contact with the radial neck in some patients, so great care must be exercised. For middle or distal third fractures, the pronator teres, flexor digitorum superficialis, flexor pollicis longus, or pronator quadratus is elevated as necessary based on the fracture location.

The posterior Thompson approach can be used if the surgeon prefers to directly visualize and protect the PIN, especially in proximal third radial fractures. A longitudinal incision is made in a line just anterior to the lateral epicondyle proximally down to the ulnar side of Lister's tubercle distally. Proximally, the internervous plane is between the extensor carpi radialis brevis (ECRB-radial nerve) and the extensor digitorum communis (PIN). This interval may be more obvious at the midshaft level, as the muscles have a common tendon origin. At the midshaft level, the plane is between the ECRB and the abductor pollicis longus (PIN). At the distal end of the radius, the plane lies between the ECRB and the extensor pollicis longus (PIN). The PIN must be identified, as it emerges between the superficial and deep heads of the supinator muscle about 1 cm proximal to the distal edge of the muscle, and carefully dissected to maintain its motor branches to the supinator itself. After the PIN is fully identified and protected, the forearm is fully supinated and the supinator insertion is subperiosteally dissected off the radius. For middle or distal third fractures, the abductor pollicis longus or extensor pollicis brevis is elevated as needed based on the fracture location.

The ulna is relatively subcutaneous and the approach is fairly straightforward. The internervous plane lies between the extensor carpi ulnaris (PIN) and the flexor carpi ulnaris (ulnar nerve). The periosteum is incised and elevated, and plates may be placed on either the flexor or extensor surface as desired. Plating is carried out on both the radius and ulna with 3.5 dynamic compression plates.

Ulnar shaft fractures ("nightstick fractures") do occur in isolation from a direct blow, but the proximal radioulnar joint must be scrutinized to ensure the patient does not have a Monteggia injury (ulnar shaft fracture with dislocation of the radial head). The radial head usually reduces with anatomic reduction of the ulnar shaft, but annular ligament repair may need to be performed if the radial head remains subluxed. Similarly, radial shaft fractures do occur in isolation, but the distal radioulnar joint (DRUJ) must be scrutinized to ensure the patient does not have a Galeazzi injury (radial shaft fracture and DRUJ disruption), especially if the fracture occurs within 7.5 cm of the radiocarpal joint. If the DRUJ remains unstable after anatomic reduction of the radius, the ulnar styloid fracture or the triangular fibrocartilage complex (TFCC) tear must be repaired.

Post-surgical Precautions/Rehabilitation: Early range of motion is encouraged if stable fixation is achieved intraoperatively. If a Monteggia fracture–dislocation is present and the radial head is stable, a splint can be used for the first 7 to 10 days, followed by early range of motion. If a Galeazzi fracture–dislocation is present and the DRUJ is stable after fixation, immediate range of motion is encouraged. If the DRUJ is unstable and requires repair, the forearm is immobilized in midsupination. Once mobilization is allowed, focus should be on the proximal and DRUJs, facilitating pronation and supination, as well as elbow extension. Grip strength exercises can begin from the onset, and shoulder range of motion should be maintained throughout the rehabilitation phase.

Expected Outcomes: Typically, elbow flexion will return to normal limits with activities of daily living. A full return to work and recreational activity may take up to 3 to 4 months. Postoperative complications may occur and include pain, loss of total forearm range of motion, and decreased functional abilities. Synostosis may also occur, with crush injury, same-level fracture, single incision, head injury, bone grafting, and excessive dissection around the interosseous membrane as risk factors.

Return to Play: With complete healing and restoration of normal anatomy, return to play within 4 to 6 months is possible. Protective padding is reasonable for contact athletes and hardware removal should be avoided because of risk of refracture.

Recommended Readings

Moss JP, Bynum DK. Diaphyseal fractures of the radius and ulna in adults. *Hand Clin.* 2007;23(2):143–151.

Ortega R, Loder RT, Louis DS. Open reduction and internal fixation of forearm fractures in children. *J Pediatr Orthop.* 1996;16(5):651–654.

Ring D, Jupiter JB, Waters PM. Monteggia fractures in children and adults. *J Am Acad Orthop Surg.* 1998;6(4):215–224.

Smith VA, Goodman HJ, Strongwater A, Smith B. Treatment of pediatric both-bone forearm fractures: A comparison of operative techniques. *J Pediatr Orthop.* 2005;25(3):309–313.

Wilson FC, Dirschl DR, Bynum DK. Fractures of the radius and ulna in adults: An analysis of factors affecting outcome. *Iowa Orthop J.* 1997;17:14–19.

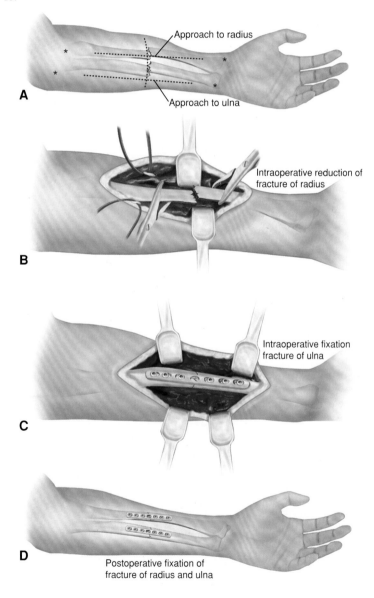

Figure 34. Open Reduction and Internal Fixation of Both Bone Forearm Fractures. A. Separate approaches can be made for the ulna and radius. **B.** Once exposed the fracture is reduced. **C.** The ulna is shown following plate and screw fixation. **D.** Final fixation with restoration of radial bow and length.

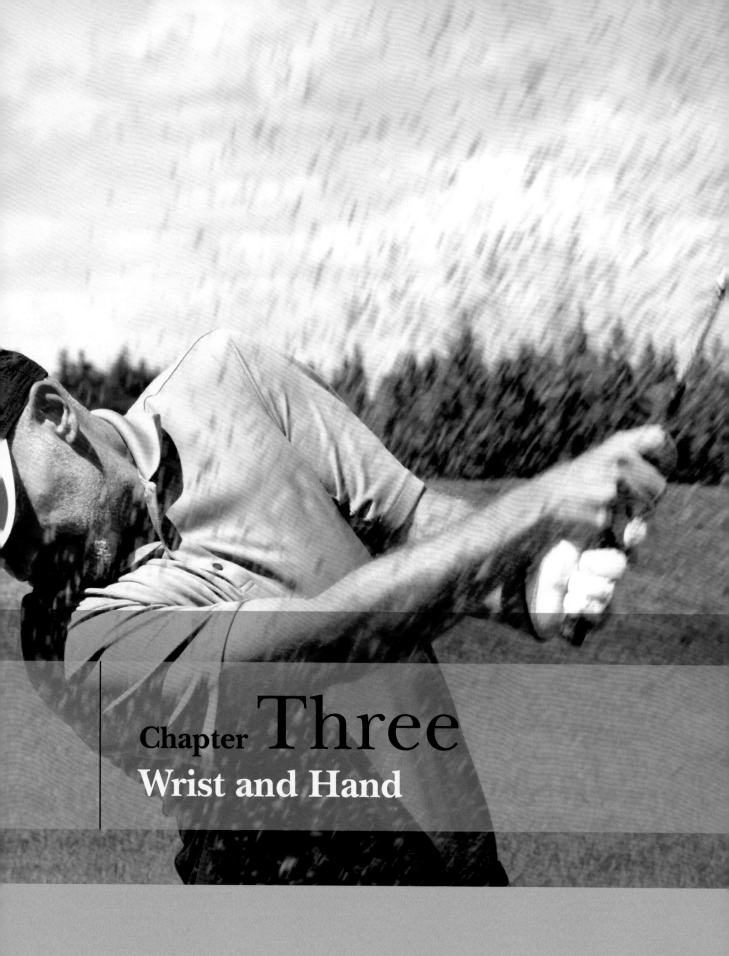

Chapter Three
Wrist and Hand

Wrist Arthroscopy

Indications and Goals: Wrist arthroscopy is becoming more widespread, with the realization that it is extremely valuable for a variety of diagnostic and therapeutic purposes. Indications include assessment of ligamentous injuries of the wrist, especially the scapholunate and lunotriquetral ligaments, debridement and repair of triangular fibrocartilage complex (TFCC) tears, assessment and debridement of chondral defects, removal of loose bodies, synovectomy, lavage of septic arthritis, arthroscopic-assisted reduction of intraarticular distal radius fractures, distal ulnar resection, and ganglion excision.

Procedure and Technique: A traction tower is used for positioning and distraction, with the index and long fingers in finger traps with 10 to 15 lbs of longitudinal traction applied. A small-joint 2.7 mm arthroscope is typically used. Portals are based on the dorsal wrist compartments. There are 10 described dorsal portals for the wrist: 5 at the radiocarpal joint, 2 at the midcarpal joint, 1 at the scaphotrapeziotrapezoid (STT) joint, and 2 at the distal radioulnar joint (DRUJ). The 3-4 portal (between extensor pollicis longus and extensor digitorum communis) is usually created first, 1 cm distal to Lister's tubercle. The joint is insufflated with 5 to 10 mL of fluid, then a small superficial skin incision is made. A blunt trochar is used to access the joint to avoid transection of the extensor tendons and is angled to follow the anatomical 12-degree palmar tilt of the distal radius. The 4-5 portal (between the extensor digitorum communis and extensor digiti minimi) is usually created next. The 6-R portal is immediately radial to the extensor carpi ulnaris tendon, while the 6-U portal is immediately ulnar to it. These are often used as outflow portals. The dorsal branch of the ulnar nerve is particularly at risk for injury with creation of the 6-U portal. The 1-2 portal (between the extensor pollicis brevis and extensor carpi radialis longus), has limited utility due to its proximity to the branches of both the lateral antebrachial cutaneous nerve and the sensory branch of the radial nerve as well as the deep branch of the radial artery. The radiocarpal joint is inspected in a systematic fashion beginning radially and working ulnarly. Debridement is carried out as necessary, and ligamentous structures including the scapholunate ligament are inspected. The TFCC should be taut, with a trampoline-like effect when probed. Midcarpal arthroscopy is critical to evaluate the integrity of the scapholunate and lunotriquetral ligaments, and a probe pushed between the scaphoid and lunate can assess for laxity. The midcarpal radial portal is located 1 cm distal to the 3-4 portal, in line with the radial margin of the third metacarpal, while the midcarpal ulnar portal is located approximately 1 cm distal to the 4-5 portal, in line with the fourth metacarpal.

Post-surgical Precautions/Rehabilitation: The type of rehabilitation involved following a wrist arthroscopy depends upon whether or not tissue was repaired or removed. If the procedure involves removing or debriding tissue without any repair, then acute rehabilitation can focus on pain relief and scar management at the portal sites. A wrist splint is usually applied at the time of arthroscopy, and is removed at the first postoperative visit, at which time range of motion exercises can begin. A splint may be used for strenuous activity for approximately 4 weeks. If the procedure involved a repair, then care should be taken to avoid placing too much stress on the repaired tissue until adequate and safe healing has occurred. The timeframe for rehabilitation progression will depend upon the specific tissue that is repaired and the stability of the repair.

Expected Outcomes: Outcomes for wrist arthroscopy certainly vary based upon the procedure being performed. Overall, however, general benefits associated with wrist arthroscopy include minimal damage to surrounding soft tissue, less postoperative pain, shorter recovery times, and fewer surgical complications. Potential complications include injuries to the extensor tendons, radial artery, and the superficial branches of the radial and ulnar nerves. The tendon most at risk for arthroscopy is the extensor pollicis longus, with both acute and late rupture of this tendon being reported. Neurovascular complications are related to the more ulnar portals.

Return to Play: Return to activity is totally dependent upon the procedure done. If the structural integrity of the wrist is not compromised, return within weeks is possible. The majority of patients are able to perform activities of daily living by 2 weeks, and full recovery is anticipated by 6 weeks.

Recommended Readings

Atzei A, Luchetti R, Sgarbossa A, Carità E, Llusà M. [Set-up, portals and normal exploration in wrist arthroscopy] *Chir Main.* 2006;25(suppl 1):S131–S144. Review.

Chloros GD, Shen J, Mahirogullari M, Wiesler ER. Wrist arthroscopy. *J Surg Orthop Adv.* 2007;16(2):49–61. Review.

Culp RW, Osterman AL, Kaufmann RA. Wrist Arthroscopy: Operative Procedures. In: Green DP, et al., eds. *Green's Operative Hand Surgery.* 5th ed. Philadelphia, PA: Elsevier; 2005:781–804.

McGinty JB, et al. eds. *The Wrist, in Operative Arthroscopy*. 3rd ed. Baltimore, MD: Lippincott Williams and Wilkins; 721–818.

Ricks E. Wrist arthroscopy. *AORN J.* 2007;86(2):181–188; quiz 189–192. Review.

Ruch DS, Poehling GG. Wrist Arthroscopy: Anatomy and Diagnosis. In: Green DP, et al., eds. *Green's Operative Hand Surgery*. 5th ed. Philadelphia, PA: Elsevier; 769–780.

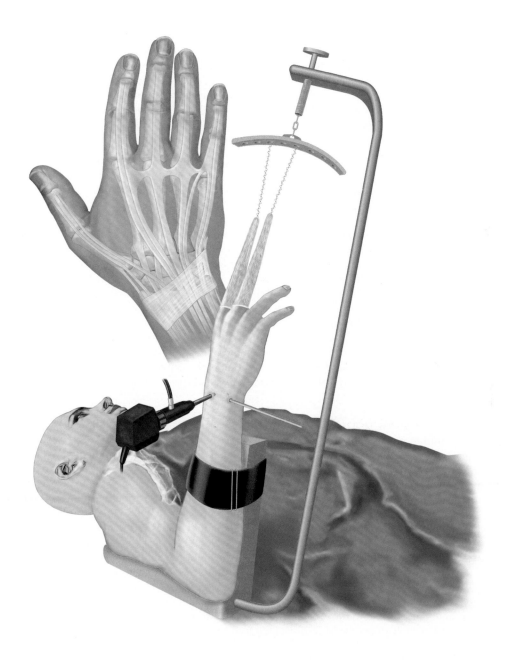

Figure 35. Scope Portals and Views from OSA

Scapholunate Ligament Repair

Indications and Goals: Scapholunate ligament disruption is a potentially devastating injury if left untreated, yet the initial injury is often unrecognized and dismissed as merely a "wrist sprain." Scapholunate ligament injury can lead to significant alteration of normal wrist kinematics and resultant carpal instability, characterized by wrist pain, loss of motion, weakness, degenerative arthritis, and disability. Static instability shows abnormal carpal alignment on standard radiographs, while dynamic instability requires stress radiographs for abnormal carpal alignment to become apparent. Scapholunate ligament disruption leads to the dorsal intercalated segmental instability (DISI) type of deformity. Loss of the normal ligamentous constraints leads to scaphoid hyperflexion and lunate hyperextension. This is evident on lateral radiographs showing a scapholunate angle greater than 70 degrees (normal being 47 degrees). AP views may show a widened scapholunate interval (>3 mm), and bilateral clenched fist stress views can confirm a scapholunate diastasis. Pathologic scaphoid hyperflexion may also manifest as a "cortical ring sign" on the PA view. A positive Watson's test is when a palpable clunk is felt while applying dorsal pressure to the volar scaphoid tubercle as the wrist is moved from ulnar to radial deviation. MRI has become more sensitive for the detection of scapholunate ligament disruption, but wrist arthroscopy remains the gold standard for diagnosis.

If left untreated, the injury will progress along a predictable pattern of degenerative arthritis, known scapholunate advanced collapse (SLAC). This stepwise degenerative process involves radial styloid and scaphoid arthritis early due to edge-loading, followed by proximal capitate migration, and finally pancarpal arthritis. The primary goal, therefore, is early diagnosis and treatment of this injury.

Procedure and Technique: Treatment depends on the stage and type of instability. In cases of partial scapholunate ligament injury and occult instability, arthroscopic debridement and a period of postoperative immobilization may be sufficient. Some authors recommend arthroscopic pin fixation for 6 to 8 weeks. Acute complete scapholunate ligament ruptures without evidence of arthritic degeneration may be amenable to primary open repair by passing nonabsorbable suture through drill holes. The scapholunate interval is then pinned with K-wires, and the primary repair is often augmented by a dorsal capsulodesis procedure, such as the Blatt capsulodesis or the dorsal intercarpal capsulodesis. Many other repair techniques have been described, such as tenodesis, bone–ligament–bone autograft reconstruction, and intercarpal fusion. Cases of chronic, static instability that have progressed to SLAC require a different approach. The radioscaphoid and capitolunate joints are affected, but the radiolunate joint is spared. Treatment is dependent on the condition of the capitate articular surface and the radioscaphocapitate ligament. Options include radial styloidectomy, proximal row carpectomy, scaphoid excision and four-corner fusion, and total wrist fusion.

Post-surgical Precautions/Rehabilitation: Postoperative protocols obviously depend on the procedure performed, with more involved reconstructive and repair procedures requiring longer periods of immobilization. However, for scapholunate ligament repair procedures, the wrist is immobilized in neutral position in an above elbow thumb spica cast for 8 weeks, following which time the pins are removed and active motion is initiated. Some follow the approach of using a long arm splint of 2 weeks and a Muenster cast for 6 weeks more. Once the pins are removed, a short arm cast is used for another 4 weeks. Range of motion should focus on regaining only functional movement that is necessary for activities of daily living, without aggressively forcing end range wrist flexion as it could adversely affect the stabilizing repair. Grip strengthening exercises should be delayed until satisfactory healing has occurred.

Expected Outcomes: Results vary as reported in the literature. Grip strength deficits, range of motion deficits (wrist flexion and radial deviation), and ongoing pain up to 30 months postoperative with activities of daily living may persist. Decrease in symptoms of pain and clunking as well as improvement of functional status have also been reported. The most common complication of the dorsal capsulodesis involves limited wrist flexion. This loss of wrist flexion is inherently related to the procedure and not due to scarring after immobilization and attempts at regaining the last 12 to 20 degrees of wrist flexion could lead to disruption or weakening of the reconstruction.

Return to Play: Return to participation requires complete healing and restored stabilization of the joint(s) involved. This may take up to 4 to 6 months conservatively.

Recommended Readings

Dagum AB, Hurst LC, Finzel KC. Scapholunate dissociation: An experimental kinematic study of two types of indirect soft tissue repairs. *J Hand Surg [Am]*. 1997;22(4):714–719.

Deshmukh SC, Givissis P, Belloso D, Stanley JK, Trail IA. Blatt's capsulodesis for chronic scapholunate dissociation. *J Hand Surg [Br]*. 1999;24(2):215–220.

Garcia-Elias M, Geissler WB. Carpal Instability. In: Green DP, et al., eds. *Green's Operative Hand Surgery*. 5th ed. Philadelphia, PA: Elsevier; 535–604.

Walsh JJ, Berger RA, Cooney WP. Current status of scapholunate interosseous ligament injuries. *J Am Acad Orthop Surg*. 2002;10(1):32–42.

Wintman BI, Gelberman RH, Katz JN. Dynamic scapholunate instability: Results of operative treatment with dorsal capsulodesis. *J Hand Surg [Am]*. 1995;20(6):971–979.

Wyrick JD, Stern PJ, Kiefhaber TR. Motion-preserving procedures in the treatment of scapholunate advanced collapse wrist: Proximal row carpectomy versus four-corner arthrodesis. *J Hand Surg [Am]*. 1995;20(6):965–970.

Wyrick JD, Youse BD, Kiefhaber TR. Scapholunate ligament repair and capsulodesis for the treatment of static scapholunate dissociation. *J Hand Surg [Br]*. 1998;23(6):776–780.

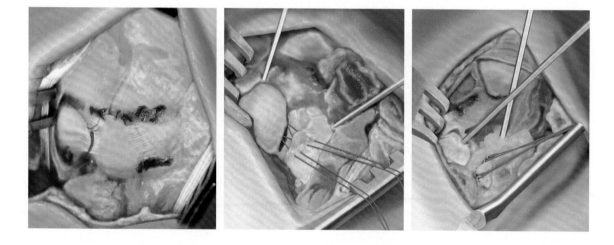

Figure 36. **Acute Scapholunate Ligament Repair**

Wrist Fusion

Indications and Goals: Wrist fusion is most commonly performed for patients with severe post-traumatic or degenerative arthritis that cannot be improved by another motion-saving procedure. Arthrodesis may also be performed in patients with joint destruction, bone loss, or contractures such as in inflammatory arthritis, infection, paralytic or spastic conditions, trauma, or tumor resection. Fusion may also be required in late stages of complex carpal instability or after failure of a limited intercarpal arthrodesis, proximal row carpectomy or arthroplasty. The goal is to provide predictable pain relief and a stable wrist for power grip.

Procedure and Technique: Current techniques favor rigid internal plate fixation, in an attempt to avoid prolonged cast immobilization and decrease rates of pseudarthrosis. Rod or pin fixation may be used for patients with inflammatory arthritis or a connective tissue disorder, but plates are becoming more commonly used in these conditions as well. A recent development is the precontoured, low-contact, dynamic-compression titanium plate, which was specially designed for wrist arthrodesis. It gives a lower profile to reduce the incidence of hardware prominence and resultant tenderness and extensor tendon irritation. It also eliminates the need for time-consuming precontouring of the plate into slight wrist extension and ulnar deviation. Bone graft is often used to increase fusion rates, and may be taken from the distal radius. Larger defects may be filled with iliac crest graft, but this involves significant donor site morbidity including persistent pain, hematoma formation, infection, and nerve injury.

The procedure is carried out by making a longitudinal incision from the distal third of the index–middle finger interosseous space, across Lister's tubercle, and over the radial shaft to the proximal border of the abductor pollicis longus. Full-thickness skin flaps are elevated while preserving as many cutaneous nerves and dorsal veins as possible. The third dorsal extensor compartment is opened, and the extensor pollicis longus tendon is transposed. The second and fourth dorsal compartments are elevated subperiosteally. Dissection is then continued to expose the dorsal aspect of the third metacarpal, carpometacarpal, capitolunate, and radiocarpal articulations. Articular cartilage is removed with a curette, rongeur, or burr, and the joints are denuded to cancellous bone. The triquetrohamate, capitohamate, and scaphotrapeziotrapezoid joints may be included if indicated by preoperative examination or radiographs. Lister's tubercle is removed, and the dorsal surfaces of the scaphoid, lunate, and capitate are decorticated to provide a flat surface for plate application. Cancellous bone graft is harvested from within the distal metaphyseal region of the radius through a cortical window created 2 cm proximal to the distal radial articular surface and radial to the intended plate position. One centimeter of subchondral and metaphyseal bone should be preserved during harvesting to prevent fracture. Bone graft is inserted into the prepared joint spaces that will lie beneath the plate. An appropriate plate is then selected and contoured, or the precontoured plates may be used. The plate is fixed to the third metacarpal shaft with bicortical screws. Alternatively, the plate may be fixed to the second metacarpal to position the wrist in slight ulnar deviation, thus enhancing power grip. The holes must be drilled exactly from dorsal to volar in the sagittal plane or rotational malalignment of the finger will occur when the plate is secured to the radius. The plate should be placed as far proximally as possible on the metacarpal shaft to avoid irritation of the overlying extensor tendons by the distal edge of the plate. An additional bicortical screw is placed into the capitate. The plate is fixed to the radius with bicortical screws in a compression technique. The extensor pollicis longus is transposed above the extensor retinaculum as the third dorsal compartment is closed.

Post-surgical Precautions/Rehabilitation: Postoperative rehabilitation will initially focus on pain management and incisional wound healing. No range of motion is expected to be gained at the site of the fusion. However, adjacent joints should undergo mobilization exercises as soon as tolerated by the patient, beginning with passive digital motion. Strengthening exercises were begun 6 weeks after surgery. Splinting is discontinued at 6 to 8 weeks, and full unrestricted use of the extremity is usually permitted by 10 to 12 weeks postoperatively when healing is complete and radiographs confirm successful fusion.

Expected Outcomes: Dorsal plating techniques with autologous bone graft have been shown to be superior to various other techniques, with fusions rates exceeding 90%. Wrist arthrodesis results in high subjective patient satisfaction with respect to pain relief and correction of deformity. Grip strength, digital range of motion, and forearm rotation do not significantly change from preoperative values. Improvements in pinch and grip strengths have been reported following wrist arthrodesis in patients with osteoarthritis, but not in those with rheumatoid arthritis. Most patients will be able to perform activities of daily living and return to work, though modifications may be required. The ability to achieve full supination or pronation may not be realistic and should be shared with the patient prior to the procedure so that a clear picture of functional abilities is understood. Maximum improvement may take over a year to achieve. Complications from this procedure include non-union, extensor tendon adhesions or tenosynovitis, intrinsic muscle contracture, plate tenderness, carpal tunnel syndrome, infection, neuroma formation, ulnocarpal impaction, and distal radioulnar joint arthritis.

Return to Play: Unlikely for most athletes. After complete bony fusion, return to activities as tolerated may occur within 4 months postoperatively.

Recommended Readings

Jebson PJ, Adams BD. Wrist arthrodesis: Review of current technique. *J Am Acad Orthop Surg.* 2001;9(1):53–60.

Hayden RJ, Jebson PJ. Wrist arthrodesis. *Hand Clin.* 2005;21(4):631–640. Review.

Honkanen PB, Mäkelä S, Konttinen YT, Lehto MU. Radiocarpal arthrodesis in the treatment of the rheumatoid wrist. A prospective midterm follow-up. *J Hand Surg Eur Vol.* 2007;32(4):368–376. Epub 2007 Jun 4.

Markiewitz AD, Stern PJ. Current perspectives in the management of scaphoid nonunions. *Instr Course Lect.* 2005;54:99–113. Review.

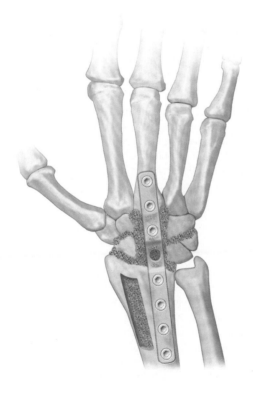

Figure 37. Wrist Fusion

TFCC Debridement/Repair

Indications and Goals: The triangular fibrocartilage complex (TFCC) is a meniscus homologue in the wrist at the distal end of the ulna, and acts to stabilize the distal radioulnar joint (DRUJ). It is bordered and anchored by the dorsal and volar radioulnar ligaments that run from the sigmoid notch to the base of the ulnar styloid. It is a load-bearing structure and in patients with neutral ulnar variance the TFCC bears about 20% of the load across the wrist. Patients with ulnar positive variance will have relatively more load placed on the TFCC and thinning of its central portion. The central and radial aspects of the TFCC are relatively avascular and are amenable to debridement, whereas the ulnar and peripheral portions are more vascular and amenable to repair.

Injuries to the TFCC can be either traumatic or degenerative. Acute traumatic injuries will present with ulnar-sided wrist pain after a rotatory injury and are classified according to the location of the tear. Chronic degenerative tears are usually a result of ulnar positive variance, which can be idiopathic or post-traumatic, such as in malunion, growth arrest, or radial head excision.

Procedure and Technique: TFCC tears are usually evaluated and repaired arthroscopically. Palpation of the TFCC is important, because it normally has a "trampoline" effect when probed. In the acute traumatic setting, central tears without instability can be debrided as long as 2 mm of the peripheral rim remains to maintain stability. Peripheral tears at the base of the ulnar styloid are often associated with DRUJ instability and should be repaired. If there is an associated ulnar styloid fracture, it should undergo internal fixation or excision of the fragment followed by TFCC repair. Peripheral repairs can be performed either through an inside-out or an outside-in technique. The outside-in technique may have a lower incidence of irritation of the dorsal ulnar sensory nerve. A 1 cm incision is made just volar to the extensor carpi ulnaris and distal to the ulnar styloid. The tendon is retracted ulnarly, and two needles are passed through the capsule and across the tear under direct arthroscopic visualization. A wire loop is passed through one needle to grab a 2-0 nonabsorbable suture introduced into the joint through the other needle. The suture is then tied over the dorsal wrist capsule, securing the tear. If the TFCC is avulsed from the ulnolunate or ulnotriquetral ligaments or from the sigmoid notch (as in distal radius fractures), repair can be carried out either open or arthroscopically.

In the chronic setting, ulnar positive variance must be treated in addition to the TFCC pathology. The ulnocarpal impaction may be addressed either through an open extraarticular ulnar shortening osteotomy, or arthroscopically with a wafer procedure, where a burr is used to remove the distal 1 to 4 mm of the ulna through an associated central TFCC tear. Wearing of the TFCC without perforation can be treated by ulnar shortening osteotomy alone. If there is perforation of the TFCC with associated lunate chondromalacia, the TFCC can be debrided and an ulnar shortening procedure can be performed.

Post-surgical Precautions/Rehabilitation: For debridement procedures, range of motion exercises can be initiated relatively early after a short period of immobilization. For repair procedures, a sugar-tong splint for 2 weeks followed by a short arm or Munster cast for 4 weeks can be used. Range of motion has begun thereafter with strengthening started at 10 weeks. For ulnar shortening osteotomies, the area must be protected until there is evidence of healing across the osteotomy site on radiographs.

Expected Outcomes: Outcomes following a TFCC repair depend upon the size of the tear, the ability to accomplish a repair, and the age-related degenerative change in the wrist. A majority of patients experience a reduction in pain after surgery, with improvement in grip strength and daily activities. Acute tears repaired within 3 months of the injury usually regain about 80% of their range of motion and strength. Arthroscopic repairs usually have better recovery of range of motion and strength than open repairs. Loss of wrist rotation, loss of grip strength, and an ulnar positive variance are factors that are correlated with poor outcomes. Stiffness is a common long-term complaint.

Return to Play: Return to participation varies upon whether debridement of repairs performed, and is usually between 6 to 12 weeks.

Recommended Readings

Chen AC, Hsu KY, Chang CH, Chan YS. Arthroscopic suture repair of peripheral tears of triangular fibrocartilage complex using a volar portal. *Arthroscopy.* 2005;21(11):1406.

Conca M, Conca R, Dalla Pria A. Preliminary experience of fully arthroscopic repair of triangular fibrocartilage complex lesions. *Arthroscopy.* 2004;20(7):e79–e82.

Estrella EP, Hung LK, Ho PC, Tse WL. Arthroscopic repair of triangular fibrocartilage complex tears. *Arthroscopy.* 2007;23(7):729–737, 737.e1.

Gupta R, Bozentka DJ, Osterman AL. Wrist arthroscopy: Principles and clinical applications. *J Am Acad Orthop Surg.* 2001;9(3):200–209.

Ruch DS, Papadonikolakis A. Arthroscopically assisted repair of peripheral triangular fibrocartilage complex tears: Factors affecting outcome. *Arthroscopy.* 2005;21(9):1126–1130.

Yao J, Dantuluri P, Osterman AL. A novel technique of all-inside arthroscopic triangular fibrocartilage complex repair. *Arthroscopy.* 2007;23(12):1357.e1–e4.

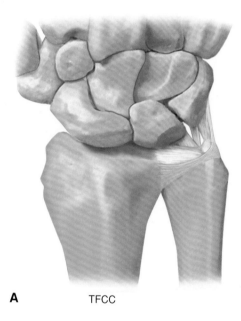

A   TFCC

Figure 38. Arthroscopic TFCC Debridement and Repair (*continued*)

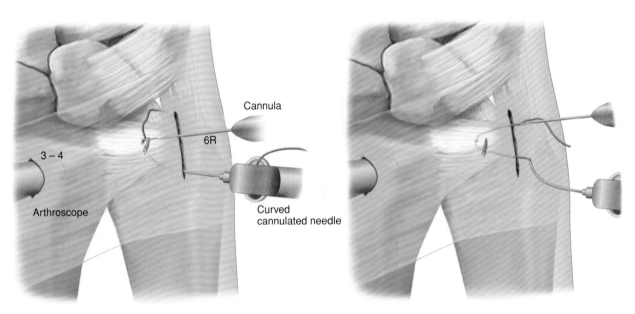

TFCC REPAIR: Whipple outside – in technique

Figure 38. (*continued*)

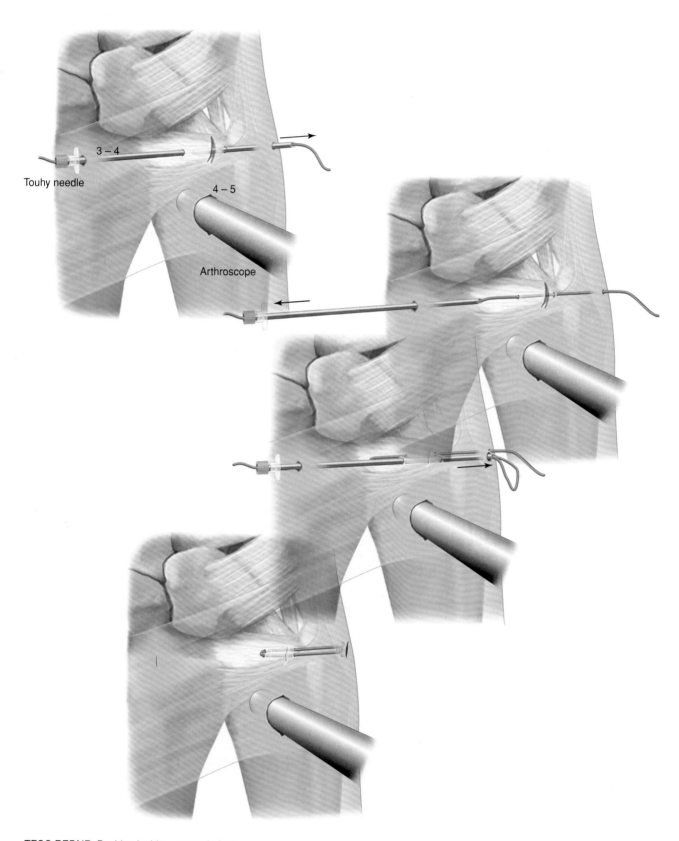

TFCC REPAIR: Poehing inside – out technique

Figure 38. (*continued*)

Tenosynovitis Decompression

Indications and Goals: Tenosynovitis should be insersene of the second and first compartment typically involves the first dorsal wrist compartment (APL and EPB) (de Quervain's syndrome) and the intersection of the second (ECRL and ECRB) and first (APL, EPB) compartments (intersection syndrome). The diagnosis of de Quervain's syndrome is confirmed with Finkelstein's test (thumb is place in the fist and the wrist is ulnarly deviated) and pain with resisted thumb metacarpophalangeal joint extension. de Quervain's is six times more common in women than in men, and often affects the dominant hand in middle age. It is worsened by repetitive activities involving simultaneous thumb abduction and wrist ulnar deviation. Over time this can cause narrowing of the fibro-osseous canal through the extensor retinaculum. A subset of patients who will have new onset but self-limited disease is pregnant and lactating women.

Intersection syndrome is commonly diagnosed in rower's ("oarsman's wrist") and golfers, and presents with a history of wrist pain and crepitance or "squeaking" approximately 5 cm proximal to Lister's tubercle. Both conditions are initially treated conservatively with activity modification, nonsteroidal anti-inflammatories, injections, and thumb spica splinting. Intersection syndrome is more likely to respond to these conservative measures than de Quervain's. Surgical intervention is indicated in patients who have failed a prolonged trial of nonoperative measures.

Procedure and Technique: For both procedures, the patient is placed supine on the operating table with a hand table. For de Quervain's, a 2 cm transverse incision is made over the first dorsal compartment, 1 cm proximal to the radial styloid. Branches of the lateral (should be lateral antebrachial cutaneous) antebrachial cutaneous and superficial radial sensory nerve are identified and protected. The sheath over the APL and EPB is incised in a longitudinal fashion. The APL may have multiple slips (2 to 4), and the EPB is in a separate compartment in many individuals. A small portion of the dorsal retinaculum is excised. For intersection syndrome, a 4 cm longitudinal incision is made proximal to the wrist and the second compartment is released and the bursa at the intersection of the two compartments is debrided.

Post-surgical Precautions/Rehabilitation: Range of motion for the thumb started early while the wrist is splinted in 10 degrees of extension for 2 weeks to prevent a volar tendon prolapse. Sutures will be removed between 1 and 2 weeks, at which time gentle hand and finger strengthening exercises can be initiated. Supervised rehabilitation should emphasize scar management and tendon gliding to prevent against postoperative scarring. Full recovery could take several months. Pain and symptoms generally begin to improve after surgery, but tenderness in the area of the incision may last for several months.

Expected Outcomes: Surgical release of tendons of first dorsal compartment of the wrist has excellent results in patients with de Quervain's tenosynovitis. However, patients may have incomplete relief or persistent pain if a separate EPB compartment is not identified and released intraoperatively, or the superficial radial sensory nerve is irritated or injured. Debate exists regarding the type of incision. The use of a longitudinal incision may be associated with complications such as poor cosmesis, superficial radial nerve injury, and poor wound healing. Advantages of using a longitudinal incision versus a transverse incision include ease in recognition of compartment variations and superficial branches of the radial nerve.

Return to Play: A return to basic activities of daily living can occur within 3 to 4 weeks. More involvement with resistive type work and sport activity may take up to 3 to 4 months.

Recommended Readings

Gundes H, Tosun B. Longitudinal incision in surgical release of de Quervain disease. *Tech Hand Up Extrem Surg.* 2005;9(3):149–152.

Ilyas AA, Ast M, Schaffer AA, Thoder J. de Quervain tenosynovitis of the wrist. *J Am Acad Ortho Surg.* 2007;15(12):757–764.

Jackson WT, Viegas SF, Coon TM, Stimpson KD, Frogameni AD, Simpson JM. Anatomical variations in the first extensor compartment of the wrist. A clinical and anatomical study. *J Bone Joint Surg Am.* 1986;68(6):923–926.

Mellor SJ, Ferris BD. Complications of a simple procedure: de Quervain's disease revisited. *Int J Clin Pract.* 2000;54(2):76–77.

Wolfe SW. Tenosynovitis. In: Green DP, et al., eds. *Green's Operative Hand Surgery.* 5th ed. Philadelphia, PA: Elsevier; 2005:2137–2158.

Yuasa K, Kiyoshige Y. Limited surgical treatment of de Quervain's disease: Decompression of only the extensor pollicis brevis subcompartment. *J Hand Surg [Am].* 1998;23(5):840–843.

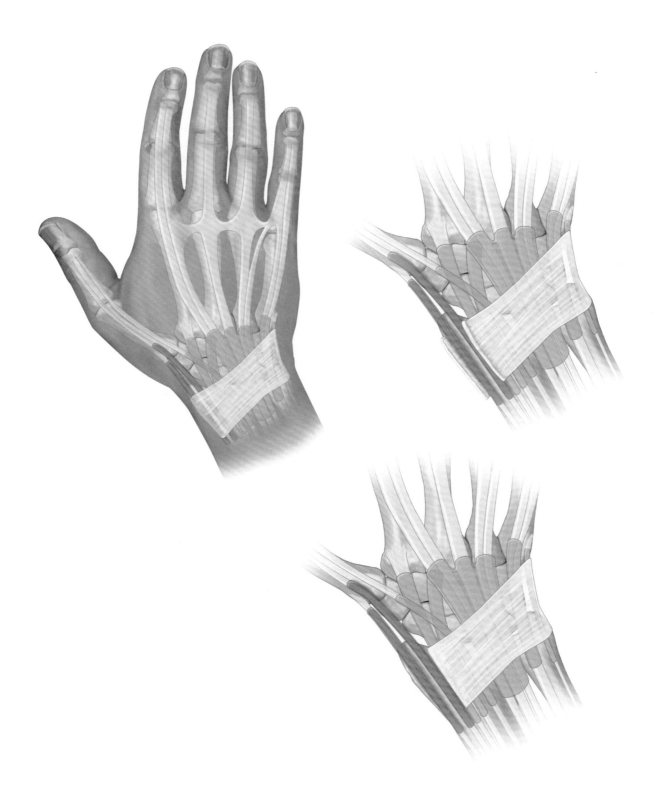

Figure 39. Surgical Decompression of de Quervain's Tenosynovitis

Wrist Ganglion Excision

Indications and Goals: Ganglion cysts are the most common soft tissue tumors of the hand. These mucin-filled cysts are usually attached to the adjacent underlying joint capsule, tendon, or tendon sheath, and can cause pain from compression of surrounding structures. They are most prevalent in women and usually occur between the second and fourth decades of life. Patients usually seek medical attention due to cosmetic appearance of the mass, pain, weakness, and concern of potential malignancy. A specific antecedent traumatic event is present in at least 10% of cases, and repeated minor trauma may be an etiologic factor in their development. A one-way valvular mechanism has been postulated to connect the wrist joint to the cyst. Ganglions usually occur singly and in very specific locations but have been reported to arise from almost every joint of the hand and wrist. The dorsal wrist ganglion accounts for 60% to 70% of all ganglions of the hand and wrist. The main cyst is most often directly over the scapholunate ligament, but may protrude elsewhere between the extensor tendons and can be connected to the ligament through a long pedicle. Failure to identify this pedicle and excise its scapholunate ligament attachment increases the likelihood of recurrence. Transillumination or aspiration confirms the diagnosis preoperatively. Aspiration and injection may provide long-term relief and has been reported to be effective in 20% to 30% of patients. Volar wrist ganglions may be in close proximity to the radial artery, so aspiration should be done with extreme care or simply avoided. Surgical excision of ganglions is performed for persistent pain.

Procedure and Technique: Most dorsal ganglions may be approached through a transverse incision over the proximal carpal row, but a modified incision or second transverse incision may be necessary for ganglions not directly over the scapholunate ligament. The diagnosis of ganglion cyst should be confirmed before commitment to a transverse incision because this type of incision is not readily incorporated into a limb-sparing incision in the event of a subsequent diagnosis of a malignant soft tissue tumor. Typically, a dorsal ganglion appears between the extensor pollicis longus and extensor digitorum communis tendons, which are retracted radially and ulnarly, respectively. The main cyst and its pedicle are mobilized down to the underlying joint capsule. With the wrist in volar flexion, the joint capsule is opened along the border of the radius and proximal pole of the scaphoid. The capsule is elevated and retracted distally to expose the capsular attachments to the scapholunate ligament. Smaller intraarticular cysts are often seen attached to the scapholunate ligament. The capsular incision is then continued around the ganglion, but all capsular attachments to the ligament are left intact. The ganglion and its capsular attachments are then tangentially excised off the scapholunate ligament. Arthroscopic dorsal wrist ganglion excision is becoming more popular with lower recurrence rates and smaller rehabilitation.

Post-surgical Precautions/Rehabilitation: A bulky dressing extending from the proximal forearm to the MP joints is applied and the hand elevated. Early finger motion is encouraged. The dressing and sutures are removed between 7 and 10 days postoperatively. Wrist motion should be initiated and encouraged, especially volar flexion. Hand therapy is continued until a full range of motion has been obtained. Essentially no restrictions need to be placed on the individual apart from assuring adequate wound healing and a gradual increase in activity level and usage of the wrist.

Expected Outcomes: While ganglion excision appears to be an effective treatment method with minimal to no impairment of wrist motion and function, it is not without complications. Volar ganglia resection complication rates are significantly higher versus dorsal, including damage to the superficial radial sensory nerve, the palmar cutaneous branch of the median nerve, and the radial artery. Early recurrences, the most common complication of ganglion surgery, are usually due to inadequate and incomplete excisions. Stiffness of the wrist can be avoided by early motion, physical therapy if necessary, and splinting of the wrist in slight flexion in the immediate postoperative period. It is imperative to stress early volar flexion. To avoid keloid or hypertrophic scars, longitudinal incisions across the wrist joint should be avoided. Awareness and respect for the sensory branches of the radial and ulnar nerves prevent neuroma formation, which often defies effective treatment.

Return to Play: Under optimum circumstances, return to participation should occur between 6 and 8 weeks to minimize the likelihood of a return of the cyst. With some athletes, functional ability may be restored much sooner than this timeframe.

Recommended Readings

Athanasian EA. Bone and Soft Tissue Tumors, In: Green DP, et al., eds. *Green's Operative Hand Surgery*. 5th ed. Philadelphia, PA: Elsevier; 2211–2264.

Dias J, Buch K. Palmar wrist ganglion: Does intervention improve outcome? A prospective study of the natural history and patient-reported treatment outcomes. *J Hand Surg [Br]*. 2003;28(2):172–176.

Dias JJ, Dhukaram V, Kumar P. The natural history of untreated dorsal wrist ganglia and patient reported outcome 6 years after intervention. *J Hand Surg Eur Vol*. 2007;32(5):502–508. Epub 2007 Aug 6.

Geissler WB. Arthroscopic excision of dorsal wrist ganglia. *Tech Hand Up Extrem Surg*. 1998;2(3):196–201.

Ho PC, Law BK, Hung LK. Arthroscopic volar wrist ganglionectomy. *Chir Main*. 2006;25(suppl 1):S221–S230. Review.

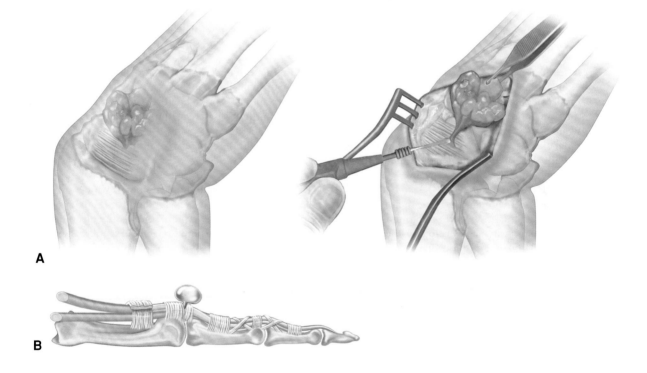

A

B

Figure 40. (A) Open Dorsal Wrist Ganglion Excision. (B) Flexor Tendon Ganglion Cyst

Carpal Tunnel Release

Indications and Goals: Carpal tunnel syndrome is the most common type of compressive neuropathy. The median nerve is impinged in the carpal tunnel by direct trauma, repetitive use, or anatomic anomalies. Paresthesias result from early microvascular compression and neural ischemia. Large sensory fibers (light touch, vibration) are affected before small fibers (pain and temperature). Continued compression may lead to structural changes such as demyelination, fibrosis, and axonal loss. These changes may cause weakness or paralysis of the motor nerve. Abnormal two-point discrimination may also be evident after prolonged compression. Patients report paresthesias and pain (often at night) in the palmar aspect of the radial 3½ digits. Weakness and loss of fine motor control are late findings. The most sensitive provocative test is the carpal tunnel compression test (Durkin's test). Other provocative tests include the Tinel and Phalen signs. Semmes Weinstein monofilament testing is sensitive for diagnosing early CTS. Thenar atrophy may be present in severe denervation. It often affects cyclists, racket sport participants and wheelchair athletes. Risk factors include female sex, obesity, pregnancy, diabetes, hypothyroidism, chronic renal failure, inflammatory arthritis, storage diseases, smoking, alcoholism, advanced age, and repetitive wrist flexion during occupational activity. Electromyography and nerve conduction studies are not necessary for diagnosis of CTS, but they may help to confirm the diagnosis in equivocal cases. Acute CTS occurs in the setting of high-energy trauma, such as distal radius fractures and fracture-dislocations of the radiocarpal joint. Nonoperative treatment includes activity modification, night splints and nonsteroidal anti-inflammatory drugs (NSAIDs). Steroid injections yield transient relief in 80% of patients; only 22% of patients are symptom-free at 12 months but 40% are symptom-free for more than 12 months if symptoms have been present for less than 1 year and they have normal two-point discrimination, no thenar atrophy, less than 1 to 2 ms prolongation sensory/motor latencies, and no denervation potentials on EMG. Failure to improve after corticosteroid injection is a poor prognostic factor, and surgery is less successful in these cases.

Procedure and Technique: The patient is placed supine with the hand on a hand table. An incision is made along a line extending from the radial side of the ring finger, usually in a palmar crease. Structures within Guyon's canal can be injured if the incision is too ulnar, and the recurrent motor branch of the median nerve can be injured if the incision is too radial. The subcutaneous tissue and palmar fascia is dissected to expose the transverse carpal ligament. Typically, a retractor is placed into the tunnel to protect the nerve and the ligament is released on the ulnar side of the nerve (to protect the recurrent motor branch). Endoscopic carpal tunnel release is an option as well for those experienced with this technique.

Post-surgical Precautions/Rehabilitation: The wrist is placed in an immobilizer for 3 to 4 days and patients are encouraged to move their fingers and wrist as soon as possible. There should be minimal postoperative pain, and the pre-operative symptoms should have subsided. Though not common, some minimal swelling may be present and it will usually resolve within a week. Use of the involved wrist should be encouraged for light activities of daily living, and an individual may return to work relatively soon with some consideration given to their work environment in terms of occupational safety and ergonomically sound equipment.

Expected Outcomes: Most patients have immediate relief but long-standing symptoms may take longer to resolve. Endoscopic carpal tunnel release (ECTR) is an alternative to the standard open procedure, but its most common complication is incomplete division of the transverse carpal ligament. ECTR is associated with an earlier return to work and better early patient satisfaction scores; however, the complication rate appears higher. The long-term results of open CTR and ECTR are equivalent. Complication rates are most closely associated with the experience of the operating surgeon, rather than the operative technique. After standard open release, pinch strength returns to the preoperative level in 6 weeks and grip strength returns in 3 months. Pillar pain in the palm adjacent to the incision is common for 3 to 4 months in open CTR. Persistent symptoms after CTR may be secondary to incomplete release of the transverse carpal ligament, iatrogenic median nerve injury, missed double crush phenomenon, concomitant peripheral neuropathy, or a space-occupying lesion. The success of revision CTR relies on identifying the underlying cause of the failure.

Return to Play: Return to work or play can occur immediately with restricted use of the wrist and hand. Under optimum circumstances, full return to restored function may occur within 6 to 8 weeks postoperative.

Recommended Readings

Adams BD. Endoscopic carpal tunnel release. *J Am Acad Orthop Surg.* 1994;2(3):179–184.

Benson LS, Bare AA, Nagle DJ, Harder VS, Williams CS, Visotsky JL. Complications of endoscopic and open carpal tunnel release. *Arthroscopy.* 2006;22(9):919–924, 924.e1–e2. Review.

Cranford CS, Ho JY, Kalainov DM, Hartigan BJ. Carpal tunnel syndrome. *J Am Acad Orthop Surg.* 2007;15(9):537–548.

Pomerance J, Fine I. Outcomes of carpal tunnel surgery with and without supervised postoperative therapy. *J Hand Surg [Am].* 2007;32(8):1159–1163; discussion 1164–1165.

Scholten RJ, Mink van der Molen A, Uitdehaag BM, Bouter LM, de Vet HC. Surgical treatment options for carpal tunnel syndrome. *Cochrane Database Syst Rev.* 2007;(4):CD003905. Review.

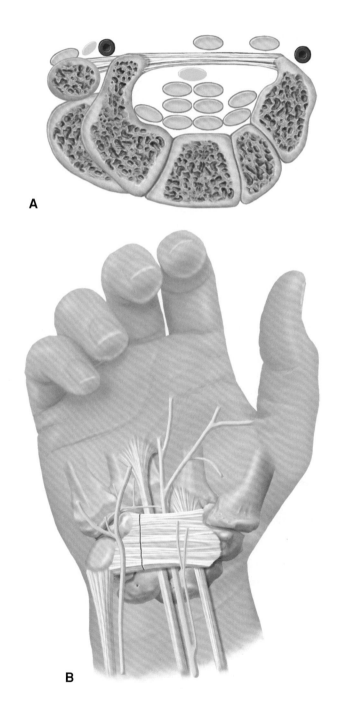

A

B

Figure 41. Anatomy of Transverse Carpal Ligaments (A) Incision for Open CTR (B)

Guyon's Canal (Ulnar Nerve Compression at the Wrist) Release

Indications and Goals: Ulnar tunnel syndrome is a compression neuropathy of the ulnar nerve in Guyon's canal and is less common than carpal tunnel syndrome. The borders of Guyon's canal are the volar carpal ligament (roof), the transverse carpal ligament (floor), the hook of the hamate (radial) and the pisiform and the abductor digiti minimi muscle belly (ulnar). The canal is approximately 4 cm long, and it is divided into three zones: (1) located proximal to the bifurcation of the nerve; (2) surrounding mostly the deep motor branch; and (3) surrounding mostly the superficial sensory branch. The most common cause of ulnar tunnel syndrome is a ganglion cyst (80% of nontraumatic cases). Other causative factors include hook of hamate nonunion, ulnar artery thrombosis, direct compression (cyclists-handlebar palsy), palmaris brevis hypertrophy, or anomalous muscle. Success of treatment is dependent on identifying the cause. Useful adjunctive tests include computed tomography (CT) for hook of hamate fracture, magnetic resonance imaging (MRI) for ganglion cyst or other space-occupying lesion, Doppler ultrasound for ulnar artery thrombosis, and so on. Symptoms may be pure motor, pure sensory or mixed, based on the zone of compression. Pain and paresthesias can occur in the ulnar 1½ digits and intrinsic muscle weakness may be present. Nerve conduction studies are helpful in confirming the diagnosis. Nonoperative treatment includes activity modification, splints and NSAIDs. Operative treatment involves decompressing the ulnar nerve by addressing the underlying cause. Guyon's canal is adequately decompressed by release of the transverse carpal ligament when concurrent CTS exists.

Procedure and Technique: The patient is placed supine with the hand on a hand table. A 5-cm incision is made just radial to the flexor carpi ulnaris (FCU) tendon and curvilinear across the wrist crease. After dissection of the subcutaneous tissue and palmar fascia, the FCU is retracted ulnarly and the pisiform bone and pisohamate ligament identified. The motor branch is identified as it dives deep and it is protected. The volar carpal ligament and pisohamate ligament is then incised and the nerve is decompressed.

Post-surgical Precautions/Rehabilitation: A bulky dressing is applied to maintain a wrist neutral position, and this dressing is removed 2 days after surgery. The patient is instructed in range-of-motion exercises for the fingers, wrist, and arm. A wrist splint in a neutral position is used at night for patient comfort. The sutures are removed 10 to 14 days postoperatively.

Expected Outcomes: Similar to carpal tunnel release, most patients have immediate relief, but long-standing symptoms may take longer to resolve. Complete relief is dependent on correctly identifying the underlying cause. Persistent symptoms may be due to failure to identify and release the deep motor branch of the ulnar nerve, or continued compression from a deep unidentified ganglion cyst.

Return to Play: Patients are allowed full activity and return to work or play without restrictions 6 to 8 weeks after surgery.

Recommended Readings

Black S, Hofmeister E, Thompson M. A unique case of ulnar tunnel syndrome in a bicyclist requiring operative release. *Am J Orthop.* 2007;36(7):377–379.

Capitani D, Beer S. Handlebar palsy–a compression syndrome of the deep terminal (motor) branch of the ulnar nerve in biking. *J Neurol.* 2002;249(10):1441–1445.

Cobb TK, Carmichael SW, Cooney WP. Guyon's canal revisited: An anatomic study of the carpal ulnar neurovascular space. *J Hand Surg [Am].* 1996;21(5):861–869.

Elhassan B, Steinmann SP. Entrapment neuropathy of the ulnar nerve. *J Am Acad Orthop Surg.* 2007;15(11):672–681.

König PS, Hage JJ, Bloem JJ, Prosé LP. Variations of the ulnar nerve and ulnar artery in Guyon's canal: A cadaveric study. *J Hand Surg [Am].* 1994;19(4):617–622.

Mackinnon SE, Novak CB. Compression Neuropathies. In: Green DP, et al., eds. *Green's Operative Hand Surgery.* 5th ed. Philadelphia, PA: Elsevier; 2005:998–1046.

Posner MA. Compressive neuropathies of the ulnar nerve at the elbow and wrist. *Instr Course Lect.* 2000;49:305–317. Review.

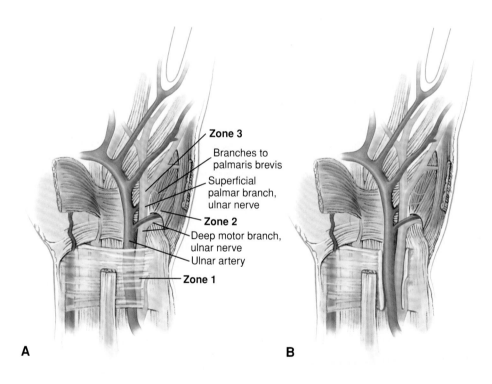

Figure 42. Release of Guyon's Tunnel (A and B)

Trigger Finger Release

Indications and Goals: Stenosing tenosynovitis (trigger finger) is caused by inflammation of the flexor tendon sheath which inhibits the smooth gliding motion of flexor tendons in the digits or thumb. This common condition is initially characterized by pain and tenderness at the distal palm near the A1 pulley. If left untreated, stenosing tenosynovitis may lead to catching and locking of the digit as the space available for the flexor tendon narrows. The most widely used classification scheme was developed by Green. Stage 1 is pain and tenderness at the A1 pulley. Stage 2 is catching of the digit during motion. Stage 3 presents with actual locking of the digit, but it is passively correctable by the patient. Stage 4 is a fixed, locked digit. The ring finger is the most commonly affected digit in adults (thumb in children). It occurs more frequently in middle-aged females, diabetics and patients with rheumatoid arthritis. It may result from repetitive grasping activities. A great majority of patients, excluding the diabetic population, will respond favorably to corticosteroid injection into the flexor tendon sheath. Surgical release is indicated for those who fail nonoperative management.

Procedure and Technique: A small transverse incision is made over the A1 pulley (usually at the level of the distal palmar crease). The subcutaneous tissues are dissected and care is taken to protect the adjacent digital neurovascular bundles. The pulley is identified and it is simply released with a longitudinal incision. Care is taken to not violate the proximal edge of the A2 pulley so as to prevent the potential for bowstringing and loss of digital flexion. The digit is passively moved to ensure that no more triggering occurs. A length of the tendon may be pulled through the incision and inspected for damage or attrition. Percutaneous techniques done in the office setting with various instruments have been reported with good initial results.

Post-surgical Precautions/Rehabilitation: Typically, supervised rehabilitation is not required for patients following a trigger finger release. A home exercise program may suffice to restore range of motion following surgery. In addition, education and instructions for completing activities of daily living can be helpful. Scar management can also be taught from the onset. However, home exercise programs are only successful with compliant patient.

Expected Outcomes: The overall complication rate is low, approximately 1%, consisting of adverse wound healing, extension lag, and possibly residual stiffness. Open release of the A1 pulley yields a less than 10% recurrence rate. Incomplete relief of triggering has been reported in a higher percent of patients with grade 4 trigger digits and fixed flexion contractures.

Return to Play: Return to participation is usually possible 4 to 6 weeks postoperative, and in some cases sooner.

Recommended Readings

Bae DS, Sodha S, Waters PM. Surgical treatment of the pediatric trigger finger. *J Hand Surg [Am]*. 2007;32(7):1043–1047.

Lim MH, Lim KK, Rasheed MZ, Narayanan S, Beng-Hoi Tan A. Outcome of open trigger digit release. *J Hand Surg Eur Vol*. 2007;32(4):457–459. Epub 2007 May 4.

Saldana MJ. Trigger digits: Diagnosis and treatment. *J Am Acad Orthop Surg*. 2001;9(4):246–252.

Wolfe SW. Tenosynovitis. In: Green DP, et al., eds. *Green's Operative Hand Surgery*. 5th ed. Philadelphia, PA: Elsevier; 2005:2137–2158.

Draganich LF, Greenspahn S, Mass DP. Effects of the adductor pollicis and abductor pollicis brevis on thumb metacarpophalangeal joint laxity before and after ulnar collateral ligament reconstruction. *J Hand Surg [Am]*. 2004;29(3):481–488.

Firoozbakhsh K, Yi IS, Moneim MS, Umada Y. A study of ulnar collateral ligament of the thumb metacarpophalangeal joint. *Clin Orthop Relat Res*. 2002;(403):240–247.

Glickel SZ. Thumb metacarpophalangeal joint ulnar collateral ligament reconstruction using a tendon graft. *Tech Hand Up Extrem Surg*. 2002;6(3):133–139.

Harley BJ, Werner FW, Green JK. A biomechanical modeling of injury, repair, and rehabilitation of ulnar collateral ligament injuries of the thumb. *J Hand Surg [Am]*. 2004;29(5):915–920.

Heyman P. Injuries to the ulnar collateral ligament of the thumb metacarpophalangeal joint. *J Am Acad Orthop Surg*. 1997;5(4):224–229.

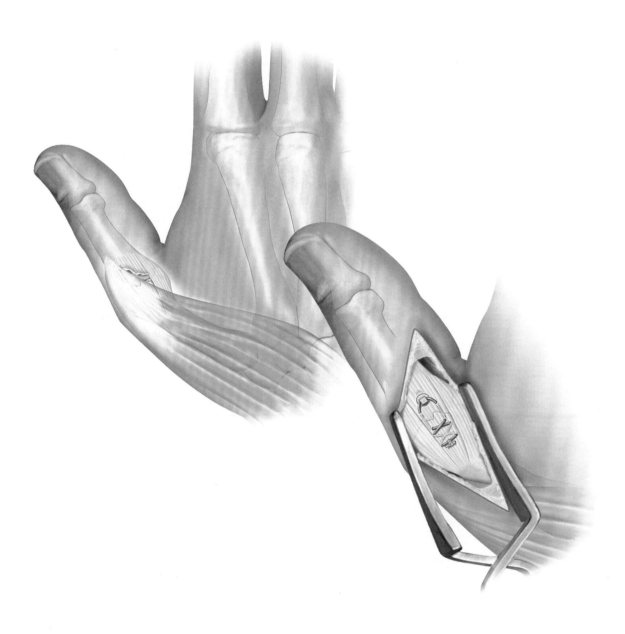

Figure 46. UCL Repair

ORIF Distal Radius Fractures

Indications and Goals: Distal radius fractures are the most common fractures of the upper extremity. They typically result from high-energy trauma in young individuals and low-energy falls in older individuals with osteoporosis. Patients will present with pain, swelling, and deformity at the wrist. Median nerve function should be assessed before and after closed reduction. Acute carpal tunnel syndrome may develop in a small percentage of cases and requires emergent median nerve decompression.

Radiographs should be scrutinized for the amount of deformity to help guide operative versus nonoperative treatment. Intraarticular fractures with more than 1 mm of articular stepoff can lead to early post-traumatic radiocarpal arthrosis. On the AP view, normal radial height is 11 to 13 mm, and is measured as the distance between two parallel horizontal lines, one drawn tangential to the tip of the radial styloid and the other drawn tangential to the distal surface of the ulna. An attempt should be made to correct greater than 5 mm of radial shortening. Radial inclination is measured on the AP view and is normally about 22 degrees. It is the angle between a horizontal line drawn tangential to the distal radius articular surface and another line drawn from the most ulnar aspect of the distal radius articular surface to the tip of the radial styloid. Greater than 15 degrees is acceptable. Volar tilt is measured on the lateral view. A line is drawn tangential to the volar and dorsal aspects of the lunate fossa. The angle between this tangential line and a line perpendicular to the radial shaft averages 11 degrees volar. Up to 10 degrees of dorsal tilt or within 20 degrees of the opposite side is generally accepted. Greater than 20 degrees of initial dorsal angulation may correlate with instability and failure of closed treatment. The distal radioulnar joint (DRUJ) should be evaluated for injury on the lateral view, indicated by subluxation of the ulna in a dorsal or volar direction. The carpal bones should also be evaluated. Scaphoid fractures or scapholunate ligament disruption, indicated by diastasis of the scapholunate interval by greater than 3 mm, are commonly associated with the radial styloid or "chauffeur's" fracture.

Initial closed reduction is indicated in displaced fractures with unacceptable radiographic parameters. At the very least, an attempt should be made to restore radial height and volar tilt. A hematoma block of 1% plain lidocaine can be administered dorsally to aid in patient comfort during the procedure. A combination of finger traps and an upper arm counterweight is a commonly employed method of achieving ligamentotaxis prior to manipulation. The reduction maneuver requires initial recreation and exaggeration of the deformity. The distal fragment is then manipulated on top of the radial shaft. A sugar-tong plaster splint is applied with a three-point mold. The splint should not compromise MCP motion.

Goals for treatment include maintaining reduction until union, restoring hand and wrist function and preventing early radiocarpal arthritis. Factors such as age, general medical condition, activity demands, bone stock, fracture stability and other associated injuries must be considered. Definitive closed treatment with cast immobilization is sufficient in low-energy injuries that are nondisplaced or minimally displaced after closed reduction, especially in functionally low-demand patients. Radiographs should be obtained weekly for the first several weeks to make sure reduction is maintained. Recent literature shows that loss of reduction correlates with increasing age. Immobilization continues for approximately 6 to 8 weeks. Indications for surgery include a large amount of initial displacement, inadequate reduction, or loss of reduction over time.

Procedure and Technique: There are many options for surgical intervention. Closed reduction and percutaneous pinning with 0.062-inch K-wires may be sufficient for extraarticular fractures. Kapandji intra-focal pinning employs K-wires as reduction tools to manipulate the distal fragment into anatomic alignment, but is contraindicated in intraarticular fracture patterns and osteoporotic bone. These techniques may be supplemented by external fixation. Both bridging (distal pins in the second metacarpal) and nonbridging (distal pins in the distal fragment) external fixation methods have been advocated, either used alone or in combination with other treatment methods. Restoration of volar tilt and avoidance of joint distraction are technical challenges in bridging external fixation.

Open reduction and internal fixation is used for complex, unstable intraarticular fractures. A well-performed ORIF most reliably restores articular congruity. Dorsal, volar, and fragment-specific fixation methods have been employed, each with specific advantages and disadvantages. The main advantage of performing ORIF is to allow early wrist motion.

Dorsal plating is performed through a relatively simple approach between the third and fourth extensor compartments. The articular reduction is directly visualized. Although newer lower profile plates are now available, the historical disadvantages of this approach are extensor tendon irritation, potential tendon rupture and frequent need for hardware removal. These problems are avoided through a volar Henry approach between the FCR and radial artery. The classic indications for volar plating are the Smith and volar Barton fracture patterns. Newer fixed-angle locking plates allow for reduction and stabilization of dorsally displaced fractures. The fragment-specific fixation method, popularized by Medoff, uses low-profile constructs to restore anatomy, but requires multiple incisions and is technically challenging. Intramedullary nails have been developed to allow for simple, percutaneous fixation of minimally comminuted extraarticular fracture patterns, but no long-term data exists to determine their efficacy.

Wrist arthroscopy can be used to assist with reduction in intraarticular fracture patterns, and also to evaluate and treat associated injuries, such as TFCC tears and scapholunate or lunotriquetral ligament injuries. Care must be taken with inflow pressure in these cases, as the wrist capsule is disrupted and irrigation fluid will infiltrate into surrounding soft tissues.

Post-surgical Precautions/Rehabilitation: Postoperative protocols depend on degree of stability achieved intraoperatively. If locking plates are used and fixation is deemed to be adequate, a volar plaster wrist splint is applied for 5 to 7 days. Finger motion and hand elevation to reduce swelling is encouraged immediately postoperatively. The splints and dressings are removed at the first postoperative visit. Supervised hand therapy is started for gentle range of motion, and a removable wrist splint is worn for protection at all other times. The splint can be discontinued after radiographic evidence of healing at 8 weeks, but should be worn for activities for 5 months.

Expected Outcomes: Restoration of normal anatomic relationships and articular surface congruity correlate with good outcomes. Complications include nonunion, malunion, post-traumatic arthritis, carpal instability, EPL rupture, hardware failure, stiffness and complex regional pain syndrome. Nonunion is uncommon. Asymptomatic malunion in a functionally low-demand patient does not require treatment. Low-demand patients with pain from ulnocarpal impaction may benefit from a distal ulna resection (Darrach's procedure). Otherwise, a corrective radius osteotomy with ORIF and bone grafting may be indicated for higher demand patients. Radiocarpal arthrosis is present in over 90% of patients with residual articular stepoff of 1 mm and in 100% of patients with over 2 mm. Jupiter has determined that approximately 2/3 of these patients will be symptomatic. EPL ruptures occur in approximately 3% of distal radius fractures during the course of treatment. When primary repair is not possible, a palmaris longus graft or EIP to EPL transfer is used.

Return to Play: Complete bony healing, restoration of range of motion, and return of symmetric grip strength should occur before return to play. Typically this will be at least 3 to 4 months postoperatively.

Recommended Readings

Fernandez DL, Wolfe SW. Distal Radius Fractures. In: Green DP, et al., eds. *Green's Operative Hand Surgery*. 5th ed. Philadelphia, PA: Elsevier; 2005:645–710.

Guofen C, Doi K, Hattori Y, Kitajima I. Arthroscopically assisted reduction and immobilization of intraarticular fracture of the distal end of the radius: Several options of reduction and immobilization. *Tech Hand Up Extrem Surg*. 2005;9(2):84–90. Review.

Putnam MD, Fischer MD. Treatment of unstable distal radius fractures: Methods and comparison of external distraction and ORIF versus external distraction-ORIF neutralization. *J Hand Surg [Am]*. 1997;22(2):238–251.

Westphal T, Piatek S, Schubert S, Winckler S. Outcome after surgery of distal radius fractures: No differences between external fixation and ORIF. *Arch Orthop Trauma Surg*. 2005;125(8):507–514. Epub 2005 Oct 22.

Wright TW, Horodyski M, Smith DW. Functional outcome of unstable distal radius fractures: ORIF with a volar fixed-angle tine plate versus external fixation. *J Hand Surg [Am]*. 2005;30(2):289–99. Erratum in: *J Hand Surg [Am]*. 2005;30(3):629.

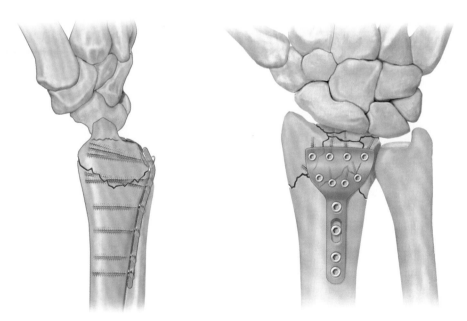

Figure 47. Open Reduction and Internal Fixation of Distal Radius Fracture—Dorsal and Volar

ORIF Scaphoid Fractures

Indications and Goals: The scaphoid is the most commonly fractured carpal bone, accounting for up to 15% of all acute wrist injuries. Approximately 75% of the scaphoid is covered by articular cartilage. Its main blood supply enters dorsally at the waist and flows retrograde toward the proximal pole, and additional branches perfuse the distal one-third. Because of this tenuous vascular anatomy, fractures of the waist and proximal pole are at risk for nonunion and post-traumatic avascular necrosis. The most common mechanism for fracture is a forced hyperextension and radial deviation of the wrist. Patients may have tenderness in the anatomic snuffbox dorsally, but is more reliably elicited over the scaphoid tubercle volarly. A standard radiographic wrist trauma series, including PA, lateral, oblique and scaphoid (30-degree wrist extension, 20-degree ulnar deviation) views, will be nondiagnostic in over 30% of cases on initial presentation. When standard radiographs are negative and a high clinical suspicion exists, patients can be placed in a thumb spica cast and imaging repeated 2 to 3 weeks after injury, at which time a radiolucent line may be more evident from bone resorption at the fracture site. Bone scan, CT, and MRI have all been utilized for early diagnosis, with MRI appearing to provide the most accurate and cost-effective method. Waiting over 4 weeks to initiate treatment increases the overall nonunion rate from 5% to 45%. Nonoperative treatment is best for nondisplaced fractures and consists of cast immobilization. Expected time to union increases and the overall union rates decrease as the fracture becomes more proximal. Consequently, the length of immobilization should be greater for more proximal fractures. Distal third fractures can be immobilized for 2 months, waist fractures for 3 to 4 months, and proximal third fractures for 4 to 5 months. The indications for surgery include fractures with greater than 1 mm of displacement, angulation greater than 15 degrees (humpback deformity), and trans-scaphoid perilunate dislocations. Proximal pole fractures represent another relative indication for acute surgical intervention.

Procedure and Technique: Acute fractures with minimal displacement may be treated compression screw fixation techniques, especially in patients in higher demand activities. Setup for compression screw fixation is similar to that for wrist arthroscopy using the hand table and traction tower, except that the thumb alone is placed in the finger traps. This allows rotation of the forearm around a fixed axis for easier fluoroscopic imaging to confirm hardware placement. A K-wire is placed percutaneously in a retrograde fashion from the distal pole. Fluoroscopic imaging is used to confirm center–center placement on orthogonal views. Another K-wire can be placed to prevent rotation or displacement of the fragments during drilling and instrumentation. A small 5 mm incision is then made around the K-wire. A drill is passed over the K-wire, followed by the compression screw. The supplemental K-wire is then removed. Compression screws may also be placed antegrade with the wrist pronated and flexed.

Formal ORIF with compression screw fixation is favored for displaced or angulated fractures. The approach is dictated by the location of the fracture and surgeon preference. A volar exposure is often used in an attempt to limit injury to the dorsal blood supply of the scaphoid, but it is easier to address very proximal fractures with a dorsal exposure. The volar approach is also the preferred approach to address humpback deformities.

For the volar approach, a 4 cm longitudinal incision is made along the radial border of the flexor carpi radialis (FCR) tendon, centered at the level of the radial styloid, which usually corresponds to the level of the fracture itself. The radial artery is retracted radially and protected, and the FCR tendon is retracted ulnarly. The capsule is divided longitudinally, and the underlying deep volar radiocarpal ligaments are either divided partially and retracted or completely severed and tagged for later repair. K-wires or compression screws can be passed in a retrograde fashion. If a humpback deformity is present requiring bone graft, a cavity is created in both fracture fragments and cancellous iliac crest bone graft is impacted while correcting the deformity. Internal fixation may not be required, but K-wires can be placed if there is evidence of persistent instability after graft placement. The radiocarpal ligaments are repaired, and the hand and wrist are immobilized in a compression-type dressing incorporated into a long-arm cast.

For the dorsolateral approach, a curvilinear incision is centered over the anatomic snuff box (depression between the extensor pollicis longus (EPL) and brevis (EPB) tendons just distal and dorsal to the radial styloid), extending from the base of the thumb metacarpal to a point 3 cm proximal to the snuff box. The superficial sensory branch of the radial nerve should be identified and protected. The fascia between the EPL and EPB is opened and the radial artery is identified and protected. The joint capsule can then be longitudinally incised and the scaphoid is exposed.

Alternatively, a dorsal approach may be used by making a curvilinear dorsoradial incision paralleling the course of the EPL. Branches of the superficial radial nerve are identified and protected. The EPL tendon sheath is then incised and the tendon transposed. A transverse dorsoradial capsulotomy is made to expose the scaphoid. Compression screws or K-wires are then used for fixation as desired. This approach is also useful for vascularized bone grafting for nonunions.

Post-surgical Precautions/Rehabilitation: Postoperatively, patients are placed into a long arm thumb spica cast, which is usually changed to a short arm thumb spica cast at about 6 weeks postoperatively. If the intraoperative construct is very stable or if internal fixation was used, a short arm thumb spica cast may be used from the outset. The total immobilization time for this procedure averages 4 months. Aggressive therapy is typically delayed until radiographic union is achieved. CT may be necessary to confirm union.

Expected Outcomes: Union rates of over 90% to 95% have been consistently reported with operative treatment. Complications include nonunion, malunion, avascular necrosis and post-traumatic arthritis. Symptomatic, early-stage scaphoid nonunion may be treated with ORIF and bone grafting. Scaphoid nonunion with an accompanying humpback deformity requires an opening-wedge interposition (Fisk) graft to restore scaphoid length and angulation. The inlay (Russe) technique is best utilized in cases with minimal deformity and a vascularized proximal pole, and the bone graft may be obtained from the distal radius or iliac crest. The presence of intraoperative punctate bleeding is the most reliable sign of a vascular proximal pole. Vascularized bone grafting has become more popular in the treatment of scaphoid nonunion with an avascular proximal pole. The graft may be harvested

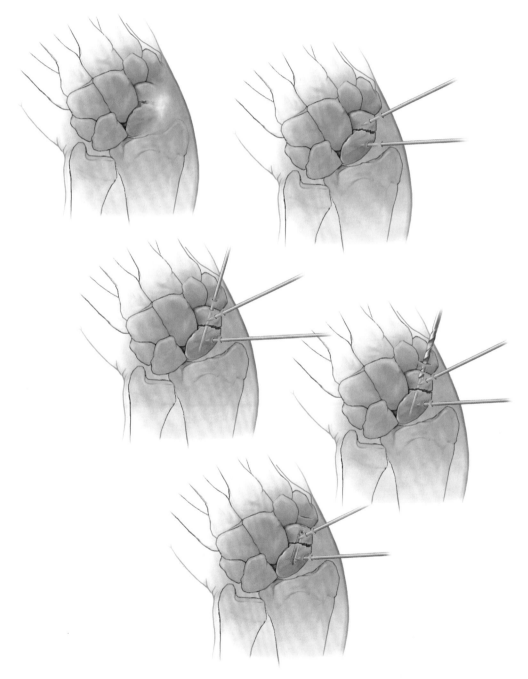

Figure 48. Open Reduction and Internal Fixation: Scaphoid Fracture

from the distal radius and is based on the 1-2 intercompartmental supraretinacular artery (1,2 ICSRA). Untreated chronic nonunions develop a dorsal intercalated segment instability (DISI) deformity and a characteristic progression of arthritis, called a scaphoid nonunion advanced collapse (SNAC) wrist. Options for treatment of a SNAC wrist include radial styloidectomy, proximal row carpectomy, scaphoid excision and four-corner fusion and total wrist fusion, depending on the stage of presentation and surgeon preference.

Return to Play: Complete evidence of bony union via radiographs, restoration of range of motion, and return of strength should be present prior to return to play. This typically will take 3 to 4 months, but protected return to play may be sooner.

Recommended Readings

Amadio PC, Moran SL. Fractures of the Carpal Bones. In: Green DP, et al., eds. *Green's Operative Hand Surgery*. 5th ed. Philadelphia, PA: Elsevier; 2005:711–768.

Bushnell BD, McWilliams AD, Messer TM. Complications in dorsal percutaneous cannulated screw fixation of nondisplaced scaphoid waist fractures. *J Hand Surg [Am]*. 2007;32(6):827–33.

Park MJ, Ahn JH. Arthroscopically assisted reduction and percutaneous fixation of dorsal perilunate dislocations and fracture-dislocations. *Arthroscopy*. 2005;21(9):1153.

Ring D, Jupiter JB, Herndon JH. Acute fractures of the scaphoid. *J Am Acad Orthop Surg*. 2000;8(4):225–231.

Rizzo M, Shin AY. Treatment of acute scaphoid fractures in the athlete. *Curr Sports Med Rep*. 2006;5(5):242–248. Review.

Excision of Hamate Hook Fractures

Indications and Goals: Patients with fractures of the hook of the hamate often present with a history of blunt trauma to the palm, frequently associated with certain sports (golf, baseball, hockey, racquet sports, etc.). Accompanying parasthesias of the ring and small fingers are common due to hemorrhage within and around Guyon's canal. Flexor tendon ruptures may also occur by attrition against the roughened edges of the fracture fragments. A carpal tunnel view may reveal the fracture, but a CT scan is the best confirmatory test. These fractures typically progress to nonunion if left untreated. This has been ascribed to its poor blood supply and to the mechanical forces of the flexor tendons in the carpal tunnel, which tend to displace the fracture fragment ulnarly with grip. Fractures detected early can be treated with a trial of cast immobilization. For those diagnosed more than a few weeks after injury or those who fail casting, excision of the fracture fragment should be performed. ORIF has been described for larger fracture fragments but has a high complication rate and little clinical benefit. Be aware of the bipartite hamate (os hamuli proprius), which may be differentiated from a fracture by smooth cortical surfaces.

Procedure and Technique: The hook of the hamate is approached through a short palmar incision directly overlying the tip. Care should be taken to preserve the integrity of the motor branch of the ulnar nerve, which is in close proximity. In some patients, there may be difficulty localizing the fracture site, but subperiosteal dissection and gentle manipulation of the tip of the hamate hook should lead to the site of nonunion. The fracture fragment is excised and the base of the hook of the hamate is rasped smooth and covered by careful repair of the overlying periosteum.

Post-surgical Precautions/Rehabilitation: Postoperative immobilization is required only until acute tenderness subsides. Gentle range of motion exercises and tendon gliding can begin when the patient is comfortable. Grip strength can be initiated once the incision is healed, and a gradual return to full activities is allowed. Scar tissue management is key to maintain pliable tissue and minimize skin breakdown at the site of the incision.

Expected Outcomes: Excision of hamate hook fractures yields excellent results with few complications. Some pain and weakness may persist, but most patients are able to return to full athletic and occupational activities.

Return to Play: Since bony healing is not required, patients may return to play relatively quickly, after soft tissue healing—even within 2 to 3 weeks.

Recommended Readings

Aldridge JM 3rd, Mallon WJ. Hook of the hamate fractures in competitive golfers: Results of treatment by excision of the fractured hook of the hamate. *Orthopedics*. 2003;26(7):717–719.

Amadio PC, Moran SL. Fractures of the Carpal Bones. In: Green DP, et al., eds. *Green's Operative Hand Surgery*. 5th ed. Philadelphia, PA: Elsevier; 2005:711–768.

Fredericson M, Kim BJ, Date ES, McAdams TR. Injury to the deep motor branch of the ulnar nerve during hook of hamate excision. *Orthopedics*. 2006;29(5):456–458.

Scheufler O, Andresen R, Radmer S, Erdmann D, Exner K, Germann G. Hook of hamate fractures: Critical evaluation of different therapeutic procedures. *Plast Reconstr Surg*. 2005;115(2):488–497.

Scheufler O, Radmer S, Erdmann D, Germann G, Pierer G, Andresen R. Therapeutic alternatives in nonunion of hamate hook fractures: Personal experience in 8 patients and review of literature. *Ann Plast Surg*. 2005;55(2):149–154. Review.

Expected Outcomes: Outcomes are generally good following an open reduction internal fixation for a phalangeal fracture. Return to activity and participation are dependent upon one's goals, and oftentimes quicker returns can be achieved with protective devices. Complications include loss of motion from joint contracture or extensor lag, nonunion, and malunions such as malrotation, angulation, and shortening. Complications of distal phalangeal fractures include numbness, cold sensitivity, hyperesthesia, restricted DIP motion, and nail growth abnormalities.

Return to Play: After complete bony healing and restoration of full range of motion—as early as 6 weeks postoperatively. Protected return to play may be possible sooner in certain athletes.

Recommended Readings

Agarwal AK, Karri V, Pickford MA. Avoiding pitfalls of the pins and rubbers traction technique for fractures of the proximal interphalangeal joint. *Ann Plast Surg*. 2007;58(5):489–495.

Cornwall R, Ricchetti ET. Pediatric phalanx fractures: Unique challenges and pitfalls. *Clin Orthop Relat Res*. 2006;445:146–156. Review.

Hamilton SC, Stern PJ, Fassler PR, Kiefhaber TR. Mini-screw fixation for the treatment of proximal interphalangeal joint dorsal fracture-dislocations. *J Hand Surg [Am]*. 2006;31(8):1349–1354.

Orbay JL, Touhami A. The treatment of unstable metacarpal and phalangeal shaft fractures with flexible nonlocking and locking intramedullary nails. *Hand Clin*. 2006;22(3):279–286.

Rafique A, Ghani S, Sadiq M, Siddiqui IA. Kirschner wire pin tract infection rates between percutaneous and buried wires in treating metacarpal and phalangeal fractures. *J Coll Physicians Surg Pak*. 2006;16(8):518–520.

Roth JJ, Auerbach DM. Fixation of hand fractures with bicortical screws. *J Hand Surg [Am]*. 2005;30(1):151–153.

Stern PJ. Fractures of the metacarpals and phalanges., In: Green DP, et al., eds. *Green's Operative Hand Surgery*. 5th ed. Philadelphia, PA: Elsevier; 2005:277–342.

Suzuki Y, Matsunaga T, Sato S, et al. The pins and rubbers traction system for treatment of comminuted intraarticular fractures and fracture-dislocations in the hand. *J Hand Surg Br*. 1994;19:98–107.

Trevisan C, Morganti A, Casiraghi A, Marinoni EC. Low-severity metacarpal and phalangeal fractures treated with miniature plates and screws. *Arch Orthop Trauma Surg*. 2004;124(10):675–680. Epub 2004 Oct 28.

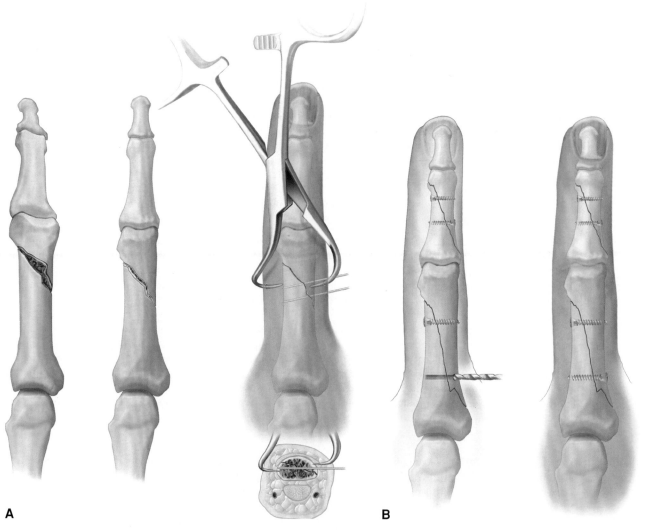

A   **B**

Figure 51. ORIF with (A) K-wires and (B) Screws

ORIF Thumb Fractures

Indications and Goals: The most common fracture pattern of the thumb metacarpal is the extraarticular epibasal (metaphyseal–diaphyseal junction) fracture. Because of the compensatory movement of the adjacent joints, the thumb is more forgiving of residual deformity than the fingers. Malrotation is rarely a problem. Angulation of 20 to 30 degrees is acceptable without functional deficit. Excessive angulation, however, may lead to MP joint hyperextension and requires fixation. A Bennett's fracture describes a fracture dislocation of the base of the thumb metacarpal. The abductor pollicis longus (APL) causes proximal, dorsal and radial displacement of the metacarpal base fragment. The adductor pollicis causes supination and adduction of the metacarpal shaft. The anterior oblique ligament keeps the volar ulnar base fragment reduced. CRPP or ORIF is chosen based on the size of the fracture fragments. A Rolando's fracture is a comminuted intraarticular fracture which may be in the shape of a "Y" or a "T." The degree of comminution guides treatment, as CRPP, ORIF and external fixation are all viable options.

Metacarpal shaft fractures are uncommon because of the lack of firm fixation of the proximal portion of the bone and because stress applied to the thumb is usually well tolerated by the strong cortical shaft and is dissipated by the soft cancellous bone at its base. Fractures of the distal and proximal phalanges are approached in a similar fashion to the analogous fractures in the digits.

Procedure and Technique: Bennett fractures with involvement of less than 15% to 20% of the articular surface can be treated with closed reduction and percutaneous pinning of the CMC joint. The thumb metacarpal is extended and pronated while the reduction is held, and a K-wire is drilled obliquely across the trapeziometacarpal joint under fluoroscopic guidance. For Bennett fractures involving greater than 25% to 30% of the articular surface, ORIF is preferred. The joint is approached with an incision starting distally between the abductor pollicis longus and the thenar muscles and extending proximally and radially to the radial border of the flexor carpi radialis. The thenar muscles are reflected subperiosteally, the joint capsule is incised, and the fracture is visualized. The Bennett fragment is held reduced and secured with a lag screw or K-wires. With K-wire fixation, it is advisable to protect the reduction with a transarticular pin.

For Rolando fractures, fixation can be performed with multiple K-wires, tension band wiring, or plate fixation. Articular reduction is most likely to be successful when there are two fragments with minimal comminution. The surgical exposure is the same as for a Bennett fracture. Plate fixation can be applied with a 2.4 to 2.7 mm "L" or "T" plate. Comminuted fractures can be difficult and frustrating to instrument adequately, and may be better treated with external fixation. A variety of methods of external fixation have been described, including a quadrilateral mini external fixation device placed between the thumb and index metacarpal, a triangular frame with pins in the distal end of the radius, thumb, and index metacarpal, or a uniplanar frame consisting of one pin in the trapezium and two pins in the thumb metacarpal. Cancellous bone grafting can be used to fill voids and K-wires or screws can be used to fix larger fragments.

If open reduction of a fracture of the proximal phalanx is required, the fracture is exposed through a dorsal "Y"-shaped incision. The distal portion of the incision is made in a curved fashion to avoid the proximal portion of the nailbed, while crossing the interphalangeal joint transversely. A longitudinal limb is then created along the dorsal P1 shaft. The extensor pollicis longus insertion left intact while exposing and reducing the fracture. Fixation is carried out with interfragmentary lag screws or a mini fragment plate.

Post-surgical Precautions/Rehabilitation: For Bennett fractures, if screw fixation is used, a short period of immobilization in a thumb spica splint is followed by active range of motion in 5 to 10 days. If pins are used, the thumb is immobilized in a thumb spica cast for 4 weeks and the transarticular pin is removed. The pins holding the fracture fragment are removed at 6 weeks. For Rolando fractures with minimal comminution and stable internal fixation, early range of motion can be initiated after a short period of thumb spica splint immobilization. Comminuted fractures require an extended period of external fixation (6 to 8 weeks) followed by a gradual increase in motion. Similarly, protocols after fixation of phalangeal fractures are based on the stability achieved intraoperatively.

Expected Outcomes: Outcomes are generally good following an open reduction and internal fixation for a thumb fracture. Return to activity and participation are dependent upon one's goals, and oftentimes quicker returns can be achieved with protective devices. Complications include wound infection, non-unions, and malunions. Malunion of Bennett and Rolando fractures may result in recurrent or persistent subluxation of the trapeziometacarpal joint. A contracture of the first web can result if the thumb metacarpal has been immobilized in an adducted position.

Return to Play: After complete healing and restoration of motion and grip strength—usually 2 to 3 months. Protected return to play may be possible sooner in some athletes. However, in some sports that require gripping with use of the thumb, such as a ski pole, hockey stick, or other device, care should be taken not to place added stress on the area too soon.

Recommended Readings

Al-Qattan MM, Cardoso E, Hassanain J, Hawary MB, Nandagopal N, Pitkanen J. Nonunion following subcapital (neck) fractures of the proximal phalanx of the thumb in children. *J Hand Surg [Br]*. 1999;24(6):693–698.

Brüske J, Bednarski M, Niedźiedź Z, Zyluk A, Grzeszewski S. The results of operative treatment of fractures of the thumb metacarpal base. *Acta Orthop Belg*. 2001;67(4):368–373.

Edmunds JO. Traumatic dislocations and instability of the trapeziometacarpal joint of the thumb. *Hand Clin*. 2006;22(3):365–392. Review.

McGuigan FX, Culp RW. Surgical treatment of intra-articular fractures of the trapezium. *J Hand Surg [Am]*. 2002;27(4):697–703.

Soyer AD. Fractures of the base of the first metacarpal: Current treatment options. *J Am Acad Orthop Surg*. 1999;7(6):403–412. Review.

Stern PJ. Fractures of the metacarpals and phalanges. In: Green DP, et al., eds. *Green's Operative Hand Surgery*. 5th ed. Philadelphia, PA: Elsevier; 2005:277–342.

Tan V, Beredjiklian PK, Weiland AJ. Intra-articular fractures of the hand: Treatment by open reduction and internal fixation. *J Orthop Trauma*. 2005;19(8):518–523.

Wiesler ER, Chloros GD, Kuzma GR. Arthroscopy in the treatment of fracture of the trapezium. *Arthroscopy*. 2007;23(11):1248.e1–e4. Epub 2007 Jan 5.

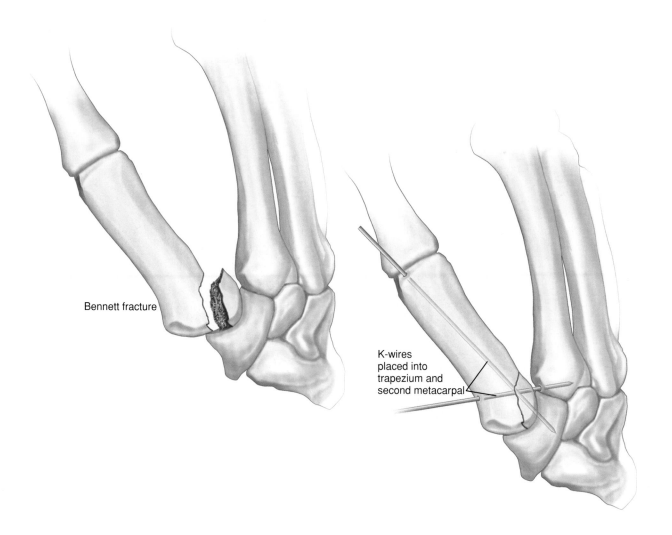

Bennett fracture

K-wires placed into trapezium and second metacarpal

Figure 52. ORIF of Thumb Fracture

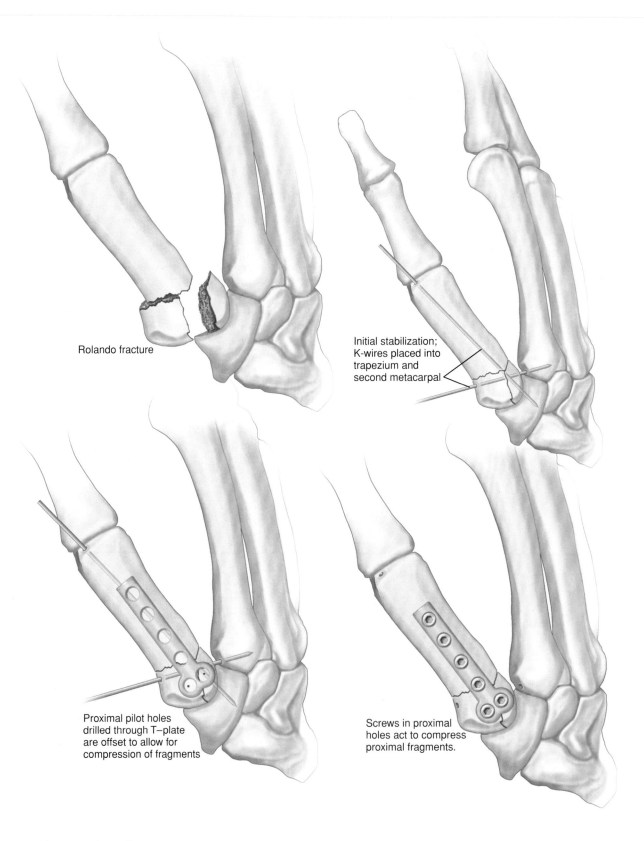

Rolando fracture

Initial stabilization;
K-wires placed into
trapezium and
second metacarpal

Proximal pilot holes
drilled through T–plate
are offset to allow for
compression of fragments

Screws in proximal
holes act to compress
proximal fragments.

Figure 52. (*continued*)

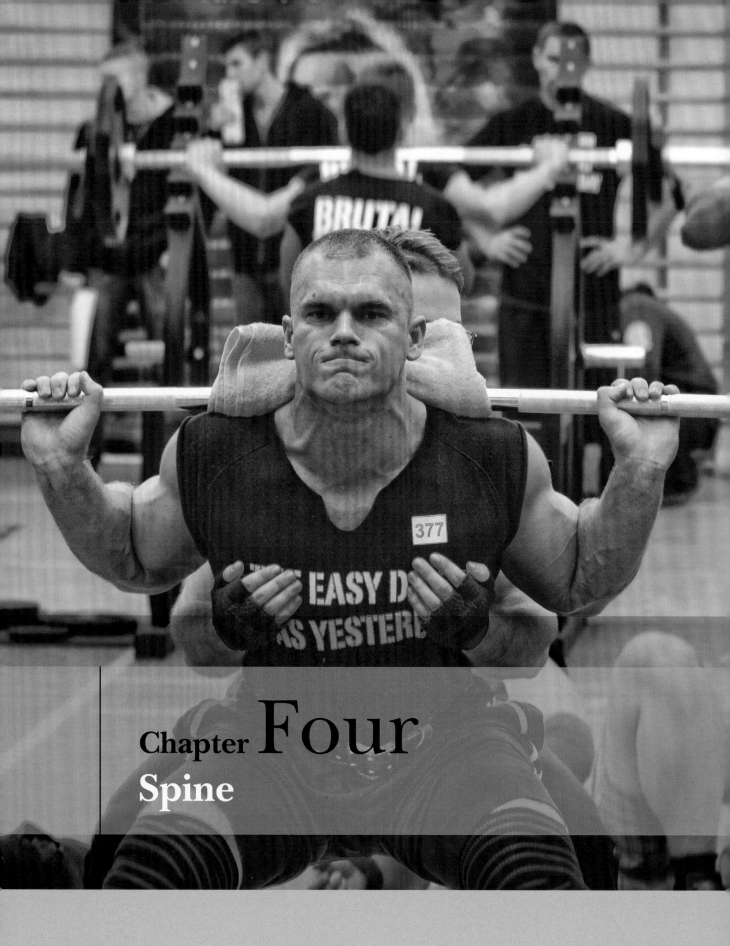

Chapter Four
Spine

Anterior Cervical Decompression/Discectomy

Indication and Goals: Anterior cervical decompression and/or discectomy is indicated in patients with symptomatic herniated and/or extruded vertebral discs (the soft cushion between the bony vertebral bodies) or cervical spondylosis (degeneration and stenosis [narrowing] of the neural foramen [windows where the nerve roots exit]) or stenosis of the spinal cord itself. Patients may have radiculopathy (nerve root dysfunction), myelopathy (spinal cord dysfunction), or long-tract signs (clumsiness, unsteadiness, bowel/bladder problems). Surgery may be indicated in patients with examination and imaging abnormalities, who have failed non-operative measures (therapy, traction, epidural injections, etc.). For symptomatic herniated discs, patients will often have radicular symptoms (pain, numbness, tingling that goes down the arm; weakness; loss of reflexes; etc.) that correspond to the level of the exiting root (the more distal level—i.e., a C5,6 herniated disc would affect the C6 nerve root on the side of the pathology). The goal of the procedure is to eliminate all symptoms and allow the athlete to return to his or her sport. This procedure is often combined with a fusion of the vertebral bodies above and below the affected disc (see Cervical Fusion). An anterior cervical approach is used for this procedure. This procedure is preferred over posterior cervical procedures in patients who have kyphosis (forward bending of the spine).

Procedure and Technique: A horizontal or oblique incision is made on the affected side of the neck based on the planned level. Landmarks are helpful in determining the location of this incision (Fig. 51A,B):

Bone/Cartilage	Level
Hyoid	C3/C4
Thyroid	C4/5
Cricoid	C7

The appropriate level is identified (usually with an intra-operative radiograph) and if needed, the two vertebral bodies can be distracted by placing temporary metal pins into the vertebral bodies or a lamina spreader between the vertebral bodies. This helps to improve access to the intervertebral discs (Fig. 51C–F). The affected disc is then removed (Fig. 51G,H) and the two vertebral levels are fused with the bone graft (Fig. 51I,J). The addition of spinal instrumentation may also be required and can help facilitate the rate of fusion and earlier return to function.

Post-surgical Precautions/Rehabilitation: Physical therapy may or may not be prescribed and will be based upon each individual patient. Hospital stay may be overnight, with early ambulation immediately following surgery. Some patients may be placed in a neck collar for comfort. Often times patients will experience some slight discomfort or pressure in the throat with swallowing and talking (dysphagia) that may last for a few weeks. Physical therapy consists of general range of motion and muscle strengthening around the shoulder and upper limb, interventions for pain reduction, localized inflammation, and education related to a safe return to work and/or activities of daily living. Patients may typically return to driving once off pain medicines and when they have regained neck motion. Restrictions on light lifting may vary, but typically may begin at 4 to 6 weeks. More aggressive lifting and sporting activity may resume at 3 to 6 months. During the course of formal rehabilitation, postural exercises can be implemented, as well as the addition of cardiovascular conditioning.

Expected Outcomes: A modification of job tasks may be suggested prior to a return to work based upon one's ability to recover from surgery and present with a good prognosis for limited recurrence of symptoms.

Return to Play: Return to play is typically based on the number of levels fused (see Cervical Fusion). Athletes with one-level fusions may return to play after complete healing—typically this is a season-ending surgery. Flexion–extension films should be taken to ensure spinal stability. Multiple-level fusions typically preclude participation.

Recommended Readings

Erickson M, Fites BS, Thieken MT, McGee AW. Outpatient anterior cervical discectomy and fusion. *Am J Orthop.* 2007;36(8):429–432.

Fountas KN, Kapsalaki EZ, Nikolakakos LG, Smisson HF, Johnston KW, Grigorian AA, Lee GP, Robinson JS Jr. Anterior cervical discectomy and fusion associated complications. *Spine (Phila Pa 1976).* 2007(1);32(21):2310–2317. Review.

Mobbs RJ, Rao P, Chandran NK. Anterior cervical discectomy and fusion: Analysis of surgical outcome with and without plating. *J Clin Neurosci.* 2007;14(7):639–642.

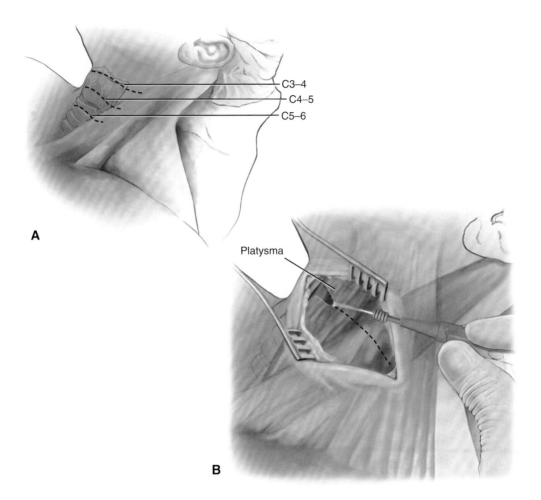

Figure 53. Anterior Approach to Cervical Spine. A: Superficial cervical spine landmarks correlate with cervical disc spaces. Hyoid bone (C3–4), thyroid cartilage (C4–5), carotid tubercle (C6) and cricoid cartilage (C7). **B:** Anterior cervical approach skin incision is most often left sided continuing through the platysma. (*continued*)

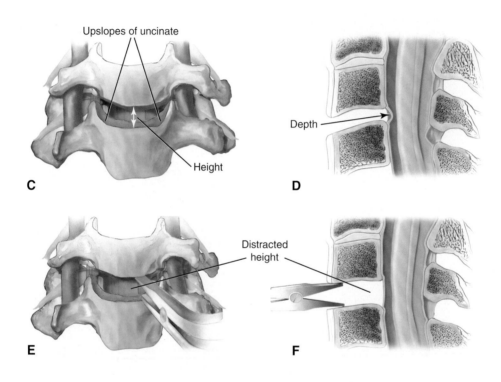

Figure 53. (*continued*) **C:** Uncinate upslope is defined during discectomy. **D:** Disc is removed to the level of the posterior longitudinal ligament (PLL). **E, F:** Distraction of the disc space can be performed to improve visualization, restore neuroforaminal height, and relieve buckling of the PLL.

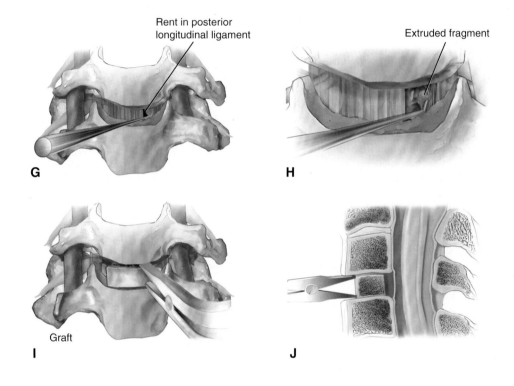

Figure 53. (*continued*) **G, H:** In cases of extruded disc herniations, a rent in the PLL can be identified and fragments removed. **I, J:** The graft is then sized and inserted with or without instrumentation.

Posterior Cervical Decompression/Discectomy

Indications and Goals: Indications for posterior cervical decompression/discectomy are similar to those for anterior cervical decompression and discectomy. A posterior approach is usually favored for cervical discs that are located more laterally without substantial bony involvement. The procedure is also more commonly utilized for patients with normal or lordotic (backward bending) cervical spine alignment. In patients with a more centrally located herniation, or if the narrowing is secondary to anteriorly located bony spurs, then an anterior cervical decompression/discectomy may be better.

Procedure and Technique: A posterior midline approach is used centered on the affected level(s) (Fig. 52A,B). Radiographic conformation of the planned level is usually done intra-operatively. The paraspinal muscles are stripped off the posterior elements of the vertebrae and the lateral aspects of the lamina and foramen are widened with various punches and gouges (laminoforaminotomy) (Fig. 52C,D). This allows inspection and decompression of the affected exiting nerve roots. Alternatively, if there is multilevel compression and/or central compression posteriorly, then removal of the entire bony arch may be necessary (laminectomy). In patients who undergo a laminoforaminotomy, if 50% of the facet (joint between two vertebrae) is preserved, then no fusion is required. In patients who undergo a laminectomy, the resulting instability typically requires fusion of the affected level(s). This is performed by adding bone graft and sometimes instrumentation (screws and rods) to stabilize the vertebral segment(s) (see Cervical Fusion).

Post-surgical Precautions/Rehabilitation: Physical therapy may or may not be prescribed and will be based upon each individual patient. The length of hospital stay may be a few days depending on the procedure; however, early ambulation immediately following surgery is still recommended. The patient will likely have a neck brace for comfort post-operatively. Formal rehabilitation may be necessary depending on the number of levels addressed and include patient education. Range of motion will be limited early on to allow for the bone graft and implants to undergo healing. Gradual and supervised range of motion may typically begin between weeks 4 and 6, but communication with the surgeon should confirm since some patients may be allowed to be mobilized earlier while others may require additional stabilization and healing time.

Expected Outcomes: Functional activities such as driving may take up to 6 weeks, and a return to work may take a few weeks to a few months based upon the physical requirements of the job or activity.

Return to Play: If no fusion is required, athletes may return to competition as soon as the soft tissue has healed, 6 to 8 weeks typically. Return to play varies on the number of levels involved in patients who require a fusion (see Cervical Fusion).

Recommended Readings

Dvorak MF, Fisher CG, Fehlings MG, Rampersaud YR, Oner FC, Aarabi B, Vaccaro AR. The surgical approach to subaxial cervical spine injuries: An evidence-based algorithm based on the SLIC classification system. *Spine (Phila Pa 1976).* 2007;32(23):2620–2629.
Liu P, Zhao J, Liu F, Liu M, Fan W. A novel operative approach for the treatment of old distractive flexion injuries of subaxial cervical spine. *Spine (Phila Pa 1976).* 2008;33(13):1459–1464.

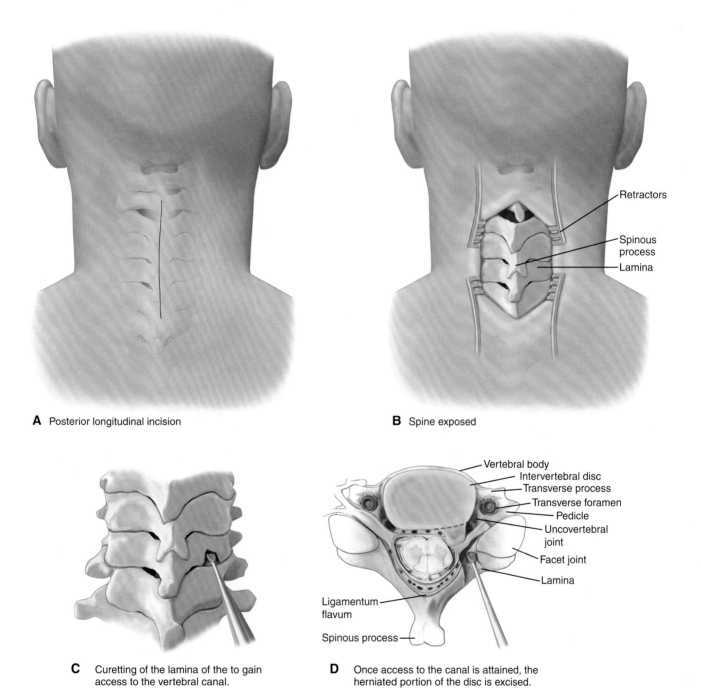

A Posterior longitudinal incision

B Spine exposed

C Curetting of the lamina of the to gain access to the vertebral canal.

D Once access to the canal is attained, the herniated portion of the disc is excised.

Figure 54. Posterior Cervical Spine Approach. A: Posterior longitudinal incision is made over the spinous processes. **B:** The posterior spine is exposed. **C:** Keyhole laminoforaminotomy is performed at the junction of the lamina and facet joint. **D:** Lateral disc herniations can be accessed posteriorly by carefully retracting the cervical nerve root. However, the spinal cord itself should not be manipulated.

Cervical Fusion

Indications and Goals: Cervical fusion is indicated for the management of spinal deformity, infection, tumor reconstruction, and stabilization of unstable vertebral segments resulting from trauma, various destructive processes (tumors, arthritides, etc.) and surgically induced instability. The goal is to achieve a solid arthrodesis between two affected vertebral bodies/segment(s) at the expense of some loss of motion. A secondary goal is to maintain spinal mobility by attempting to limit the number of levels fused whenever possible. Cervical fusion can be performed from either an anterior, posterior, or combined anterior and posterior approaches, depending on a variety of factors.

Procedure and Technique: Anterior and/or posterior approaches are made as described previously. For anterior cervical fusions, once the discectomy and/or corpectomy with the associated disc(s) have been removed, a cervical fusion is performed by placing the bone graft within the space created. During the discectomy(ies), the cartilaginous endplates of the corresponding superior and inferior discs are removed as well (Fig. 53A). The subchondral bone is preserved if possible to allow for a bony endplate for the cervical fusion and to reduce the risk of graft subsidence (Fig. 53B). This is typically performed with either structural autologous tricortical iliac crest graft (Smith-Robinson technique) or with allograft (Fig. 53C). For multilevel corpectomies, a fibular strut allograft is typically used. In unusual cases of extremely long constructs, patient request and/or surgeon preference, a structural cage filled with autograft bone can be used instead. The use of an anterior cervical plate is individualized (Fig. 53D) on the basis of the patient and pathology addressed, but is more common in the case after multilevel decompressions; however, its use even in single-level fusions can help patients return to activity more quickly and reduce or eliminate the need for post-operative external immobilization.

For posterior fusions, the posterior elements, in particular the facet joints and intervening spinous process and lamina, are decorticated and the graft is laid onto the opposing surfaces. Segmental fixation with instrumentation either in the lateral masses or spinous processes and less commonly in the lamina or pedicle may be added in selected cases (Fig. 54).

Post-surgical Precautions/Rehabilitation: A fusion can take a few months to demonstrate early healing, and a few years for complete fusion to take place. Post-operative care of the cervical spine procedure is individualized to both the patient and the procedure performed. Patients may have to wear a halo-type vest or a rigid external neck brace for 2 to 3 months based upon surgeon preference and the stability of the fusion. However, the use of internal fixation may eliminate or reduce the need for additional external immobilization. Hospitalization could last up to a week, during which time cervical bending and rotation are limited. Supervised rehabilitation should address reducing the pain and localized inflammation, and initiating gradual cervical mobility as tolerated for the first 6 to 8 weeks. Advancement to more resistive cervical movements will depend upon how the patient progresses and will require close communication between the therapist and physician.

Expected Outcomes: The goal during the post-operative period is to achieve a solid fusion, maintain alignment, and restore function. Although remodeling of a fusion and fracture can take up to 1 to 2 years, early fusion typically occurs around 12 to 16 weeks. However, this can be delayed in smokers, diabetics, and in patients on steroids or with other associated morbidities. Return to activity may be potentially quicker in cases where instrumentation is included with the fusion.

Return to Play: Athletes with one-level fusions may return to play after complete healing—typically, this is a season-ending surgery. Flexion–extension films should be taken to ensure spinal stability. Multiple-level fusion typically precludes participation.

Recommended Readings

Floyd T, Ohnmeiss D. A meta-analysis of autograft versus allograft in anterior cervical fusion. *Eur Spine J*. 2000;9(5):398–403.

Fraser JF, Härtl R. Anterior approaches to fusion of the cervical spine: A metaanalysis of fusion rates. *J Neurosurg Spine*. 2007;6(4):298–303.

Liu P, Zhao J, Liu F, Liu M, Fan W. A novel operative approach for the treatment of old distractive flexion injuries of subaxial cervical spine. *Spine (Phila Pa 1976)*. 2008;33(13):1459–1464.

van Limbeek J, Jacobs WC, Anderson PG, Pavlov PW. A systematic literature review to identify the best method for a single level anterior cervical interbody fusion. *Eur Spine J*. 2000;9(2):129–136. Review.

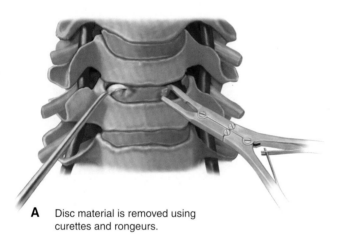

A   Disc material is removed using curettes and rongeurs.

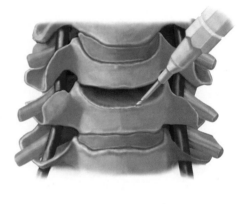

B   Endplates drilled away, creating anterior and posterior lips.

Figure 55. Anterior Cervical Decompression and Fusion (ACDF). A: Disc material removed anteriorly with curettes and rongeurs. **B:** Endplates are prepared for graft placement. (*continued*)

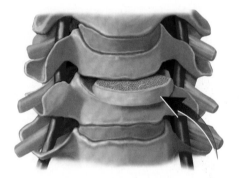

C Graft from the iliac crest is shaped and placed into the created disc space.

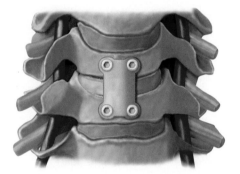

D A titanium plate is secured over the grafts with four screws.

Figure 55. (*continued*) **C:** Graft material is placed into the disc space. **D:** Anterior plate and screws are placed for stabilization.

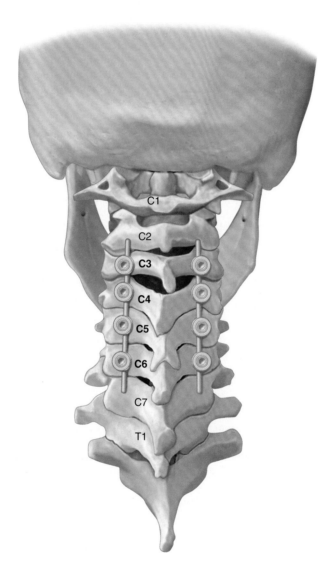

Figure 56. **Posterior Cervical Instrumented Fusion from C3 to C6**

Open Reduction and Internal Fixation (ORIF) of Cervical Fractures

Indications and Goals: ORIF is indicated in certain cervical fractures and dislocations that fail attempts at closed reduction or in patients in whom a closed reduction is contraindicated (disc herniation or bony fragments that may displace following a closed reduction maneuver or in cases that place the spinal cord at risk). The goal is to reduce, or restore to normal, the bones that are fractured (broken) and to stabilize them with some form of internal fixation (screws, plates, etc.). Fusion is sometimes necessary to further stabilize the fracture. Fractures and dislocations include a wide variety of injuries, and so it is difficult to generalize. Reduction can sometimes be done with indirect methods (traction will distract the fracture/dislocation and it can sometimes be reduced by the ligaments themselves [ligamentotaxis]). In other cases, open reduction may be necessary. Direct visualization, protection, and/or decompression of the neural elements (spinal cord and nerve roots) whenever possible is one of the primary goals of ORIF.

Procedure and Technique: Anterior, posterior, and combined approaches are based on location, pattern, and individual characteristics of the fracture dislocation, presence of associated neural element compression, associated injuries, and surgeon preference. Both anterior and posterior approaches were described previously.

Open reduction can be performed by either indirect methods (through traction above and below the site of injury with subsequent distraction and relocation of the fracture and/or dislocation, also known as ligamentotaxis) or by directly decompressing the neural elements by direct surgical removal of the offending lesion and reducing the fracture/dislocation (Fig. 55A,B).

Once spinal reduction, decompression, and realignment have been completed, stabilization can be performed with screws and/or plates, rods, and/or wires depending on the pathology being addressed (Fig. 55C,D). The use of external halo immobilization in addition, or instead of internal immobilization may be indicated or necessary in selected cases.

Post-surgical Protection and Rehabilitation: Management of cervical spine open reduction internal fixation vary depending on location, pathology, and surgical reconstruction performed. Rigid internal fixation may allow for the elimination of the use of halo immobilization; however, in extremely unstable fractures or when internal immobilization is not possible then the use of a halo vest for 2 to 3 months followed by a rigid cervical collar for another 1 to 2 months may be necessary.

Expected Outcomes: Solid fusion with elimination of the need for long-term external immobilization is expected. Return of neurologic function varies greatly on injury pattern, duration, and location. However, even in patients with complete spinal cord injuries (permanent loss of motor, sensory, and proprioception), the ability to achieve a solid fusion is critical for allowing early rehabilitation. Possible complications include subluxation (loss of anatomic alignment), wound infection, muscle weakness, dysphagia, and nasal phonation.

Return to Play: Often not possible or reasonable, depending on the sport and the injury. For lesser injuries, return should only be considered after complete healing and maintenance of stability is expected.

Recommended Readings

Scapinelli R, Balsano M. Traumatic enucleation of the body of the sixth cervical vertebra without neurologic sequelae: A case report. *Spine (Phila Pa 1976)*. 2002;27(13):E321–E324.

Shapiro SA. Management of unilateral locked facet of the cervical spine. *Neurosurg.* 1993;33(5):832–837; discussion 837. Review.

Wang C, Yan M, Zhou HT, Wang SL, Dang GT. Open reduction of irreducible atlantoaxial dislocation by transoral anterior atlantoaxial release and posterior internal fixation. *Spine (Phila Pa 1976)*. 2006;31(11):E306–E313.

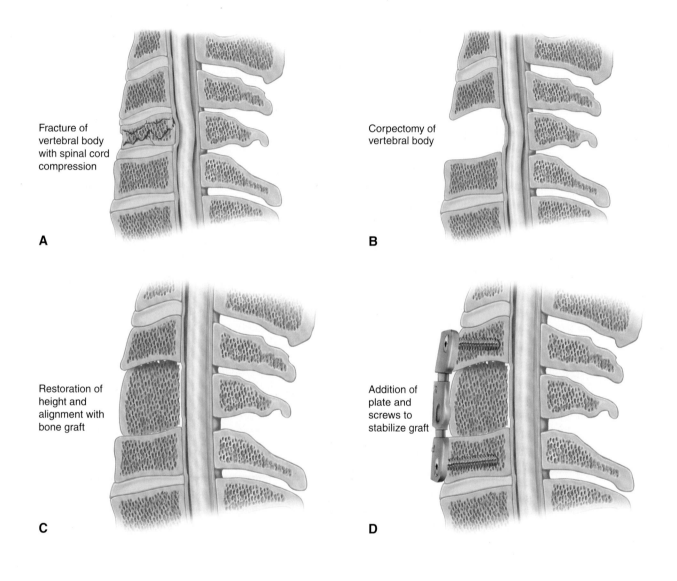

Fracture of
vertebral body
with spinal cord
compression

A

Corpectomy of
vertebral body

B

Restoration of
height and
alignment with
bone graft

C

Addition of
plate and
screws to
stabilize graft

D

Figure 57. Anterior Cervical Corpectomy and Instrumented Fusion. A: Cervical spine fracture
is identified with spinal cord compression. **B:** Following anterior approach a cervical corpectomy is performed. **C:** Graft size is measured and bone graft inserted into
defect. **D:** Anterior plate and screws placed for stabilization.

Thoracolumbar Decompression

Indications and Goals: Surgical decompression of the thoracolumbar spine with/without stabilization is indicated for patients with symptomatic spondylosis (spinal degeneration) and stenosis of either the central spinal canal and/or neuroforamen. Presenting symptoms depend on the neural elements under compression. In the thoracic spine, patients may present with either myelopathy (spinal cord compression) and/or radiculopathy (nerve root compression). Signs and symptoms consistent with myelopathy include clumsiness, ataxia, bowel and bladder, and other long tract signs, while patients with radiculopathy (nerve root compression) may present with localized pain/numbness or weakness along a specific nerve root distribution. Because the spinal cord typically ends at the thoracolumbar junction (T12 to L1), patients with symptomatic lumbar stenosis will present with symptoms consistent with radiculopathy. In rare cases, with either severe stenosis or a large disc herniation, the patient may present with a cauda equina (bowel and bladder dysfunction, saddle numbness, loss of rectal tone and function). In these unusual cases, urgent/emergent medical evaluation by a spinal specialist is indicated.

The goal of any surgical procedure for symptomatic stenosis is to decompress the affected neural structures to halt progression and attempt to reduce or eliminate symptoms. The surgical approach selected is based on the symptoms present, location of the pathology, and existing co-morbidities. In the thoracic spine, typically the compressive lesion is the result of a herniated disc. Because removal of the disc from a direct posterior approach would require manipulation of the spinal cord, it is typically not recommended. In these instances, an anterior approach through a transthoracic approach is more common. In selected cases, particularly for far-lateral disc herniations, consideration for a far-lateral/extracavitary approach may be an option; however, it is typically utilized only by the experienced surgeon. In cases of multilevel stenosis occurring from posterior compression, a posterior thoracic laminectomy usually with fusion and instrumentation is also an option.

In the lumbar spine, careful manipulation of the nerve roots for access to the herniated disc is possible and therefore lumbar herniated discs are most commonly addressed from a posterior approach.

Procedure and Technique: For anterior transthoracic approaches to the thoracic spine, the patient is placed in a lateral decubitus position and standard thoracotomy incision centered on the rib of the superior affected vertebra (Fig. 56). Careful correlation with preoperative imaging is imperative to ensure that herniated or sequestered disc fragments are retrieved from the spinal canal. Varying degree of rib is resected to achieve sufficient access and visibility. The lung is protected and the pleura entered. The rib is followed back to the thoracic spine and an intraoperative radiograph is obtained to confirm the level (Fig. 57). A discectomy is then performed by making an annulotomy in the affected disc and the fragments removed. Depending on the degree of decompression, typically a fusion using the resected rib with or without instrumentation is included. Depending on the degree of resection and the pathology involved, supplemental posterior fusion with or without instrumentation may be necessary.

For posterior approaches to the thoracolumbar spine, a standard midline incision is made and the paraspinal muscles are stripped off of the posterior elements of the vertebrate to be addressed (Fig. 58A,B). An intraoperative radiograph is obtained to verify the appropriate level (Fig. 58C). In the thoracic spine, a laminectomy is performed by removing the posterior elements and is typically combined with an instrumented fusion to reduce the risk of iatrogenic instability with subsequent deformity (see Thoracic Fusion). As discussed previously, manipulation of the spinal cord is not advised in the thoracic spine; therefore, if substantial spinal cord compression remains from anterior spinal compression (herniated disc, anterior osteophytes, etc.) then a separate anterior approach should be included. Far-lateral/extracavitary approaches to thoracic discs is an option; however, it should be performed by experienced spine surgeons and is beyond the scope of this discussion.

In the lumbar spine, bony landmarks can be established through manual palpation to help localize the skin incision (Fig. 59). A standard posterior approach is performed with a midline incision and subperiosteal dissection of the paraspinous muscles and exposure of the vertebra of interest (Fig. 60A). A laminotomy (partial removal of the lamina to make a "window" into the spinal canal) or a laminectomy (complete removal of the lamina) can be used to decompress the offending lesions (Fig. 60B). If necessary, the nerve roots can be gently retracted to allow for access to the intervertebral disc space. If 50% of the facet joint is preserved during the completion of the decompression, then a fusion can be avoided (Fig. 60C). However, if the pars is resected, or greater than 50% of bilateral facet joints, or 100% of one of the facet joints is resected, then a fusion with or without instrumentation should be strongly considered.

The use of the microscope and/or specialized retractors has helped to develop the concept of minimally invasive spine surgery (MISS). These techniques continue to evolve, however are gaining more use, especially in the lumbar spine. In selected cases, these techniques can help reduce the degree of soft tissue dissection and reduce the length of post-operative recovery and facilitate earlier return to activities. However, it should be emphasized that the goals of decompressing neural elements, preserving bony and ligamentous structures, and preserving mobility whenever possible still remains the primary goal of spinal surgery and should not be compromised by the use of the microscope and specialized retractors.

Post-surgical Precautions/Rehabilitation: Rehabilitation following a thoracolumbar decompression has become much more progressive than in years past. Early ambulation as tolerated and with assistive devices as needed are encouraged, though a spinal support is not necessary. Appropriate posture is emphasized, and long car rides, bending and twisting activities, and being seated for an extended period of time are discouraged for the first month post-operative. During the next 2 months, supervised flexibility and strengthening exercises are implemented using pain tolerance as a guide for progression.

Expected Outcomes: Relatively newer techniques for surgical stabilization of the fracture and decompression of the neural elements allow for a quicker recovery time due to immediate stability of the spine that reduces the need for prolonged post-operative bedrest. This in turn allows for earlier general mobilization and re-conditioning.

Return to Play: Much more likely for single-level microdiscectomy (90%). Sufficient pain relief and range of motion without increased risk of injury—typically 6 to 8 weeks for noncontact sports and at least 3 months for contact sports.

Recommended Readings

Cengiz SL, Kalkan E, Bayir A, Ilik K, Basefer A. Timing of thoracolomber spine stabilization in trauma patients; impact on neurological outcome and clinical course. A real prospective (rct) randomized controlled study. *Arch Orthop Trauma Surg.* 2008;128(9):959–966.

Chow GH, Nelson BJ, Gebhard JS, Brugman JL, Brown CW, Donaldson DH. Functional outcome of thoracolumbar burst fractures managed with hyperextension casting or bracing and early mobilization. *Spine (Phila Pa 1976).* 1996;21(18):2170–2175.

Heary RF, Salas S, Bono CM, Kumar S. Complication avoidance: Thoracolumbar and lumbar burst fractures. *Neurosurg Clin N Am.* 2006;17(3):377–388, viii. Review.

Mikles MR, Stchur RP, Graziano GP. Posterior instrumentation for thoracolumbar fractures. *J Am Acad Orthop Surg.* 2004;12(6):424–435. Review.

Seybold EA, Sweeney CA, Fredrickson BE, Warhold LG, Bernini PM. Functional outcome of low lumbar burst fractures. A multicenter review of operative and nonoperative treatment of L3-L5. *Spine (Phila Pa 1976).* 1999;24(20):2154–2161.

Singh K, Heller JG, Samartzis D, Price JS, An HS, Yoon ST, Rhee J, Ledlie JT, Phillips FM. Open vertebral cement augmentation combined with lumbar decompression for the operative management of thoracolumbar stenosis secondary to osteoporotic burst fractures. *J Spinal Disord Tech.* 2005;18(5):413–419.

Yi L, Jingping B, Gele J, Baoleri X, Taixiang W. Operative versus non-operative treatment for thoracolumbar burst fractures without neurological deficit. *Cochrane Database Syst Rev.* 2006;18(4):CD005079. Review.

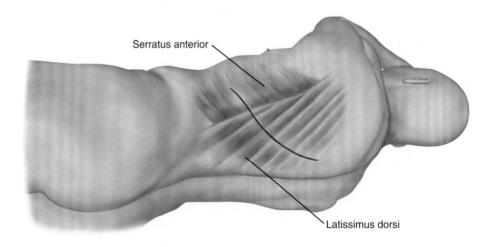

Serratus anterior

Latissimus dorsi

Figure 58. **Anterior approach to the thoracoabdominal spine is typically approached from the left lateral decubitus position; however, either side can be utilized depending on the pathology to be addressed**

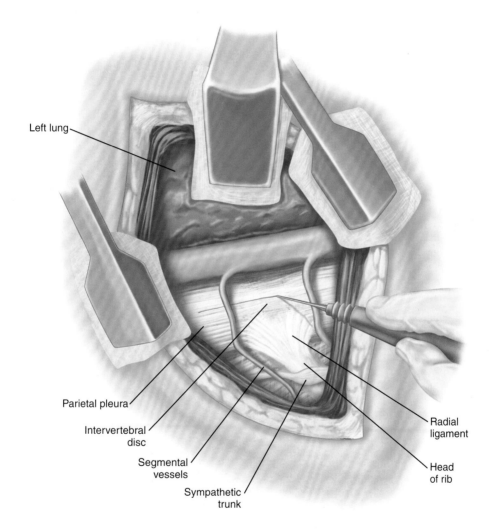

Left lung

Parietal pleura

Intervertebral
disc

Segmental
vessels

Sympathetic
trunk

Radial
ligament

Head
of rib

Figure 59. The chest is entered and the lung is retracted, exposing the lateral aspect of the thoracic spine. The intervertebral disc space lies between the segmental vessels.

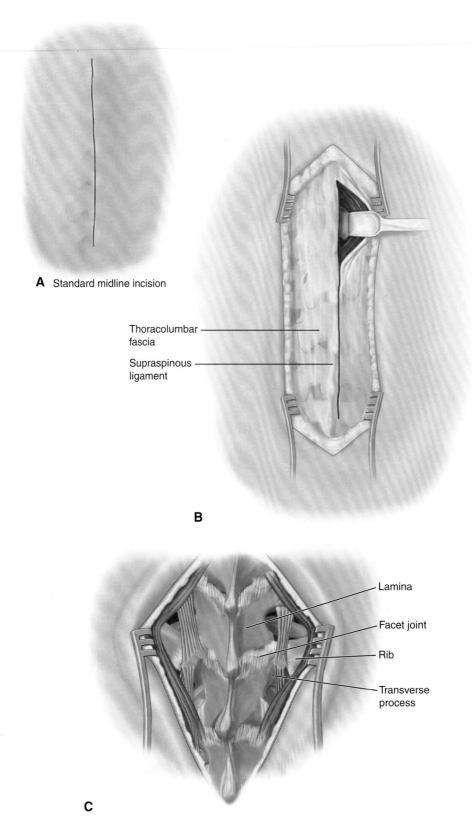

A Standard midline incision

Thoracolumbar fascia

Supraspinous ligament

B

Lamina

Facet joint

Rib

Transverse process

C

Figure 60. Posterior Midline Thoracic Approach. A: Midline incision is made overlying the spinous processes. **B:** Fascia is exposed, followed by subperiosteal elevation off the paraspinal musculature laterally. **C:** Landmarks are identified following exposure for decompression or fusion.

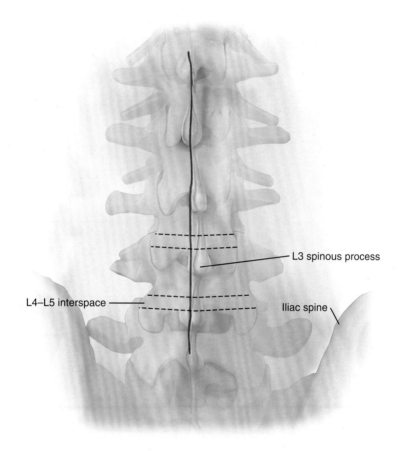

Figure 61. Posterior Midline Lumbar Spine Approach. Palpable landmarks for identification of underlying disc spaces. The L4–L5 interspace is associated with the iliac crest (intercrestal line)

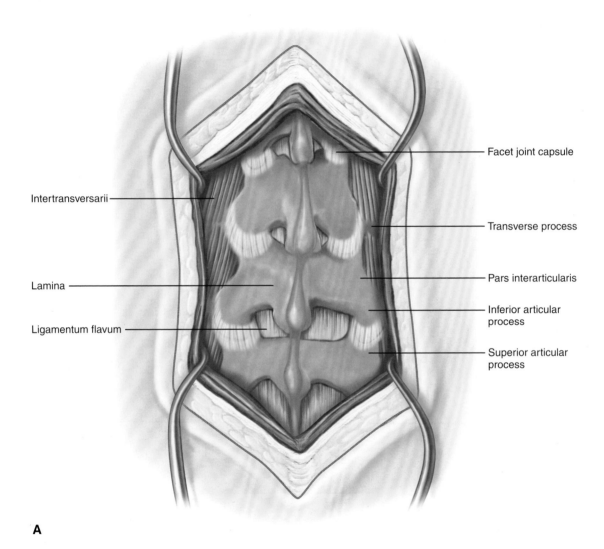

Intertransversarii

Lamina

Ligamentum flavum

Facet joint capsule

Transverse process

Pars interarticularis

Inferior articular process

Superior articular process

A

Figure 62. Pedicle Screw Insertion. A: Once exposed lumbar spine landmarks are identified for decompression or pedicle screw insertion. (*continued*)

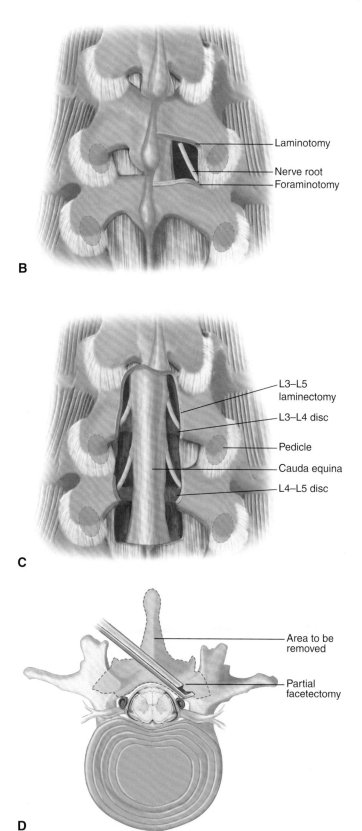

Figure 62. (*continued*) **B:** Lumbar hemilaminotomy or **C:** laminectomy. Note the relationship of the intervertebral disc to the pedicle. Note the relationship of the disc with the exiting and traversing nerve roots. Pedicle location is noted by dashed lines. **D:** Preservation of the facet joints will allow for avoidance of spinal fusion.

Thoracolumbar Fusion

Indications and Goals: Thoracolumbar fusion is the indication for the management of symptomatic spinal deformity, infection, tumor reconstruction, and stabilization of unstable vertebra segments resulting from trauma, various destructive processes (tumors, arthritides, etc.), and surgically induced instability. Frequently, the addition of instrumentation may increase fusion rates, while facilitating return to activity at a quicker rate. The goal is to achieve a solid arthrodesis between the affected vertebral bodies/segment(s) or prevent/reduce/halt progressive spinal deformity, while preserving neural function. A secondary goal is to maintain spinal mobility by attempting to limit the number of levels fused whenever possible.

Procedure and Technique: Anterior and posterior approaches are made as described previously.

For anterior approaches, once the discectomy and/or corpectomy with the associated disc(s) have been removed, a spinal fusion is performed by placing bone graft within the space created. During the discectomy(ies), the cartilaginous endplates of the corresponding superior and inferior discs are removed as well. The subchondral bone is preserved if possible to allow for a bony endplate for the fusion and to reduce the risk of graft subsidence. This may be performed with either auto or allograft. For multilevel corpectomies, a femoral strut allograft or a structural cage filled with autograft bone can be used instead. The use of an anterior spinal instrumentation is individualized on the basis of the patient and pathology addressed, but may be provided for a higher fusion rate, decreased risk of graft subsidence and dislodgement, and facilitate faster return to activity.

For posterior fusions, the posterior elements, in particular the facet joints and intervening spinous process and lamina are decorticated (if still present), and the graft is laid onto the opposing surfaces (Fig. 61A,B). Segmental fixation either the form of hooks or screws with longitudinal rods may be added in selected cases (Fig. 61C).

Post-surgical Precautions/Rehabilitation: Early ambulation as tolerated and with assistive devices as needed are encouraged. The need for external spinal support varies depending on the pathology and procedure performed. Appropriate posture is emphasized, and long car rides, bending and twisting activities, and being seated for an extended period of time are discouraged for the first month post-operative. During the next 2 months, supervised flexibility and strengthening exercises are implemented using pain tolerance as a guide for progression.

Expected Outcomes: The goal during the post-operative period is to achieve a solid fusion, maintain alignment, and restore function. Although remodeling of a fusion and fracture can take up to 1 to 2 years, early fusion typically occurs around 12 to 16 weeks. However, this can be delayed in smokers, diabetics, and in patients on steroids or with other associated morbidities. Return to activity may be potentially quicker in cases where instrumentation is included with the fusion.

Return to Play: Often is not possible, especially for multilevel fusions. If return is contemplated, complete fusion, restoration of strength and range of motion must be present and will take at least 6 months.

Recommended Readings

Acosta FL Jr, Buckley JM, Xu Z, Lotz JC, Ames CP. Biomechanical comparison of three fixation techniques for unstable thoracolumbar burst fractures. Laboratory investigation. *J Neurosurg Spine.* 2008;8(4):341–346.

Kuhns CA, Bridwell KH, Lenke LG, Amor C, Lehman RA, Buchowski JM, Edwards C 2nd, Christine B. Thoracolumbar deformity arthrodesis stopping at L5: Fate of the L5-S1 disc, minimum 5-year follow-up. *Spine (Phila Pa 1976).* 2007;32(24):2771–2776.

Tan GH, Goss BG, Thorpe PJ, Williams RP. CT-based classification of long spinal allograft fusion. *Eur Spine J.* 2007;16(11):1875–1881. Epub 2007 May 12.

Wang T, Zeng B, Xu J, Chen H, Zhang T, Zhou W, Kong W, Fu Y. Radiographic evaluation of selective anterior thoracolumbar or lumbar fusion for adolescent idiopathic scoliosis. *Eur Spine J.* 2008;17:1012–1018.

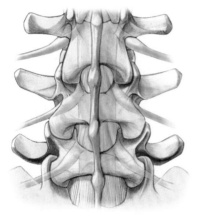 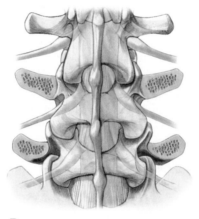 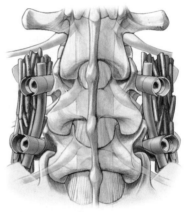

A Posterior approach to lumbar spine   **B** Decortication of tranverse processes   **C** Bone grafts with rods and screw to stabilize

Figure 63. Posterolateral Instrumented Fusion. A: Posterior approach is performed midline. **B:** Landmarks are identified and prepared for screw insertion. Transverse processes and lateral pars are decorticated. **C:** Pedicle screws and rods are inserted followed by bone graft placed for a posterolateral fusion.

Open Reduction and Internal Fixation of Thoracolumbar Fractures

Indications and Goals: Surgical indications for open reduction and internal fixation (ORIF) of the thoracolumbar spine is indicated in cases of fractures and dislocations that fail closed reduction, or a closed reduction is contraindicated (patient has associated disc herniation or bony fragment that may worsen with the reduction maneuver, or significant ligamentous injury where a closed reduction places the spinal cord at traction risk, etc.). It is also indicated in patients who undergo successful closed reduction, however have failed closed treatment, or are at risk for potentially having recurrent deformity with closed treatment. In addition to plain radiographs, the use of computerized tomography (CT) imaging and/or magnetic resonance imaging (MRI) can help assist in determining indications for surgery and surgical plan. The goal is to reduce the dislocation, decompress the neural elements, restore normal alignment, and to stabilize the fracture while minimizing the number of normal segments fused.

Procedure and Technique: Anterior, posterior, and combined approaches are based on the location, pattern, and individual characteristics of the fracture dislocation, presence of associated neural element compression, associated injuries, and surgeon preference. Both anterior and posterior approaches were well described previously.

The open reduction can be performed by either indirect methods (through traction above and below the site of injury with subsequent distraction and relocation of the fracture and/or dislocation, also known as ligamentotaxis) (Fig. 62A–D), or by directly decompressing the neural elements by direct surgical removal of the offending lesion and reducing the fracture/dislocation.

Once spinal reduction, decompression, and realignment have been completed, stabilization can be performed with screws and/or rods, and/or wires depending on the pathology being addressed. The use of external immobilization such as thoracolumbosacral orthosis (TLSO) in addition, or instead of internal immobilization may be indicated or necessary in selected cases.

Post-surgical Precautions/Rehabilitation: Early ambulation as tolerated and with assistive devices as needed are encouraged, though a spinal support may be necessary depending upon surgeon preference. Long car rides, bending and twisting activities, and being seated for an extended period of time are discouraged for the first few months post-operative.

Expected Outcomes: Reported complications include implant failures and wound infection. Prognosis and expected outcome is directly related to location, pathology, and surgical reconstruction performed. However, patients who are neurologically intact at the time of presentation are typically associated with a fairly high rate of preservation of neurologic function. However, in multilevel fusions, return to contact sports is not typically recommended.

Return to Play: Usually not possible unless there is a relatively minor fracture. In some cases, return can be contemplated after complete healing and restoration of motion—6 months minimum.

Recommended Readings

Benson DR, Burkus JK, Montesano PX, Sutherland TB, McLain RF. Unstable thoracolumbar and lumbar burst fractures treated with the AO fixateur interne. *J Spinal Disord.* 1992;5(3):335–343.

Nadeem M, Ghani E, Zaidi GI, Rehman L, Noman MA, Khaleeq-uz-Zaman. Role of fixateur interne in thoracolumbar junction injuries. *J Coll Physicians Surg Pak.* 2003;13(10):584–587.

Yosipovitch Z, Robin GC, Makin M. Open reduction of unstable thoracolumbar spinal injuries and fixation with Harrington rods. *J Bone Joint Surg Am.* 1977;59(8):1003–1015.

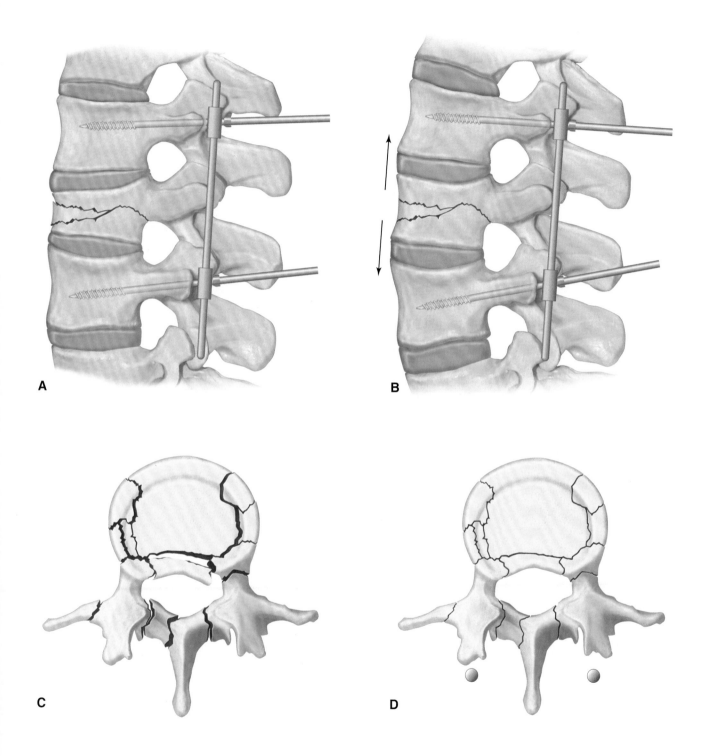

Figure 64. Open Reduction Internal Fixation of Burst Fracture. A: Lumbar Schanz pins and
longitudinal rods are inserted above and below the level of fracture. **B:** Sagittal
plane correction is restored through cantilever compression against the rod.
C: Comminuted vertebral body fracture with retropulsion of the middle column
into the canal. The presence of a lamina fracture may occasionally result in nerve
root entrapment with resulting neurologic deficit. **D:** Post-reduction demonstrates
indirect reduction of the retropulsed fragment through ligamentotaxis.

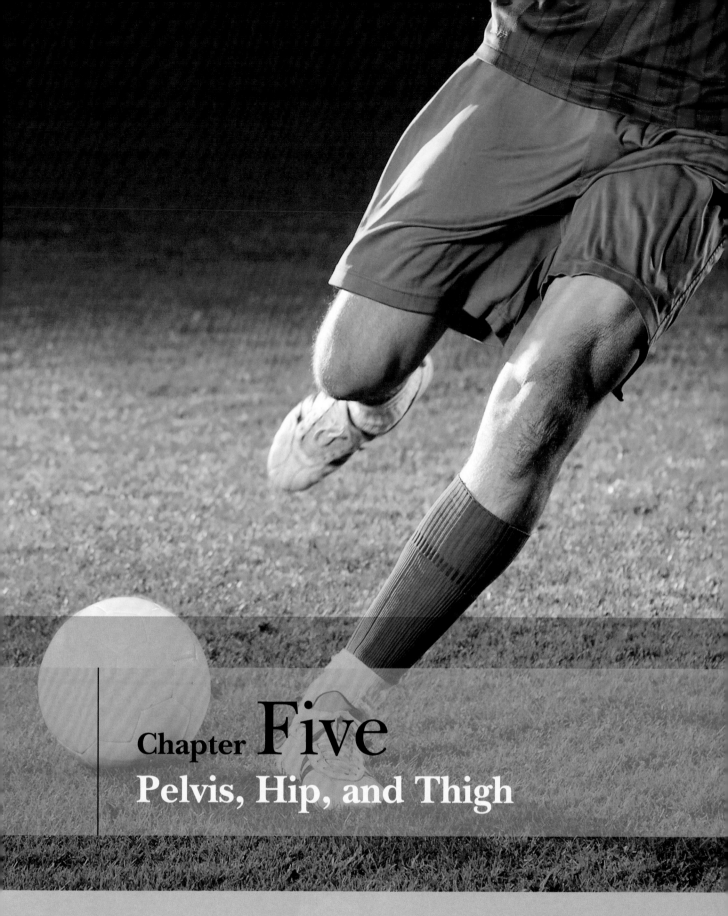

Chapter Five
Pelvis, Hip, and Thigh

Hip Arthroscopy

Indications and Goals: Hip arthroscopy can be useful for both diagnostic and therapeutic purposes. Indications have expanded as techniques improve. Common indications include labral tears, synovial diseases, chondral injuries, early osteonecrosis, hip infection, ligamentum teres injuries, and internal snapping hip. Contraindications include ankylosed hips, advanced arthritis, open wounds, and inability to undergo traction.

Procedure and Technique: Hip arthroscopy can be done in either the supine or lateral decubitus position. Traction is applied using a fracture table or with a commercially available traction device. Fluoroscopy is used to facilitate the procedure. Time is monitored as traction is applied. Traction force is included until the hip is distracted enough to allow the arthroscopic cannula and instruments to be inserted into the joint. Both 30- and 70-degree arthroscopes are used. After distention of the joint, a pertrochanteric portal (usually anterior trochanteric, i.e., 1 to 2 cm anterior and superior to the greater trochanter) is used to insert the arthroscope. An anterior portal is then established (at the intersection of a line from the anterior superior iliac spine extending inferiorly and from the greater trochanter extending medially) using a spinal or colposcopy needle for localization. Special instruments and shavers are used to carry out the indicated procedure.

Post-surgical Precautions/Rehabilitation: Post-operative rehabilitation following arthroscopic surgery of the hip joint should emphasize range-of-motion and strengthening exercises, with a close monitoring of weight-bearing activities. Since many varied procedures can be performed arthroscopically, tissue healing and the loads placed upon joint structures should be the main determinants of the rate of progression with rehabilitation. Additional considerations may include addressing associated swelling and pain, muscle atrophy and neuromuscular control, cardiovascular conditioning, and gait training.

Expected Outcomes: The goals associated with rehabilitation following a hip arthroscopy are to maintain the overall function of the hip joint, return the individual to pre-injurious activity levels, and minimize the development of premature arthrosis. Adverse affects associated with hip arthroscopy are few, occurring in <5% of patients.

Return to Play: This depends entirely on the procedure performed. For soft tissue involvement, a return to participation may be within 1 month, whereas for bony work (FAI, etc.), a return to sport participation may be delayed for up to 6 months.

Recommended Readings

Enseki KR, Martin RL, Draovitch P, Kelly BT, Philippon MJ, Schenker ML. The hip joint: Arthroscopic procedures and postoperative rehabilitation. *J Orthop Sports Phys Ther.* 2006;36(7):516–525. Review.

Khanduja V, Villar RN. Arthroscopic surgery of the hip: Current concepts and recent advances. *J Bone Joint Surg Br.* 2006;88(12):1557–1566. Review.

McCarthy JC, Lee JA. Hip arthroscopy: Indications, outcomes, and complications. *Instr Course Lect.* 2006;55:301–308. Review.

Philippon MJ. New frontiers in hip arthroscopy: The role of arthroscopic hip labral repair and capsulorrhaphy in the treatment of hip disorders. *Instr Course Lect.* 2006;55:309–316. Review.

Robertson WJ, Kadrmas WR, Kelly BT. Arthroscopic management of labral tears in the hip: A systematic review of the literature. *Clin Orthop Relat Res.* 2007;455:88–92. Review.

Shetty VD, Villar RN. Hip arthroscopy: Current concepts and review of literature. *Br J Sports Med.* 2007;41(2):64–68; discussion 68. Epub 2006 Nov 30. Review.

Shindle MK, Voos JE, Heyworth BE, Mintz DN, Moya LE, Buly RL, Kelly BT. Hip arthroscopy in the athletic patient: Current techniques and spectrum of disease. *J Bone Joint Surg Am.* 2007;89(suppl 3):29–43. Review.

Smart LR, Oetgen M, Noonan B, Medvecky M. Beginning hip arthroscopy: Indications, positioning, portals, basic techniques, and complications. *Arthroscopy.* 2007;23(12):1348–1353. Epub 2007 Oct 3. Review.

Stalzer S, Wahoff M, Scanlan M. Rehabilitation following hip arthroscopy. *Clin Sports Med.* 2006;25(2):337–357, x. Review.

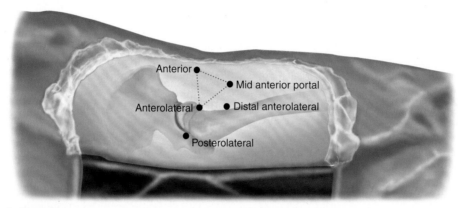

A. Portals

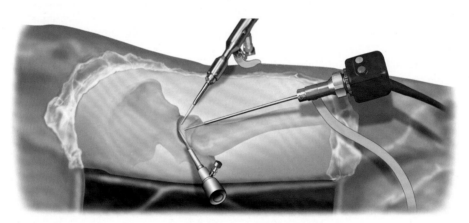

B. Placement

Figure 65. Standard Hip Arthroscopy Portals. Image **A:** The most common arthroscopic portal sites including the anterolateral viewing portal, the anterior portal, (just posterior to anterior line of ASIS), and mid-anterior portal. The distal anterolateral portal is effective for accessing the peritrochanteric compartment. Image **B:** Common set up, with the arthroscope in the anterolateral viewing portal and an instrument through the anterior portal. An accessory posterolateral portal in place.

Sports Hernia Repair

Indications and Goals: Sports hernia, also known as athlete's hernia, Gilmore's groin, and athletic pubalgia, refers to chronic inguinal or pubic area exertional pain in the absence of a true hernia. This may be a result of a hyperextension injury and can also affect the adductors. Affected athletes may have localized groin pain, adductor tightness or pain and pain with resisted sit-ups or crunches. Imaging is rarely helpful, but can be sued to rule out other diagnoses including osteitis pubis. Conservative treatment can include medication, physical therapy, and fluoroscopic guided injection.

Procedure and Technique: Pelvic floor repair involves reattaching the inferolateral edge of the rectus abdominis muscle to the pubis and adjacent anterior ligaments. The transversalis fascia can also be imbricated. Often, the adductors are also released about 2 to 3 cm from their pubic insertion.

Post-surgical Precautions/Rehabilitation: Post-operative rehabilitation depends solely upon the type of procedure performed and the preferences and guidelines of the surgeon. Acute ambulation can range from 1 day to 1 week, and a period of minimized activity can sometimes last for up to 6 weeks before allowing one to initiate lower leg and abdominal training exercises. Gradual flexibility and strengthening exercises can be incorporated based upon the tissue involvement, with care taken to avoid progressive abduction movements if the adductor muscle group is released during the procedure.

Expected Outcomes: Evidence-based concensus and reporting is not available to guide clear-cut decision making following a repair. Anecdotally, some have reported a 7- to 10-recovery period, while others encourage 6 to 8 weeks of minimal activity. The literature supports both open and laparoscopic repairs with respect to producing excellent results, but a quicker return to participation with the less-invasive technique as would be expected. The surgical procedures are relatively quick to perform, and both short- and long-term complications are rarely reported. Anecdotally, clinicians have reported athletes who have undergone a sports hernia repair on one side followed by the other side requiring a repair anywhere between 6 months to 2 years later. There is no evidence to support the rationale for such cases.

Return to Play: Return to play is usually delayed for 2 to 3 months. Earlier return may be possible for newer, more limited procedures. Care should be taken to return to sport participation too soon which may result in a delayed or absent successful repair.

Recommended Readings

Ahumada LA, Ashruf S, Espinosa-de-los-Monteros A, Long JN, de la Torre JI, Garth WP, Vasconez LO. Athletic pubalgia: Definition and surgical treatment. *Ann Plast Surg.* 2005;55(4):393–396.

Diesen DL, Pappas TN. Sports hernias. *Adv Surg.* 2007;41:177–187. Review.

Edelman DS, Selesnick H. "Sports" hernia: Treatment with biologic mesh (Surgisis): A preliminary study. *Surg Endosc.* 2006;20(6): 971–973. Epub 2006 Apr 19.

Swan KG Jr, Wolcott M. The athletic hernia: A systematic review. *Clin Orthop Relat Res.* 2007;455:78–87. Review.

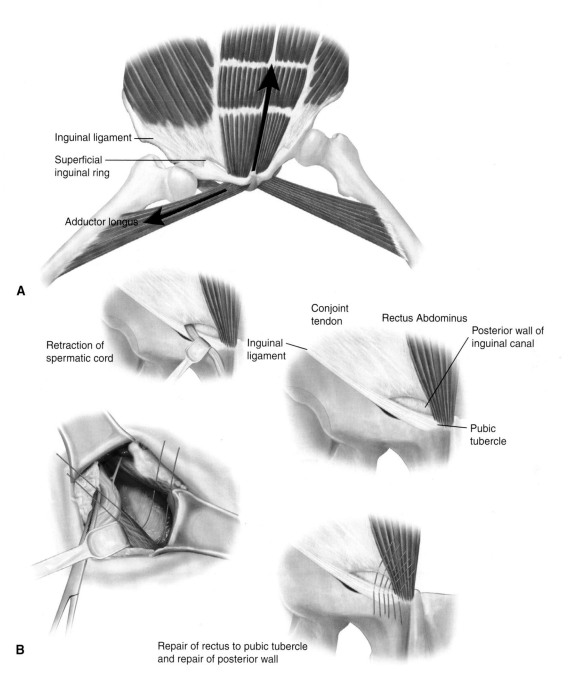

Figure 66. Sports Hernia. A: Opposing pulls of rectus abdominus and adductor longus through iliac insertion as a mechanism of injury. **B:** Direct suture repair of anterior abdominal wall. This technique involves the direct suture repair of the rectus abdominus insertion and posterior wall of the inguinal canal. Retraction of the spermatic cord and evaluation of the transversalis fascia of the posterior wall of the inguinal canal, (Figure B), as well as the insertion of the rectus abdominus to the pubic tubercle. When attenuated, these structures are repaired, utilizing only 5 to 6 nonabsorbable sutures to reapproximate the rectus tendon, conjoined tendon, and fascia back to a roughened bony bed upon the pubic tubercle insertion site and shelving portion of the ilioinguinal ligament.

Snapping Hip Release

Indications and Goals: Snapping hip, also known as coax saltans, can be caused by either the iliopsoas tendon snapping over the iliopectineal eminence (internal) or the iliotibial band and/or gluteus maximus tendon snapping over the greater trochanter (external). The snapping is often reproducible by the patient. Internal snapping can be reproduced by passively flexing and extending the hip, especially from an abducted/flexed position to an adducted/extended position. Application of pressure over the iliopsoas tendon can stop the snapping and confirm the diagnosis. Dynamic bursography or ultrasound may also be helpful. External snapping can be reproduced with hip flexion. A positive Ober's test (the patient lies on his side with the affected leg up and with the hip extended and abducted; the patient cannot adduct the hip from this position) may also be present.

Procedure and Technique: Surgery involves release of the affected tendon(s). For internal snapping, fractional release of the tendon is carried out. This can be accomplished through an open incision in the groin beginning 1 cm proximal to the lesser tuberosity or arthroscopically through an extra-articular approach. External snapping is addressed with either Z-lengthening or release of the iliotibial band/tract.

Post-surgical Precautions/Rehabilitation: Rehabilitation initially involves healing of the external wound closure, with gentle range of motion to prevent post-operative internal adhesions. A gradual progression from passive to active range of motion of the involved area will restore function within a few weeks, and return to participation is based upon the demands of the goals set forth. Care should be taken to begin passive and active hip extension, particularly with hip rotation involvement, as well as caution with active hip flexion activities.

Expected Outcomes: Results appear to be comparable between open and arthroscopic procedures, with good outcomes.

Return to Play: Since this is a soft tissue procedure, return to play can be relatively early, i.e., 4 to 6 weeks.

Recommended Readings

Byrd JW. Evaluation and management of the snapping iliopsoas tendon. *Instr Course Lect.* 2006;55:347–355. Review.

Flanum ME, Keene JS, Blankenbaker DG, Desmet AA. Arthroscopic treatment of the painful "internal" snapping hip: Results of a new endoscopic technique and imaging protocol. *Am J Sports Med.* 2007;35(5):770–779. Epub 2007 Mar 9.

Ilizaliturri VM Jr., Martinez-Escalante FA, Chaidez PA, Camacho-Galindo J. Endoscopic iliotibial band release for external snapping hip syndrome. *Arthroscopy.* 2006;22(5):505–510.

Ilizaliturri VM Jr., Villalobos FE Jr., Chaidez PA, Valero FS, Aguilera JM. Internal snapping hip syndrome: Treatment by endoscopic release of the iliopsoas tendon. *Arthroscopy.* 2005;21(11):1375–1380.

Voos JE, Rudzki JR, Shindle MK, Martin H, Kelly BT. Arthroscopic anatomy and surgical techniques for peritrochanteric space disorders in the hip. *Arthroscopy.* 2007;23(11):1246.e1–e5. Epub 2007 Apr 5.

Wettstein M, Jung J, Dienst M. Arthroscopic psoas tenotomy. *Arthroscopy.* 2006;22(8):907.e1–e4.

White RA, Hughes MS, Burd T, Hamann J, Allen WC. A new operative approach in the correction of external coxa saltans: The snapping hip. *Am J Sports Med.* 2004;32(6):1504–1508. Epub 2004 Jul 20.

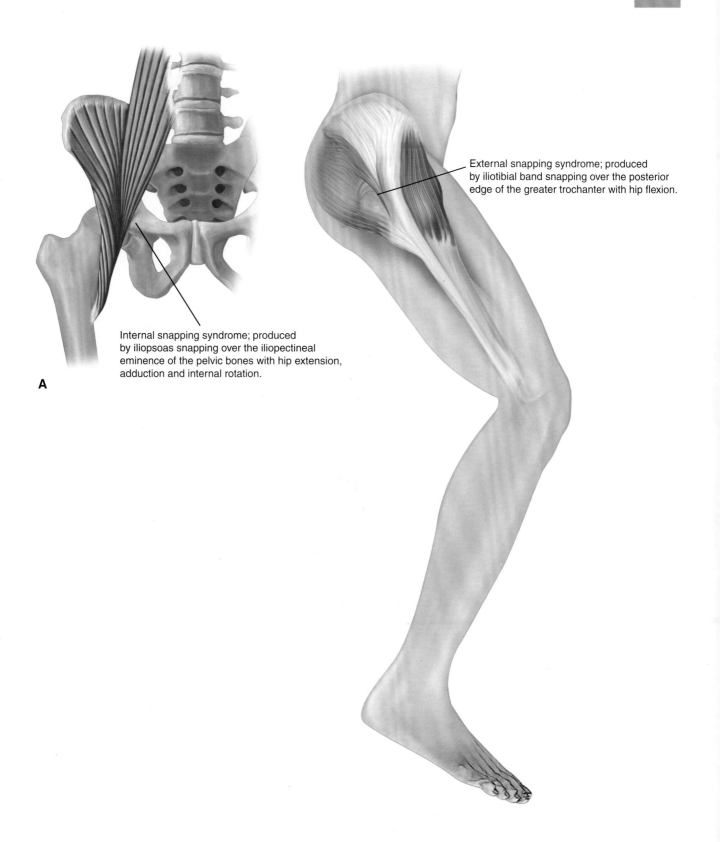

External snapping syndrome; produced by iliotibial band snapping over the posterior edge of the greater trochanter with hip flexion.

Internal snapping syndrome; produced by iliopsoas snapping over the iliopectineal eminence of the pelvic bones with hip extension, adduction and internal rotation.

A

Figure 67. **(A)** Open and **(B)** Arthroscopic Release. **(C)** External rotation of the hip aids in accessing the lesser trochanter insertion of the iliopsoas. Releases of the iliopsoas can be performed at the tendon insertion, (extra-articular release), or through the it's muscular mid-body, (intra-articular release). (*continued*)

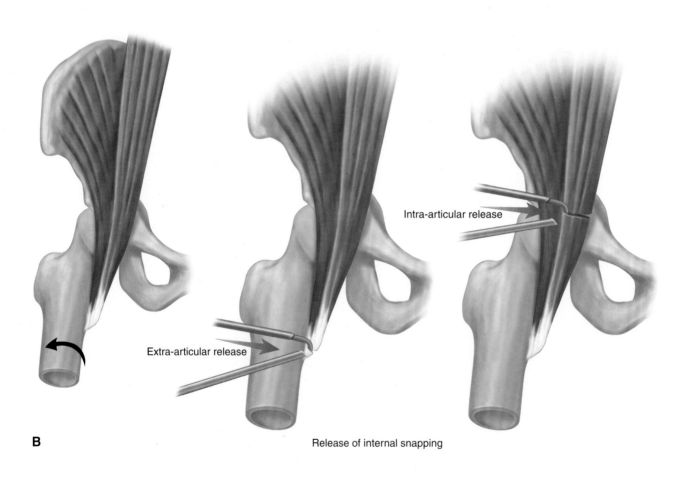

Extra-articular release

Release of internal snapping

Intra-articular release

B

Figure 67. (*continued*)

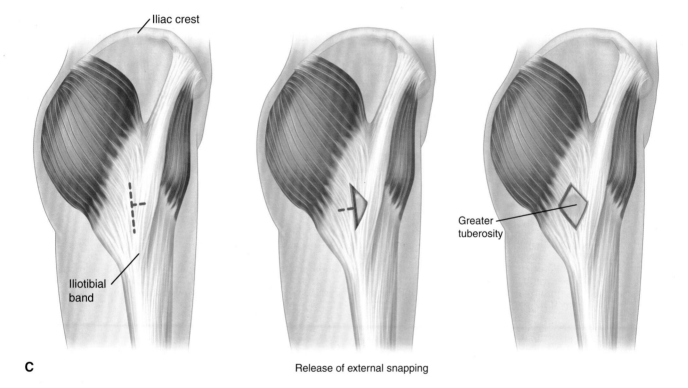

Iliac crest

Iliotibial
band

C

Release of external snapping

Greater
tuberosity

Figure 67. (*continued*)

Nerve Releases

Indications and Goals: Nerve entrapment may lead to motor and/or sensory deficits in a characteristic pattern for that nerve that is involved. Initial treatment includes removal of any external constriction, transcutaneous electrical nerve stimulation (TENS) and other conservative measures. Electrodiagnostic studies can be helpful in localizing the site of entrapment.

Procedure and Technique: Surgical release involves exploration and neurolysis of the involved nerve. The sciatic nerve can be entrapped by the piriformis muscle (piriformis syndrome). The ilioinguinal nerve can be compressed by hypertrophied abdominal muscles. The obturator nerve can be compressed in the thigh fascia. The femoral nerve can be entrapped in the groin and is seen in gymnasts, dancers, and martial arts enthusiasts. Entrapment of the lateral femoral cutaneous nerve (myalgia paresthetica) can cause anterolateral thigh numbness and paresthesias and burning pain with exertion. Release of the groin fascia and ilioinguinal ligament may be necessary.

Post-surgical Precautions/Rehabilitation: Early range of motion should begin immediately post-operative. Passive range of motion to facilitate nerve gliding and a restoration of any joint capsular accessory motion should be implemented. Scar management should also be a focus along the superficial region of the skin with attention given additionally to the subcutaneous tissue in an effort to avoid myofascial adhesions forming post-operatively.

Expected Outcomes: These nerve release techniques are useful for reducing post-operative pain immediately and they allow for an early return to activity and participation. Though a decrease in pain is noticed very soon after surgery, the results may also depend upon the underlying etiology and the duration of the symptoms prior to the surgery.

Return to Play: A full return to sport participation may be possible within 4 to 6 weeks post-operatively. Patients may require slightly longer to tolerate a less painful return to sports requiring excessive hip range of motion and strength such as soccer, basketball, or hockey.

Recommended Readings

Benezis I, Boutaud B, Leclerc J, Fabre T, Durandeau A. Lateral femoral cutaneous neuropathy and its surgical treatment: A report of 167 cases. *Muscle Nerve.* 2007;36(5):659–663.

Dezawa A, Kusano S, Miki H. Arthroscopic release of the piriformis muscle under local anesthesia for piriformis syndrome. *Arthroscopy.* 2003;19(5):554–557. Review.

Issack PS, Toro JB, Buly RL, Helfet DL. Sciatic nerve release following fracture or reconstructive surgery of the acetabulum. *J Bone Joint Surg Am.* 2007;89(7):1432–1437.

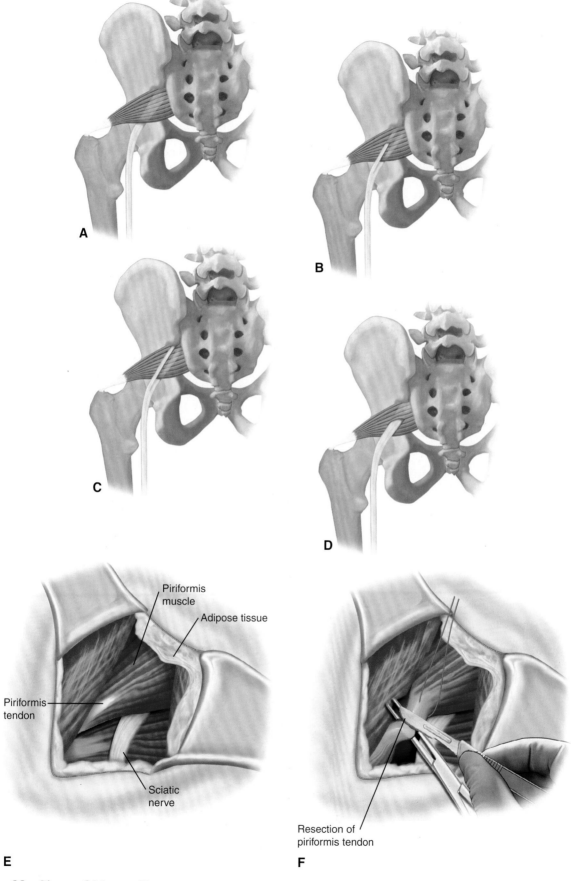

Figure 68. Sites of Nerve Entrapment

Repair of Proximal Hamstring Avulsions

Indications and Goals: These injuries can occur as a result of severe hip flexion with the knee in extension, especially during water skiing. Physical examination includes palpation of the hamstring muscle origins with the patient lying prone. Magnetic resonance imaging (MRI) can be helpful in establishing the diagnosis.

Procedure and Technique: The patient is placed in the prone position and an extended incision is made over the affected buttocks. The gluteus maximus muscle belly is split and the ischial tuberosity is exposed. The avulsed tendon is identified and repaired back to the bone using suture anchors.

Post-surgical Precautions/Rehabilitation: Typically a hip–knee–foot orthosis with the hip neutral and the knee in slight flexion is worn for 6 weeks. Avoidance of active hip extension and knee flexion exercises during this same period, with limited hip flexion movement is critical. Once the orthosis is removed, gradual progression of these activities may begin. Emphasis should be placed on range of motion as strength improvement will improve naturally with time. Once full restoration of range of motion has occurred, more sport-specific movements can be incorporated as tolerated.

Expected Outcomes: The literature states that 91% of hamstring muscle strength will return 6 months postoperatively, allowing for functional return to participation. These results are similar regardless of the timing of the repair following the tear to the proximal hamstring.

Return to Play: The return to sport participation will depend upon the healing site fixation and the ability to restore full tissue extensibility. Typical timeframe for return may be 3 to 4 months post-surgery at the earliest. Sports requiring hip flexion and extension with high tension will require additional time.

Recommended Readings

Gidwani S, Bircher MD. Avulsion injuries of the hamstring origin—a series of 12 patients and management algorithm. *Ann R Coll Surg Engl.* 2007;89(4):394–399.

Klingele KE, Sallay PI. Surgical repair of complete proximal hamstring tendon rupture. *Am J Sports Med.* 2002;30(5):742–747.

Orava S, Kujala UM. Rupture of the ischial origin of the hamstring muscles. *Am J Sports Med.* 1995;23(6):702–705.

Sallay PI, Friedman RL, Coogan PG, et al. Hamstring muscle injuries among water skiers: Functional outcome and prevention. *Am J Sports Med* 1996;24:130–136.

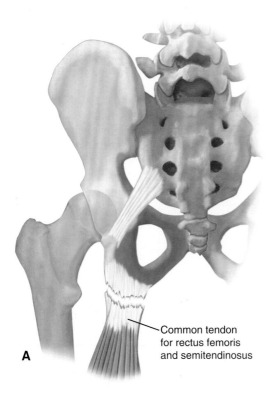 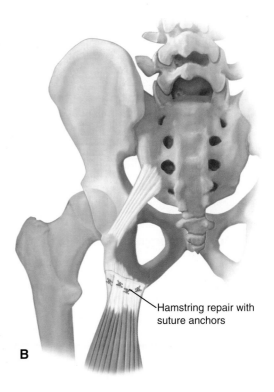

Common tendon
for rectus femoris
and semitendinosus

Hamstring repair with
suture anchors

A

B

Figure 69. **A:** Retracted tendinous avulsion of the rectus femoris and semitendinosus. **B:** Direct
repair utilizing suture anchors back to the ischial tuberosity.

Femoral Acetabular Impingement (FAI)

Indications and Goals: Femoral acetabular impingement (FAI) is a relatively new diagnosis. There are two types of FAIs described—Pincer and CAM impingements. Most cases are actually combined.

Procedure and Technique: FAI can be addressed with open or arthroscopic techniques. For Pincer impingement, osteophytes at the superior femoral neck/head junction are removed and this area is sculpted to relieve any impingement. For CAM impingement, the acetabular rim is contoured. There are several surgical approaches for hip arthroplasty. The hip joint is exposed that the femoral head is removed with a saw. The canal is prepared using reamers and rasps, and a metal stem is either pressed fit or cemented into the canal. A metal or ceramic head is attached to the stem and a special polyethylene cut is placed into a prepared acetabulum. The hip is then reduced and adjusted as necessary to provide adequate stability.

Post-surgical Precautions/Rehabilitation: Rehabilitation following surgical procedures to address FAIs requires early limited weight bearing and supervised range of motion. The amount of weight bearing and speed of progression for exercises are dependent upon the damage to the tissue structure and the amount of surgical intervention. In some cases, a person's body weight and size may also be considered in adjusting early weight bearing and ambulation status. Aside from compressive weight-bearing and landing activities being restricted, range-of-motion exercises and anti-gravity strengthening can begin early post-operatively and progress as tolerated.

Expected Outcomes: In general, good results have been reported following femoroacetabular osteoplasty and arthroscopic treatment of femoroacetabular impingement, though there appears to be a negative correlation between the severity of the cartilage lesions and post-operative outcomes. This is an uncommon procedure for athletes, and actually has resulted in the untimely end to some athletes' careers. High impact activities are discouraged following this procedure. Indications include advanced arthritis and end-stage osteonecrosis.

Return to Play: Given the likelihood of some joint sensitivity as a result of the work on the bone structure, a return to sport participation is typically at least 3 months post-operatively.

Recommended Readings

Espinosa N, Beck M, Rothenfluh DA, Ganz R, Leunig M. Treatment of femoro-acetabular impingement: Preliminary results of labral refixation. Surgical technique. *J Bone Joint Surg Am.* 2007;89(suppl 2 pt 1):36–53.

Guanche CA, Bare AA. Arthroscopic treatment of femoroacetabular impingement. *Arthroscopy.* 2006;22(1):95–106.

Jaberi FM, Parvizi J. Hip pain in young adults: Femoroacetabular impingement. *J Arthroplasty.* 2007;22(7 suppl 3):37–42.

Khanduja V, Villar RN. The arthroscopic management of femoroacetabular impingement. *Knee Surg Sports Traumatol Arthrosc.* 2007; 15(8):1035–1040. Epub 2007 May 30.

Laude F, Boyer T, Nogier A. Anterior femoroacetabular impingement. *Joint Bone Spine.* 2007;74(2):127–132. Epub 2007 Feb 5. Review.

Parvizi J, Leunig M, Ganz R. Femoroacetabular impingement. *J Am Acad Orthop Surg.* 2007;15(9):561–570.

Philippon MJ, Stubbs AJ, Schenker ML, Maxwell RB, Ganz R, Leunig M. Arthroscopic management of femoroacetabular impingement: Osteoplasty technique and literature review. *Am J Sports Med.* 2007 Sep;35(9):1571–1580. Epub 2007 Apr 9. Review.

Philippon M, Schenker M, Briggs K, Kuppersmith D. Femoroacetabular impingement in 45 professional athletes: Associated pathologies and return to sport following arthroscopic decompression. *Knee Surg Sports Traumatol Arthrosc.* 2007;15(7):908–914. Epub 2007 May 4.

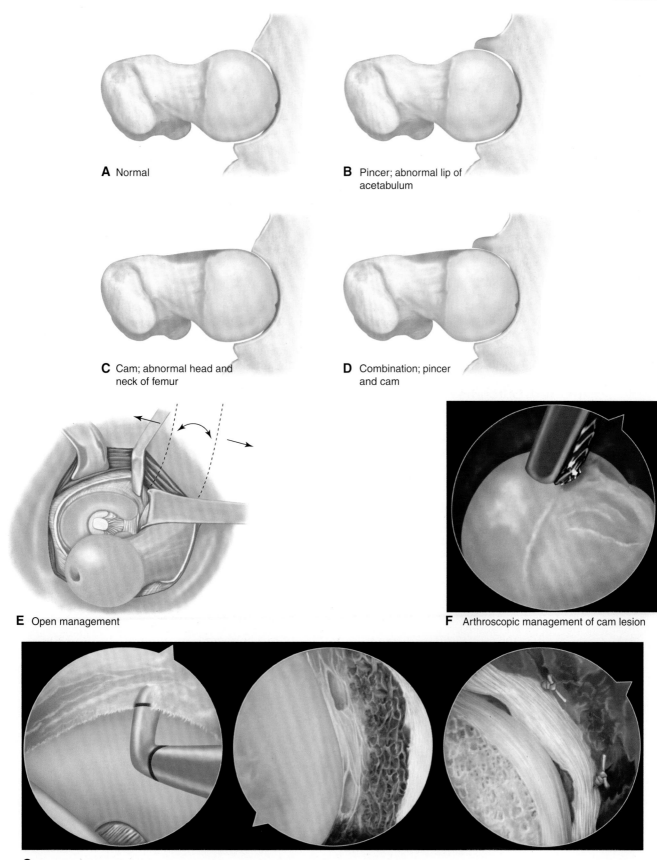

A Normal

B Pincer; abnormal lip of acetabulum

C Cam; abnormal head and neck of femur

D Combination; pincer and cam

E Open management

F Arthroscopic management of cam lesion

G Arthroscopic management of pincer lesion, acetabular rim trimming and repair

Figure 70. Arthroscopic Treatment of Combined CAM and Pincer FAI

Hip Arthroplasty

Indications and Goals: Hip arthroplasty is used to address joint failure caused mainly by arthritis (osteoarthritis, inflammatory, post-traumatic), avascular necrosis, femoral neck fractures and certain tumors. The goal is to provide a functional hip joint and pain relief. Currently available options include replacing both the femoral and acetabular ends or just the femoral side. Replacing the femoral side can be achieved either by a resurfacing procedure or by placing a femoral component fixed down the femoral canal. There are several bearing surface options including metal with plastic interface, metal on metal, ceramic on ceramic, and ceramic on plastic. Metal implants vary from chromium, cobalt, titanium, and tantalum alloys.

Procedure and Technique: Hip arthroplasty can be performed through different approaches to the hip joint (posterior, lateral, anterior). It involves making cuts in the femur in order to remove the diseased bone and fit in the prosthesis. The cup side is addressed by serial reamings on the acetabulum in order to orient it in the desired position and fit a component. Components in both sides are either press fit or cemented according to bone quality and surgeon preferences.

Post-surgical Precautions/Rehabilitation: Post-operative rehabilitation is mostly guided by the surgical approach used by the surgeon, bone quality and fit of components. Generally the patient is allowed to fully bear weight after the procedure and different hip positions are avoided according to the approach in order to prevent dislocations. Patients are usually given some type of deep venous thrombosis prophylaxis. Long-term rehabilitation for range of motion and strength of core body muscles and those around the hip joint is initiated.

Expected Outcomes: Results after hip arthroplasty have consistently been demonstrated to enhance hip function and improve pain scores. Overall quality of life improvement has also been demonstrated in multiple studies using validated quality of live assessment tools. Expected overall in-hospital and post-discharge complication rate is 7% for total hip arthroplasty (THA). The most common in-hospital complications in THA patients are fractures (0.6%) and deep vein thrombosis (DVT) (0.6%). The most common post-discharge complications in THA patients are reoperation due to bleeding, wound necrosis, and wound infection.

Recommended Readings

Cushner F, Agnelli G, FitzGerald G, Warwick D. Complications and functional outcomes after total hip arthroplasty and total knee arthroplasty: Results from the Global Orthopaedic Registry (GLORY). *Am J Orthop.* 2010;39(9 suppl):22–28.

Heisel C, Silva M, Schmalzried TP. Bearing surface options for total hip replacement in young patients. *Instr Course Lect.* 2004;53:49–65.

Saleh KJ, Kassim R, Yoon P, Vorlicky LN. Complications of total hip arthroplasty. *Am J Orthop.* 2002;31(8):485–488.

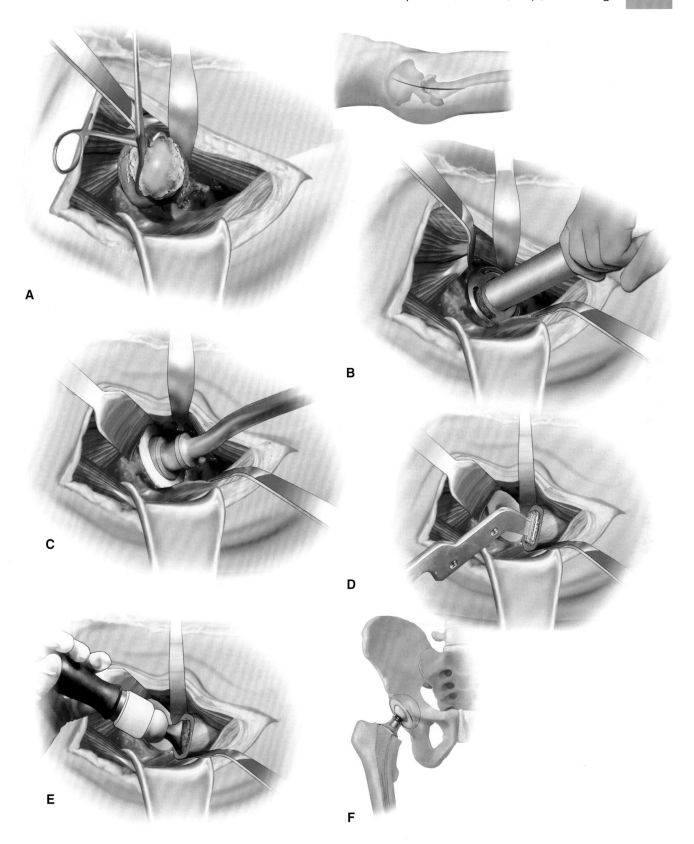

Figure 71. **A:** Lateral hip approach, with removal of the diseased femoral head. **B:** The acetabulum is prepared and reamed. **C:** The acetabular implant is impacted in place. **D:** The femoral canal is created and broached. **E:** Stem impacted into femoral canal. **F:** Completed total hip arthroplasty.

ORIF Hip Fractures

Indications and Goals: Hip fractures are unusual in athletes, but stress fractures are relatively common. Tension-sided stress fractures, which occur on the superior side of the femoral neck, are at risk for becoming complete fractures and should be fixed prophylactically. These are treated with cannulated screws. Other hip fractures, including intertrochanteric and subtrochanteric fractures are typically fixed with either compression screw/sideplate or intramedullary devices.

Procedure and Technique: Patients are placed supine on a fracture table, an incision is made over the proximal femur and guidewires are drilled into the femoral head. Usually three screws are placed in a triangular pattern. Compression screw/sideplate devices are inserted via a longer incision. A guidewire is placed in the center of the femoral head and overdrilled. A compression screw is inserted and a sideplate is attached to the screw. Intramedullary devices are inserted as described for femur fractures.

Post-surgical Precautions/Rehabilitation: Depending upon the quality of the reduction and fixation, protected weight bearing or non–weight bearing is initiated. The ability to walk and ambulate early post-operative is essential for a quick hospital discharge and reintegration into social life. Balance training and strengthening of the surrounding hip musculature can begin immediately post-operatively. Rehabilitative progression is also based upon the age and health status of the patient, as the risk of re-injury or falling increases with age and deconditioning.

Expected Outcomes: Randomized trials have yielded insufficient outcomes as evidence with open versus closed reduction of intracapsular fractures. Regardless, post-operative complications include non-unions, risk of re-fracture, and avascular necrosis. Overall, functional outcome was good for most of the patients who recovered their initial activity level. Post-operative hip musculature may take a while to restore adequate levels of strength.

Return to Play: A return to sport participation may not be possible for severely displaced or non-anatomically fixed fractures. The underlying cause of the fracture must also be corrected. After complete healing, return of strength, and gradual return to walking and eventually running without pain, it may be possible at least 6 months post-operatively for a return to low–impact-type sports.

Recommended Readings

Dobbs RE, Parvizi J, Lewallen DG. Perioperative morbidity and 30-day mortality after intertrochanteric hip fractures treated by internal fixation or arthroplasty. *J Arthroplasty.* 2005;20(8):963–966.

Macaulay W, Yoon RS, Parsley B, Nellans KW, Teeny SM; DFACTO Consortium. Displaced femoral neck fractures: Is there a standard of care? *Orthopedics.* 2007;30(9):748–749. Review.

Molnar RB, Routt ML Jr.,. Open reduction of intracapsular hip fractures using a modified Smith-Petersen surgical exposure. *J Orthop Trauma.* 2007;21(7):490–494.

Parker MJ, Banajee A. Surgical approaches and ancillary techniques for internal fixation of intracapsular proximal femoral fractures. *Cochrane Database Syst Rev.* 2005;18;(2):CD001705. Review.

Upadhyay A, Jain P, Mishra P, Maini L, Gautum VK, Dhaon BK. Delayed internal fixation of fractures of the neck of the femur in young adults. A prospective, randomised study comparing closed and open reduction. *J Bone Joint Surg Br.* 2004;86(7):1035–1040.

Wang JW, Chen LK, Chen CE. Surgical treatment of fractures of the greater trochanter associated with osteolytic lesions. Surgical technique. *J Bone Joint Surg Am.* 2006;88(suppl 1 pt 2):250–258.

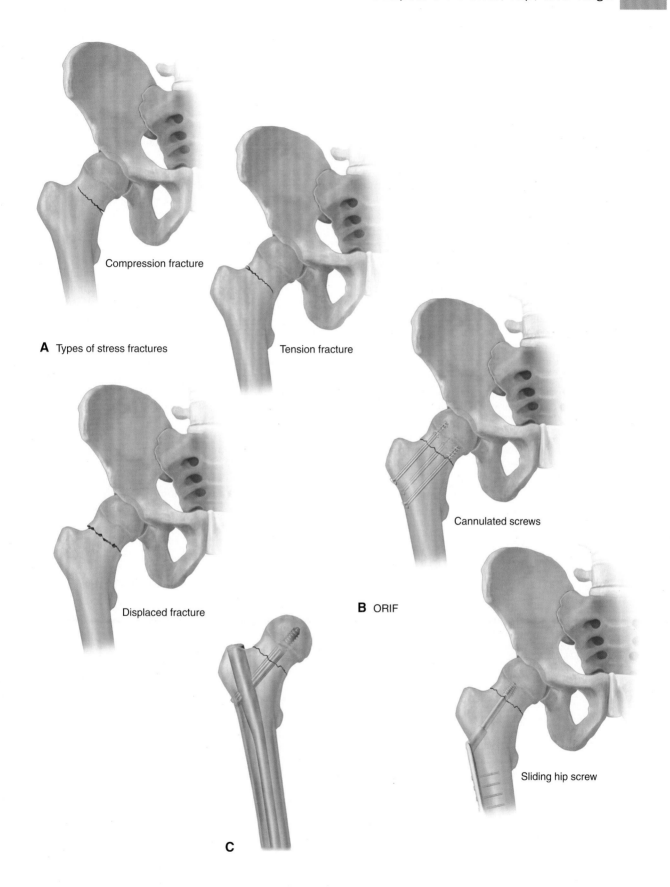

Compression fracture

A Types of stress fractures

Tension fracture

Displaced fracture

Cannulated screws

B ORIF

Sliding hip screw

C

Figure 72. Femoral Neck Fracture. (A) Cannulated Screw Fixation; **(B)** Sliding Hip Screw Construct; **(C)** Cephalomedullary Device.

ORIF Femur Fractures

Indications and Goals: Femur fractures occur as a result of blunt trauma. There is usually significant forces involved and motor vehicle accidents account for a large percentage of these injuries. Classification of these fractures is based upon the location and amount of comminution. Treatment involves restoration of length and alignment.

Procedure and Technique: The patient is placed on a fracture table and the fracture is reduced with traction. A long guidewire is placed in the intramedullary canal using either a starting point adjacent to the greater trochanter (antegrade) or through a drill hole placed just above the notch in the knee (retrograde). A flexible drill is used to ream the canal and a metal rod is inserted into the femur. The rod is then secured with interlocking screws on both ends of the femur.

Post-surgical Precautions/Rehabilitation: Initial rehabilitation consists of gentle range of motion and initiation of weight bearing as tolerated instruction with an assistive device. This phase of rehabilitation should consist of hip and knee range-of-motion activities, isometric exercises for the quadriceps and gluteal muscles as well as patella mobilization. Balance and proprioceptive exercises can be initiated in the form of weight shifting. Transition to walking over cones can be implemented with an assistive device to promote knee flexion. When the patient tolerates 50% of weight-bearing status with fair quadriceps and hip abductor strength, they progress to phase two, usually at week 4 post-operatively. Progress strengthening to 50% weight-bearing status with gait retraining. Continue with range-of-motion activity such as heel slides and wall slides until full range of motion is achieved. By week 8, full weight-bearing status should be attained. Gait activities can progress to side stepping and backward walking. Full weight bearing, strengthening, balance, proprioception, and conditioning can occur. Weight-bearing status depends on quality of reduction and fixation. Fractures typically take 3 months to heal.

Expected Outcomes: Outcomes are highly based upon the patient's age, nutritional status of the bone, and success of the fixation. Pre- and post-operative hip musculature strength and balance contributes to higher rates of success.

Return to Play: Return to sport participation should only occur after complete bony union. This may take a minimum of 6 months. Successful return to participation is also based upon the age and health status of the patient, as the risk of re-injury increases with age and deconditioning.

Recommended Readings

Haidukewych GJ, Berry DJ, Jacofsky DJ, Torchia ME. Treatment of supracondylar femur nonunions with open reduction and internal fixation. *Am J Orthop.* 2003;32(11):564–567.

Hartin NL, Harris I, Hazratwala K. Retrograde nailing versus fixed-angle blade plating for supracondylar femoral fractures: A randomized controlled trial. *ANZ J Surg.* 2006;76(5):290–294.

Paterno MV, Archdeacon MT, Ford KR, Galvin D, Hewett TE. Early rehabilitation following surgical fixation of a femoral shaft fracture. *Phys Ther.* 2006;86(4):558–572.

Zlowodzki M, Bhandari M, Marek DJ, Cole PA, Kregor PJ. Operative treatment of acute distal femur fractures: Systematic review of 2 comparative studies and 45 case series (1989 to 2005). *J Orthop Trauma.* 2006;20(5):366–371. Review.

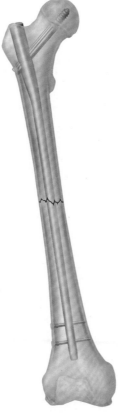

Intermeduallary
nail in femur

Figure 73. Locked IM Nail for Femoral Shaft Fracture

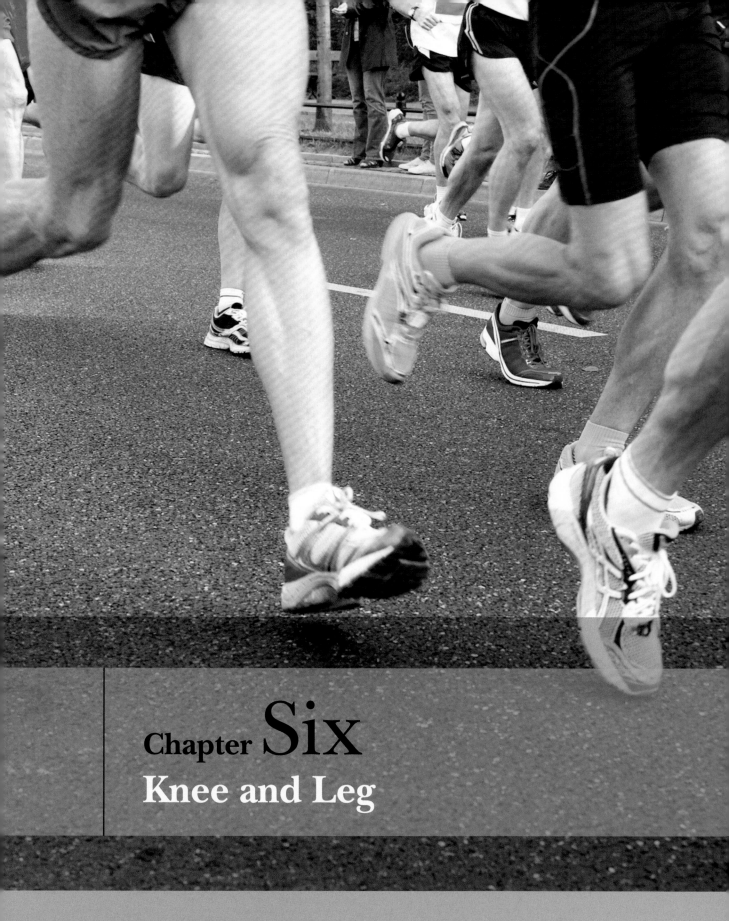

Chapter Six
Knee and Leg

Knee Arthroscopy

Indications and Goals: Knee arthroscopy is now the standard of care for treating a variety of knee problems. Arthroscopic partial meniscectomy is the most popular procedure done in orthopedics. Other arthroscopic procedures include cruciate ligament reconstruction, articular cartilage procedures, synovectomy, loose body removal, and a variety of other procedures.

Procedure and Technique: Knee arthroscopy is accomplished with the patient supine. The use of a leg holder is optional. Most procedures can be done through two portals. The main viewing portal is via an inferolateral portal just lateral the edge of the patella tendon and just superior to the joint line. The main instrumentation portal is the inferomedial portal, just medial to the edge of the patella tendon and just superior to the joint line. Accessory portals include a superolateral portal, a trans-patellar tendon portal, a posteromedial portal, and others. A systematic, thorough evaluation of the knee joint involves inspecting and probing all compartments, both gutters, the intercondylar notch, and, when indicated, the posteromedial (and posterolateral) aspects of the knee. The knee is stressed to allow access for the arthroscope and instruments. A variety of mechanical instruments (various angled biters [baskets] and grabbers) and shavers are used to carry out knee arthroscopy.

Post-surgical Precautions/Rehabilitation: Post-surgical rehabilitation varies significantly based upon the specific procedures performed. Since arthroscopic surgery of the knee can range from a minor synovectomy to a meniscal repair or an articular cartilage transplant, guidelines for rehabilitation should be closely correlated to the surgeon's preference and based upon tissue healing factors. All rehabilitative approaches, though varying in their timeline, will focus on the reduction of swelling, minimizing of quadriceps muscle atrophy, restoration of patellofemoral and tibiofemoral joint motion, and return of joint proprioceptive function.

Expected Outcomes: Generally speaking, arthroscopic procedures yield excellent results. However, specific assessment of outcomes must be procedurally based.

Return to Play: Return to sport participation can range from days in a professional athlete who simply had some soft tissue debridement or fluid aspiration to 6 months or more for anyone undergoing articular cartilage repairs.

Recommended Readings

Crawford R, Walley G, Bridgman S, Maffulli N. Magnetic resonance imaging versus arthroscopy in the diagnosis of knee pathology, concentrating on meniscal lesions and ACL tears: A systematic review. *Br Med Bull.* 2007;84:5–23.

Goodyear-Smith F, Arroll B. Rehabilitation after arthroscopic meniscectomy: A critical review of the clinical trials. *Int Orthop.* 2001;24(6):350–353. Review.

Siparsky P, Ryzewicz M, Peterson B, Bartz R. Arthroscopic treatment of osteoarthritis of the knee: Are there any evidence-based indications? *Clin Orthop Relat Res.* 2007;455:107–112. Review.

Steadman JR, Ramappa AJ, Maxwell RB, Briggs KK. An arthroscopic treatment regimen for osteoarthritis of the knee. *Arthroscopy.* 2007;23(9):948–955.

Tauber M, Fox M, Koller H, Klampfer H, Resch H. Arthroscopic treatment of a large lateral femoral notch in acute anterior cruciate ligament tear. *Arch Orthop Trauma Surg.* 2007;128(11):1313–1316.

Widuchowski W, Widuchowski J, Trzaska T. Articular cartilage defects: Study of 25,124 knee arthroscopies. *Knee.* 2007;14(3):177–182. Epub 2007 Apr 10.

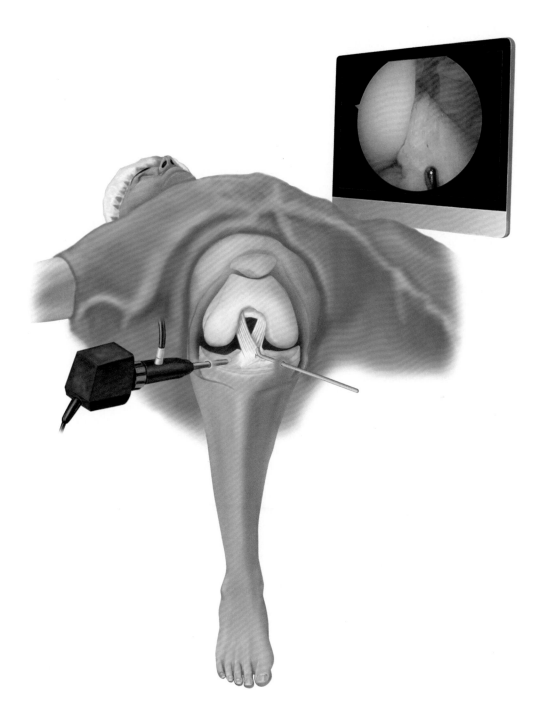

Figure 74. Knee arthroscopy with standard viewing (anterolateral) **and working** (anteromedial) **portals**

Arthroscopy Synovectomy and Lateral Release

Indications and Goals: An arthroscopy synovectomy (removal of the joint lining in the knee) can be done arthroscopically as well as open, provided that a thorough systematic approach is used through as many as six portals. Indications include pigmented villonodular synovitis (PVNS), synovial chondromatosis, rheumatoid arthritis, and a variety of other disorders. Synovial plicae, which are thickenings of the synovium, can sometimes become symptomatic and abrade the articular surfaces, especially the medial femoral condyle. Pathologic plicae, although rare, should be removed. Lateral release should also be a relatively uncommon procedure for the knee arthroscopist. Indications are limited to patients with refractory anterior knee pain and objective evidence of patellar tilting (lateral patellar compression syndrome).

Procedure and Technique: Arthroscopic synovectomy of the knee is accomplished with a large shaver. The entire synovium is shaved. Fortunately, the pathologic synovium is dark colored and it is relatively easy to see what needs to be removed. Typically, the superior joint is addressed first (using superomedial and superolateral portals), then the gutters, and then the anterior part of the knee. Additional portals are necessary to debride the posteromedial and posterolateral aspects of the knee. These portals are localized using a spinal needle as viewed through the notch. Medially, the saphenous vein and nerve branches need to be protected and laterally, the common peroneal nerve should be protected by staying anterior to these structures. Plicae can be easily resected with a combination of a biter and a shaver. A lateral release is usually accomplished under direct visualization using an electrocautery device. Care should be taken to avoid excessive bleeding (from the superolateral geniculate artery).

Post-surgical Precautions/Rehabilitation: Post-operative precautions following an isolated synovectomy involve a gradual progression to weight bearing, with range of motion exercises implemented immediately. The focus is on minimizing post-operative effusion and regaining neuromuscular control. With a lateral release performed, post-operative emphasis should be placed on quadriceps muscle activity and joint proprioception. Care should be taken early on to consider the use of a patella-stabilizing orthotic of some kind. It is also important to assess one's posture and avoid a pronated foot, thus foot orthotics may be of assistance to minimize any excessive valgus forces placed on the knee.

Expected Outcomes: Anterior knee pain has been reported to subside post-operatively in the number of patients as compared to preoperative findings as much as 2 years post-operative. However, an isolated lateral retinacular release of the patella has not proven to be effective for long-term benefit of reducing patellar instability. It is not uncommon for a person who undergoes a lateral release to have repetitive episodes of complaints of instability and pain years later if in fact continued quadriceps strengthening has not been maintained.

Return to Play: A return to sport participation can occur with days to weeks with only a synovectomy being performed. However, with the lateral release procedure, restoration of quadriceps strength and function is required prior to any competitive return to sport. This may be as early as 1 month post-operatively but is often longer.

Recommended Readings

Lattermann C, Drake GN, Spellman J, Bach BR Jr. Lateral retinacular release for anterior knee pain: A systematic review of the literature. *J Knee Surg.* 2006;19(4):278–284. Review.

Lattermann C, Toth J, Bach BR Jr. The role of lateral retinacular release in the treatment of patellar instability. *Sports Med Arthrosc.* 2007;15(2):57–60. Review.

Shannon BD, Keene JS. Results of arthroscopic medial retinacular release for treatment of medial subluxation of the patella. *Am J Sports Med.* 2007;35(7):1180–1187. Epub 2007 Mar 16.

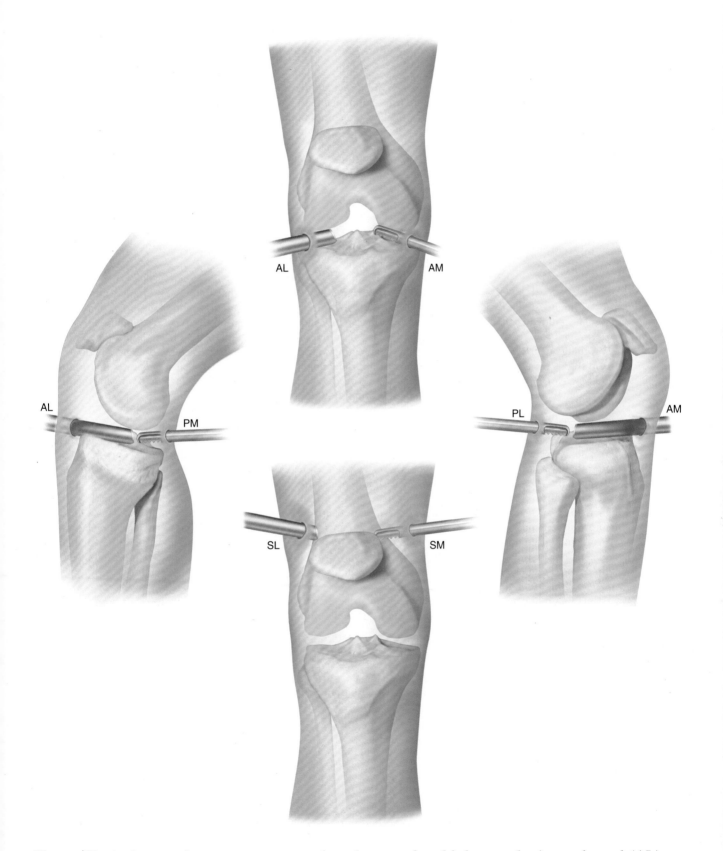

Figure 75. Arthroscopic synovectomy requires the use of multiple portals: Anterolateral (AL),
Anteromedial (AM), Posteromedial (PM), Posterolateral (PL), Superolateral (SL),
Superomedial (SM).

Meniscectomy

Indications and Goals: Meniscectomy is indicated for meniscal tears that are not repairable. These tears include complex or degenerative tears, most flap tears, and radial tears. Patients may relate a history of a twisting injury and may complain of mechanical symptoms (locking, catching, popping, etc.). Findings on examination include joint line tenderness and pain with provocative maneuvers (McMurray testing, compression testing, duck walk, etc.). Plain radiographs are helpful to evaluate the degree of associated osteoarthritis (standing radiographs are mandatory). Magnetic resonance imaging (MRI) is very helpful in confirming the diagnosis and gives some idea regarding the repairability of a meniscal tear.

Procedure and Technique: Partial meniscectomy is accomplished using a variety of biters (baskets) and shavers. Since development of late arthritis is directly related to the amount of meniscus removed, the minimal amount necessary to result in a stable rim is resected. The articular cartilage of the affected compartment should be protected by adequately stressing the joint and using careful technique and smaller shavers. Associated meniscal cysts, when present, can be debrided from inside-out.

Post-surgical Precautions/Rehabilitation: Despite the fact that some peer-reviewed literature show little evidence that formal rehabilitation is necessary to return patients to normal function following a meniscectomy, formally guided rehabilitation following a partial meniscectomy can speed up the recovery timeline for someone returning to sport participation. Emphasis is placed on minimizing joint effusion, restoring joint range of motion, regaining quadriceps control, and gradually ambulating with weight as tolerated to achieve optimal outcomes. Since no tissue is repaired in an isolated meniscectomy, rehabilitation can be progressive and integrates neuromuscular training early post-operative. Assistive devices only need to be used in some circumstances and only for the first few days. Otherwise, ambulation with full weight bearing should be promoted.

Expected Outcomes: Outcomes following partial meniscectomies are relatively good. Some resultant joint osteoarthritis may occur years post-operative, with a larger size of meniscal resection, and those performed on females, showing the most consistent associations with increased radiographic evidence of osteoarthritis. Furthermore, greater articular cartilage degeneration assessed at surgery, increased sizes of meniscal resection, greater laxity of the anterior cruciate ligament (ACL), and prior surgery on the index knee were the strongest predictors of worse functional outcomes. There appears to be no difference in functional outcome between medial or lateral meniscectomies, though radiologic results are significantly worse after lateral meniscectomy. It appears as though improved outcomes can be predicted for some patients. With an isolated medial meniscal tear, better outcomes may result, given one or more of the following: Less than 35 years old, a vertical tear, no cartilage damage, and an intact meniscal rim at the end of the meniscectomy. With an isolated lateral meniscal tear, a better prognosis can be predicted if the patient is young and has an intact meniscal rim at the end of the meniscectomy.

Return to Play: Following restoration of quadriceps tone and control of post-operative effusion, a return to activity can occur reasonably quick, ranging from weeks to months based upon one's required level of function.

Recommended Readings

Bin SI, Kim JM, Shin SJ. Radial tears of the posterior horn of the medial meniscus. *Arthroscopy.* 2004;20(4):373–378. Review.

Brindle T, Nyland J, Johnson DL. The meniscus: Review of basic principles with application to surgery and rehabilitation. *J Athl Train.* 2001;36(2):160–169.

Chatain F, Adeleine P, Chambat P, Neyret P. A comparative study of medial versus lateral arthroscopic partial meniscectomy on stable knees: 10-year minimum follow-up. *Arthroscopy.* 2003;19(8):842–849. Review.

Fabricant PD, Jokl P. Surgical outcomes after arthroscopic partial meniscectomy. *J Am Acad Orthop Surg.* 2007;15(11):647–653.

Good CR, Green DW, Griffith MH, Valen AW, Widmann RF, Rodeo SA. Arthroscopic treatment of symptomatic discoid meniscus in children: Classification, technique, and results. *Arthroscopy.* 2007;23(2):157–163.

Goodwin PC, Morrissey MC. Physical therapy after arthroscopic partial meniscectomy: Is it effective? *Exerc Sport Sci Rev.* 2003;31(2): 85–90. Review.

Hegedus EJ, Cook C, Hasselblad V, Goode A, McCrory DC. Physical examination tests for assessing a torn meniscus in the knee: A systematic review with meta-analysis. *J Orthop Sports Phys Ther.* 2007;37(9):541–550.

McDermott ID, Amis AA. The consequences of meniscectomy. *J Bone Joint Surg Br.* 2006;88(12):1549–1556. Review.

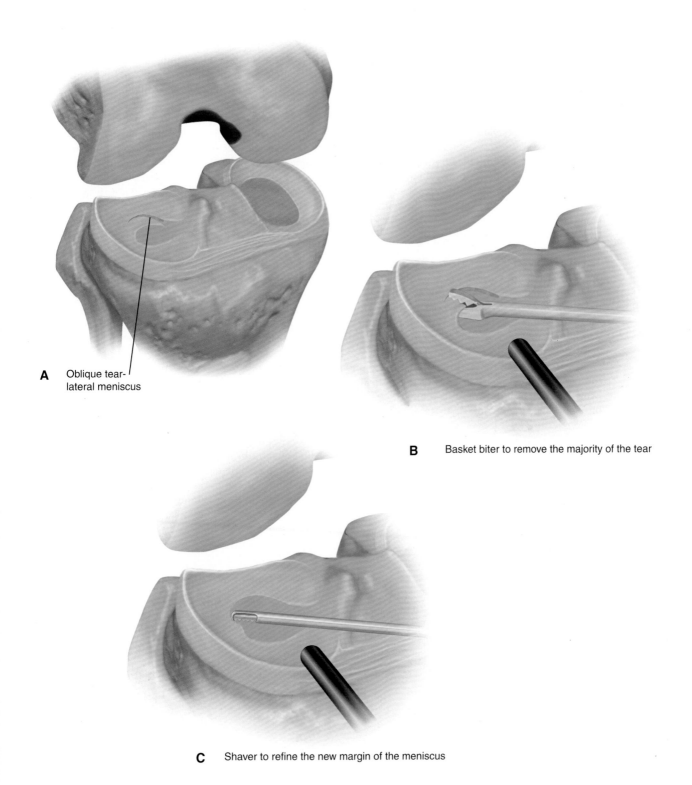

A Oblique tear-
lateral meniscus

B   Basket biter to remove the majority of the tear

C   Shaver to refine the new margin of the meniscus

Figure 76. Partial meniscectomy. A. Oblique tear of the lateral meniscus. **B.** Biter utilized for a partial meniscectomy. **C.** A shaver is used to smooth the edge of the remaining meniscus.

Meniscal Repair

Indications and Goals: Meniscal tears should be repaired rather than removed whenever there is a reasonable chance of success. The ideal candidate for meniscal repair is a peripheral longitudinal tear that is undergoing concurrent ACL reconstruction. Examination and imaging findings are similar to that described for meniscectomy. The goal is to restore meniscal integrity and function to avoid the development of late arthritis.

Procedure and Technique: There are a variety of techniques for meniscal repair including open, inside-out, outside-in, and all-inside repairs. The gold standard for meniscal repair is inside-out repair, and this should be accomplished if there is any doubt about the integrity of the repair. Inside-out repair is accomplished using long needles that are placed through special contoured cannulae. A posteromedial or posterolateral incision is made in order to "capture" the needles as they are passed through the knee. A variety of all-inside devices have been developed to make meniscal repair easier for the surgeon, but because of associate complications, not always better for the patient. Newer devices allow the surgeon to tension the repair. These new devices approach but do not equal the results of inside-out repair. The use of adjunctive techniques to improve healing rates of meniscal repair includes rasping and the use of fibrin clot.

Post-surgical Precautions/Rehabilitation: Rehabilitation following meniscal repairs should focus on minimizing joint swelling, regaining knee joint range of motion, and emphasizing quadriceps strengthening exercise—all of which can be initiated on the first day post-operatively. Excessive weight bearing and joint compressive forces that could disrupt the healing meniscus repair are avoided, oftentimes with the use of crutches for up to 4 weeks. Modifications based upon the type, size, and location of meniscal tear and other concomitant procedures may be required. Full return to weight-bearing activity may take between 4 to 6 months.

Expected Outcomes: Results vary, based upon the size of the repair, the devices used to repair the meniscus, the potential healing properties of the individual, and the overall compliance associated with a rehabilitation program that carefully monitors limited weight bearing and joint compressive forces early on. Failures, or re-tears of the repair, range from 5% to 45%, with a higher rate of failure of tears in the medial versus lateral meniscus. Although the RTP is longer, surgeons should be encouraged to repair meniscal tears whenever possible.

Return to Play: Return to sport participation may take up to 6 months safely following a meniscal repair. It is not uncommon for athletes to feel "ready" to play sooner. However, full healing of the meniscal repair may not have yet taken place, and a return to competitive sport with increased knee joint compressive loads too soon may place the repair at risk for failure. Athletes returning to sports that may involve excessive amounts of knee hyperflexion, such as soccer, may be at an increased risk for reinjury.

Recommended Readings

Farng E, Sherman O. Meniscal repair devices: A clinical and biomechanical literature review. *Arthroscopy.* 2004;20(3):273–286. Review.

Forster MC, Aster AS. Arthroscopic meniscal repair. *Surgeon.* 2003;1(6):323–327. Review.

Harris B, Miller MD. Biomedical devices in meniscal repair. *Sports Med Arthrosc.* 2006;14(3):120–128. Review.

Heckmann TP, Barber-Westin SD, Noyes FR. Meniscal repair and transplantation: Indications, techniques, rehabilitation, and clinical outcome. *J Orthop Sports Phys Ther.* 2006;36(10):795–814. Review.

Lindenfeld T. Inside-out meniscal repair. *Instr Course Lect.* 2005;54:331–336. Review.

Lozano J, Ma CB, Cannon WD. All-inside meniscus repair: A systematic review. *Clin Orthop Relat Res.* 2007;455:134–141. Review.

Miller MD, Hart JA. All-inside meniscal repair. *Instr Course Lect.* 2005;54:337–340. Review.

Voloshin I, Schmitz MA, Adams MJ, DeHaven KE. Results of repeat meniscal repair. *Am J Sports Med.* 2003;31(6):874–880.

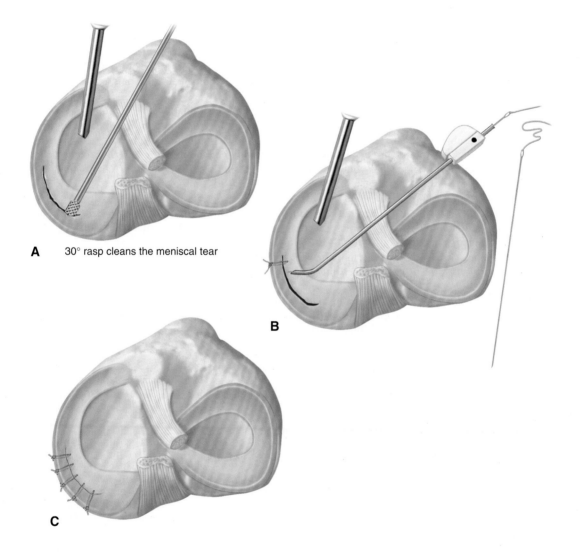

A   30° rasp cleans the meniscal tear

B

C

Figure 77. Meniscal repair. A. A rasp is used to prepare the longintudinal tear for repair.
B. Using long flexible needles, an inside-out repair is performed. **C.** Vertical mattress
sutures reapproximate tear edges.

Meniscal Transplantation

Indications and Goals: Meniscal allograft transplantation is a technically difficult procedure with few long-term results available in the literature. It appears that the transplanted meniscus may have a limited lifespan and may only delay the onset of late arthritis. Nevertheless, symptomatic younger patients following complete meniscectomy, particularly of the lateral compartment, may benefit from this procedure. It is important to make sure that mechanical alignment and knee stability is restored either before or at the same time as the transplant procedure.

Procedure and Technique: Two different surgical techniques are popular. The trough or key-hole technique (typically done for lateral meniscal transplants) involves preserving a block of bone between the horns of the meniscus and then "sliding" it into a trough created for receiving the graft. The bone-plug technique (typically done for medial meniscal transplants) involves creating separate small bone plugs for each horn and passing them into tunnels. It is important to recreate the normal anatomy of horn insertion for both techniques. After the anterior and posterior horns are secured, sutures are placed as described for meniscal repair.

Post-surgical Precautions/Rehabilitation: The rehabilitation process for a meniscal transplantation is very similar to that of a meniscal repair. The main focus is on reducing joint compression forces, while restoring range of motion and keeping effusion to a minimum. Muscular reduction can be initiated day one post-operative. Modifications based upon the type of meniscal tear and other concomitant procedures may be required. Full return to weight-bearing activity may take between 4 and 6 months. It is critical not to rush the patient through early episodes of weight bearing that will increase joint compressive loads on the healing tissue.

Expected Outcomes: Pain relief and functional improvement are often seen, and the partial restoration of meniscal function provided by this procedure may slow down the degenerative arthritic process. Continued advances with the technique may yield more long-term benefits. It appears that the success of the results are dependent upon reestablishing normal knee alignment and stability, implanting a secure fixate graft, and limiting an individual's return to light activities only.

Return to Play: This procedure is considered a salvage option and is not typically recommended for competitive athletes. Return to activities for recreational athletes should follow complete bony healing of the meniscal horns and periphery of the meniscus—which may be at least 6 months post-operatively.

Recommended Readings

Alford W, Cole BJ. The indications and technique for meniscal transplant. *Orthop Clin North Am.* 2005;36(4):469–484. Review.

Heckmann TP, Barber-Westin SD, Noyes FR. Meniscal repair and transplantation: Indications, techniques, rehabilitation, and clinical outcome. *J Orthop Sports Phys Ther.* 2006;36(10):795–814. Review.

Khetia EA, McKeon BP. Meniscal allografts: Biomechanics and techniques. *Sports Med Arthrosc.* 2007;15(3):114–120. Review.

Lubowitz JH, Verdonk PC, Reid JB 3rd, Verdonk R. Meniscus allograft transplantation: A current concepts review. *Knee Surg Sports Traumatol Arthrosc.* 2007;15(5):476–492. Epub 2007 Feb 28. Review.

Matava MJ. Meniscal allograft transplantation: A systematic review. *Clin Orthop Relat Res.* 2007;455:142–157. Review.

Sekiya JK, Ellingson CI. Meniscal allograft transplantation. *J Am Acad Orthop Surg.* 2006;14(3):164–174. Review.

Verdonk R, Almqvist KF, Huysse W, et al. Meniscal allografts: Indications and outcomes. *Sports Med Arthrosc.* 2007;15(3):121–125. Review.

Verdonk PC, Demurie A, Almqvist KF, Veys EM, Verbruggen G, Verdonk R. Transplantation of viable meniscal allograft. Surgical technique. *J Bone Joint Surg Am.* 2006;88(suppl 1 pt 1):109–118. Review.

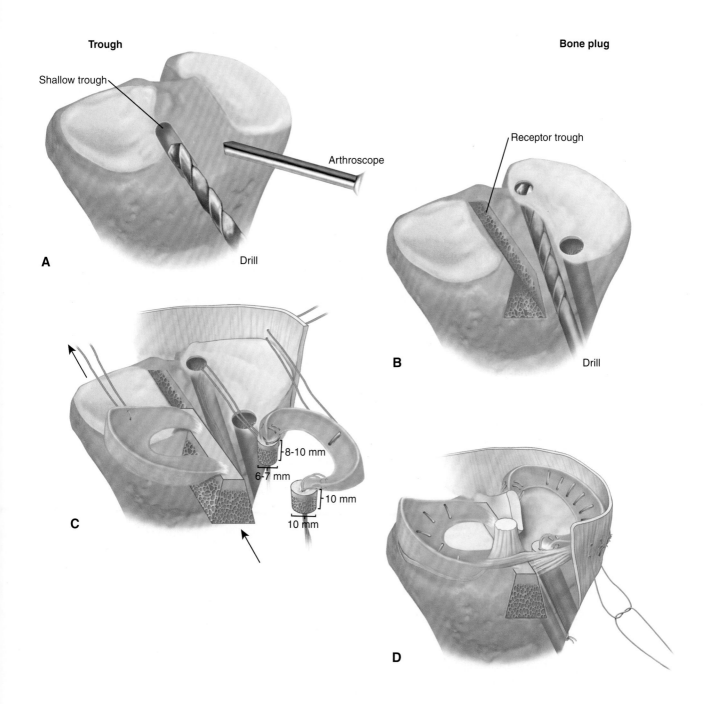

Figure 78. Meniscal transplant. A. Dovetail technique for bone bridge insertion requires drilling and later rasping for insertion of the lateral meniscus graft. **B.** Bone plug tunnels are drilled obliquely for the medial meniscus. **C.** Medial and lateral meniscus placement **D.** Final fixation and meniscal repair

Articular Cartilage Procedures

Indications and Goals: There are a variety of procedures available for treating focal chondral defects. Patients may or may not recall a specific injury. Pain, mechanical symptoms, or an effusion may be the only findings. Plain films are often normal; joint space narrowing and other findings of diffuse osteoarthritis may suggest that advanced procedures are not indicated. MRI is improving; however, it is often still difficult to diagnose focal chondral defects pre-operatively.

Procedure and Technique: There are four commonly performed procedures: Microfracture, autograft osteochondral plug transfer, autologous chondrocyte implantation (ACI), and allograft osteochondral transplantation.

Microfracture: Marrow stimulation techniques, such as microfracture, involves puncturing the subchondral bone to allow pluripotent marrow cells to escape and cover the surface of the bone with a "superclot." This will mature into fibrocartilage over time. It is important to first remove the calcified cartilage layer (usually with a curette and shaver) and then make a series of subchondral holes with angled awls at 2 to 3 mm intervals. The holes are made by aligning the awl perpendicular to the surface and inserting it deep enough to allow escape of blood and marrow elements.

Autograft Osteochondral Plug Transfer: This technique involves moving articular cartilage from an area that has less requirement for this cartilage (lower contact pressure) into an articular cartilage defect. The defect is evaluated and the geometry of the plug transferred is planned. Cylindrical cutting tools are used to harvest osteochondral plugs (typically from superolateral), a matching harvest tool is used to create a recipient site, and the plug(s) are inserted into the prepared recipient site. It is critical to have perpendicular access for both plug harvest and transfer. The defect is filled with plugs and the intervening area is microfractured or debrided to allow it to serve as "grout" for the cobblestone plugs.

ACI: This procedure involves a two-step process that includes first harvesting articular cartilage from a low-contact pressure area and then processing and culturing the chondrocytes, which are then injected under a periosteal patch at a second procedure. Periosteum is typically harvested from the proximal tibia and secured over the defect with fine absorbable suture. The chondrocyte cells are then injected under the patch which is sealed with fibrin glue. These cells then seed the resulting neocartilage.

Allograft Osteochondral Transfer: This procedure is similar to autograft plug transfer except it utilizes a matched fresh allograft, and is generally reserved for larger defects.

Post-surgical Precautions/Rehabilitation: The main goal following articular cartilage repairs is to restore full function as soon as possible by facilitating a healing response while simultaneously protecting the healing articular cartilage from excessive joint forces. Continuous passive motion (CPM) can be very beneficial in the early post-operative period, though the literature is divided as of the outcomes involving CPM units. Rehabilitation programs will vary based on the type of articular cartilage lesion or defect, the patient's overall goals and conditioning level, and the type of surgical procedure performed. In general, it may take up to 6 months before full weight-bearing running-like activities can be performed safely, and up to 1 year before complete healing has occurred. Patience compliance is critical for successful outcomes, particularly in the early post-operative phases.

Expected Outcomes: Generally, all of these procedures have reported satisfactory outcomes with success rates as high as 85% to 96% in the current literature. Microfracture appears to have the best success for smaller lesions in relatively low-demand patients as its success diminishes long-term in very active patients. Few true prospective randomized studies are available comparing techniques and to date no one procedure has been shown to be vastly superior to any of the others. The most consistent factor in determining successful outcome remains careful patient selection and individualizing treatment based on each specific patient case.

Return to Play: Typically, return to sport participation will take at the earliest 4 to 6 months post-operatively, and in many cases more like 6 to 12 months. The size of the lesion and the surgical technique used will be determining factors for return to participation timelines.

Recommended Readings

Farr J. Autologous chondrocyte implantation improves patellofemoral cartilage treatment outcomes. *Clin Orthop Relat Res.* 2007;463: 187–194.

Frisbie DD, Bowman SM, Colhoun HA, Dicarlo EF, Kawcak CE, McIlwraith CW. Evaluation of autologous chondrocyte transplantation via a collagen membrane in equine articular defects - results at 12 and 18 months. *Osteoarthritis Cartilage.* 2007;16(6):667–679.

Gill TJ, Asnis PD, Berkson EM. The treatment of articular cartilage defects using the microfracture technique. *J Orthop Sports Phys Ther.* 2006;36(10):728–738. Review.

Knutsen G, Drogset JO, Engebretsen L, Grøntvedt T, Isaksen V, Ludvigsen TC, Roberts S, Solheim E, Strand T, Johansen O. A randomized trial comparing autologous chondrocyte implantation with microfracture. Findings at five years. *J Bone Joint Surg Am.* 2007; 89(10):2105–2112.

Reinold MM, Wilk KE, Macrina LC, Dugas JR, Cain EL. Current concepts in the rehabilitation following articular cartilage repair procedures in the knee. *J Orthop Sports Phys Ther.* 2006;36(10):774–794. Review.

Siparsky P, Ryzewicz M, Peterson B, Bartz R. Arthroscopic treatment of osteoarthritis of the knee: Are there any evidence-based indications? *Clin Orthop Relat Res.* 2007;455:107–112. Review.

Vanlauwe J, Almqvist F, Bellemans J, Huskin JP, Verdonk R, Victor J. Repair of symptomatic cartilage lesions of the knee: The place of autologous chondrocyte implantation. *Acta Orthop Belg.* 2007;73(2):145–158. Review.

Wasiak J, Clar C, Villanueva E. Autologous cartilage implantation for full thickness articular cartilage defects of the knee. *Cochrane Database Syst Rev.* 2006;3:CD003323. Review.

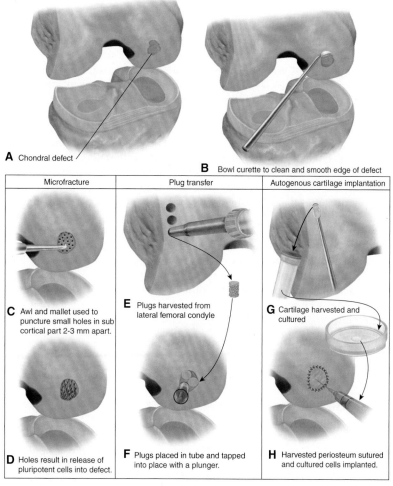

Figure 79. Options for treating full-thickness focal chondral defects. A. A chondral defect is noted and measured on the femoral condyle. **B.** A curette is used to debride the calcified cartilage layer and define edges. **C,D.** *Microfracture* is performed using and awl to puncture small holes in the subcortical bone. **E,F.** Osteochondral Autograft "plug" transfer is performed by harvesting the nonweightbearing osteochondral plugs from the superior lateral femoral condyle and placing them into the defect. Allograft plugs can be used for larger defects. **G,H.** Autogenous cartilage implantation (ACI) requires two steps. In the first surgery cartilage is harvested. Following culture, cartilage is implanted at the site of defect under a periosteal patch.

ACL Reconstruction

Indications and Goals: Anterior cruciate ligament injuries are typically a result of a non-contact pivoting injury. Patients may hear or feel a "pop" and an immediate effusion is common. If left untreated, patients may note recurrent instability (giving way), especially when attempting pivoting sports. Associated meniscal tears and chondral injuries are common. Examination typically includes a positive Lachman test and a pivot-shift test.

Procedure and Technique: Although several graft options are available, autologous hamstring and bone–patellar tendon–bone grafts are common. After debriding the ruptured ACL fibers, tunnels are drilled in the tibia and femur for the prepared graft(s). Although there is some controversy, most surgeons prefer to place the tibial tunnel in the posteromedial aspect of the ACL footprint and the femoral tunnel in the 10–10:30 position (using a clockface for orientation, right knee) with a 1 to 2 mm posterior wall. Special guides are available to assist in accurate tunnel placement. Double-bundle techniques with two tunnels in the femur (+/– two tunnels also in the tibia) have been described but have not been universally accepted.

Post-surgical Precautions/Rehabilitation: Since there are different techniques for performing an ACL reconstruction, the course of rehabilitation will depend upon the type of graft fixation utilized, whether or not the procedure was isolated at an ACL tear or involved other structural damage, and the goals of the patient. All rehabilitation interventions should also consider the physiology of tissue healing as well as the biomechanical principles of joint contact surface. Typically, ACL rehabilitation is broken into phases. The early post-operative phase focuses on pain management, scar management, the minimizing of knee joint swelling, quadriceps muscle volitional control, and gentle range of motion for the tibiofemoral and patellofemoral joints. Weight bearing can begin immediately post-operatively, with a weaning away from crutches within 1 to 2 weeks, dependent upon one's neuromuscular control and proprioceptive awareness. Once the suture wounds are closed, hydrotherapy can be initiated in an effort to gradually add weight-bearing activities with reduced joint forces from buoyancy. Exercises to improve neuromuscular control can begin gradually from the first week post-operative, with attention to not stress the graft with highly resisted knee extension exercises. Functional knee bracing is an option, with the literature reviews mixed regarding the effects of functional knee braces. However, athletes may express a sense of confidence and perception of safety while wearing a functional knee brace during the returning phases of sport specific activity.

Expected Outcomes: Overall outcomes are very good for ACL reconstructions. The differences in how outcomes are defined also play a role in how results are reported in the literature. Published studies suggest that hamstring tendon autografts are better for reducing post-operative anterior knee pain, while evidence exists, though limited in nature, that bone–patellar tendon–bone autografts provide better stability. Meanwhile, hardware removal and arthrofibrosis rates are slightly higher when using bone–patellar tendon–bone grafts. Athletes have been allowed to return to play as early as 3 to 4 months, but not without complications (e.g., patella fracture and reinjury). Delay in RTP for 6 months, or even a year, may be more prudent.

Return to Play: A return to functional activities can occur between months 4 and 6 based upon the stresses required for the activity, the individual's neuromuscular strength and proprioception, and confidence to return to activity.

Recommended Readings

Baer GS, Harner CD. Clinical outcomes of allograft versus autograft in anterior cruciate ligament reconstruction. *Clin Sports Med.* 2007;26(4):661–681. Review.

Freedman KB, D'Amato MJ, Nedeff DD, Kaz A, Bach BR Jr. Arthroscopic anterior cruciate ligament reconstruction: A metaanalysis comparing patellar tendon and hamstring tendon autografts. *Am J Sports Med.* 2003;31(1):2–11.

Lawhorn KW, Howell SM. Principles for using hamstring tendons for anterior cruciate ligament reconstruction. *Clin Sports Med.* 2007;26(4):567–585. Review.

Myer GD, Paterno MV, Ford KR, Quatman CE, Hewett TE. Rehabilitation after anterior cruciate ligament reconstruction: Criteria-based progression through the return-to-sport phase. *J Orthop Sports Phys Ther.* 2006;36(6):385–402. Review.

Poolman RW, Abouali JA, Conter HJ, Bhandari M. Overlapping systematic reviews of anterior cruciate ligament reconstruction comparing hamstring autograft with bone-patellar tendon-bone autograft: Why are they different? *J Bone Joint Surg Am.* 2007;89(7):1542–1552. Review.

Prodromos CC, Han Y, Rogowski J, Joyce B, Shi K. A meta-analysis of the incidence of anterior cruciate ligament tears as a function of gender, sport, and a knee injury-reduction regimen. *Arthroscopy.* 2007;23(12):1320–1325.e6. Review.

Schoderbek RJ Jr, Treme GP, Miller MD. Bone-patella tendon-bone autograft anterior cruciate ligament reconstruction. *Clin Sports Med.* 2007;26(4):525–547. Review.

Smékal D, Kalina R, Urban J. [Rehabilitation after arthroscopic anterior cruciate ligament reconstruction.] *Acta Chir Orthop Traumatol Cech.* 2006;73(6):421–428. Review.

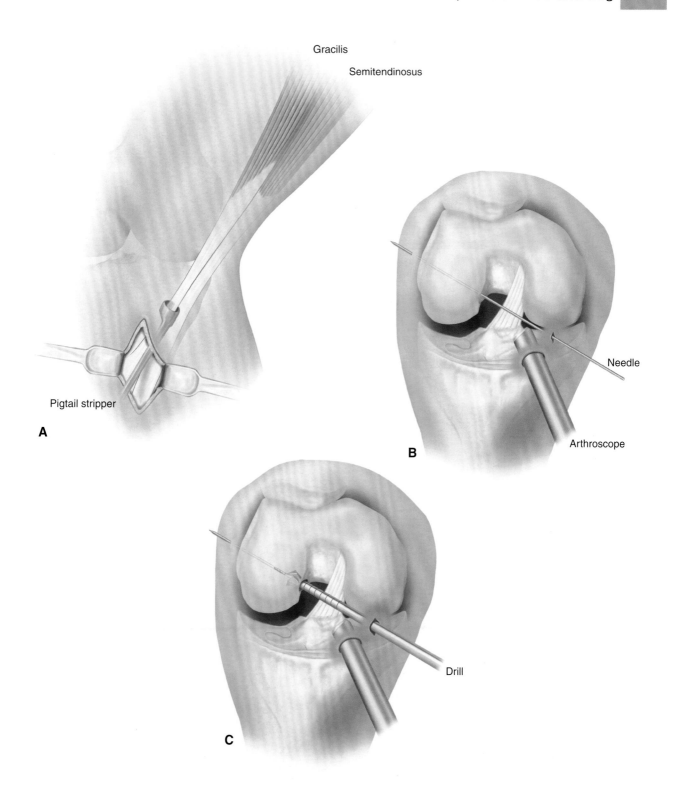

Figure 80. ACL Reconstruction. A. Autograft hamstring grafts are harvested. **B.** The ACL femoral footprint is defined and a guide pin is placed from an accessory medial portal. **C.** The Femoral tunnel is drilled. **D.** The tibial guide is used to place the tibial tunnel. **E.** Completed Femoral and tibial tunnels. **F.** The Harvested tendon is prepared and passed through the prepared tunnels. **G.** While multiple fixation options exist, endobutton fixation is shown (femoral) with tibial interference screw fixation. (*continued*)

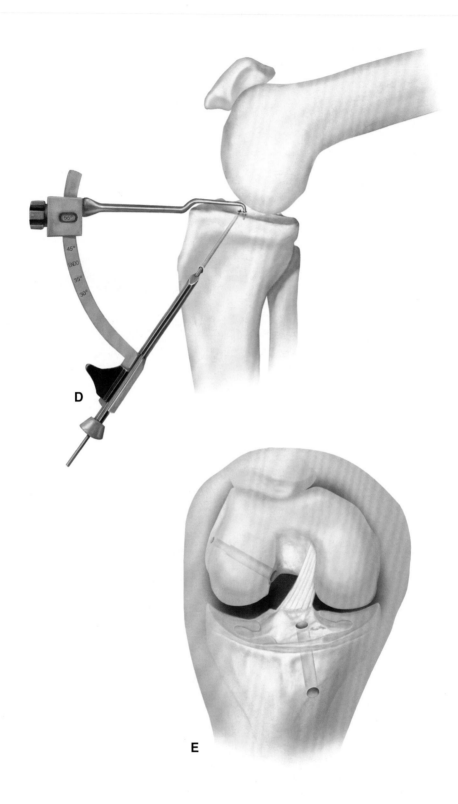

D

E

Figure 80. (*continued*)

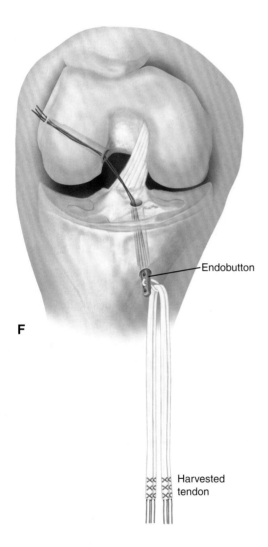

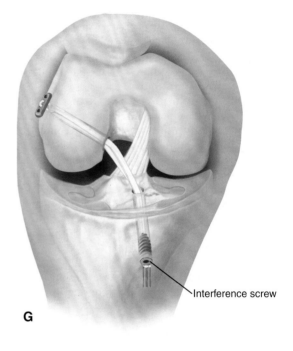

F

G

Endobutton

Harvested
tendon

Interference screw

Figure 80. (*continued*)

PCL Reconstruction

Indications and Goals: Posterior cruciate ligament (PCL) injuries are much less common than ACL injuries, and surgical indications are limited. These injuries are typically a result of a blow to the proximal tibia, but are also commonly a result of knee dislocations with other associated ligamentous injuries. The key examination is the posterior drawer test. This involves applying a posterior force to the tibia with the knee in 70 to 90 degrees of flexion. Significant posterior displacement may represent a combined PCL and posterolateral corner injury. Surgical indications included combined injuries and isolated PCL injuries that have failed non-operative treatment. Isolated PCL injuries are typically treated non-surgically.

Procedure and Technique: There are a variety of techniques for PCL reconstruction. These include the trans-tibial technique which uses an anterior to posterior tunnel, and a tibial inlay technique in which the PCL graft is placed into a trough in the back of the tibia. Either one or two tunnels can be used in the femur. The graft(s) are passed and secured with the knee in flexion while an anterior drawer force is placed on the tibia.

Post-surgical Precautions/Rehabilitation: Typically, a knee brace is applied locked in full extension immediate post-operatively for the first 2 weeks. Active knee flexion is avoided, and emphasis is on maintaining full knee extension with quadriceps control. Passively, range of motion is restored from 0 to 60 degrees, with simultaneously performed patella mobilizations. Straight leg raises may also be initiated, avoiding active hip extension. Pain control and reduction of post-operative effusion should also be addressed. At week two, the brace can be unlocked to allow for 90 degrees of motion with initiation of gentle hamstring muscle action exercises. The primary goal is to obtain approximately 110 degrees of knee flexion by week 8. At this time, weight-bearing and proprioceptive exercises are progressed, while gentle squat-like exercises can begin. The brace can be discontinued between weeks 6 and 8. With near 85% strength of the quadriceps and hamstrings demonstrated bilaterally, at week 12, single-plane running activities can begin with progression based upon one's post-operative joint stability and neuromuscular control.

Expected Outcomes: Despite the continued exploration for the optimal graft and technique to reconstruct a torn PCL, outcomes reported in the literature yield satisfactory results related to joint stability and return to function.

Return to Play: Return to sports participation varies based upon the type of fixation chosen and the demands of the activity itself that one is returning to. Typically, the return timeline can range from 6 to 9 months, though some athletes have returned as soon as 3 to 4 months and others may take up to one full year for functional readiness.

Recommended Readings

Campbell RB, Jordan SS, Sekiya JK. Arthroscopic tibial inlay for posterior cruciate ligament reconstruction. *Arthroscopy.* 2007; 23(12):1356.e1–e4. Epub 2007 Apr 24.

Höher J, Scheffler S, Weiler A. Graft choice and graft fixation in PCL reconstruction. *Knee Surg Sports Traumatol Arthrosc.* 2003;11(5): 297–306. Epub 2003 Aug 26. Review.

Johnson DH, Fanelli GC, Miller MD. PCL 2002: Indications, double-bundle versus inlay technique and revision surgery. *Arthroscopy.* 2002;18(9 suppl):40–52.

Peccin MS, Almeida GJ, Amaro J, Cohen M, Soares BG, Atallah AN. Interventions for treating posterior cruciate ligament injuries of the knee in adults. *Cochrane Database Syst Rev.* 2005;(2):CD002939. Review.

St. Pierre P, Miller MD. Posterior cruciate ligament injuries. *Clin Sports Med.* 1999;18(1):199–221.

Weiler A, Jung TM, Strobel MJ. [Arthroscopic assisted posterior cruciate ligament reconstruction and posterolateral stabilisation using autologous hamstring tendon grafts] *Unfallchirurg.* 2006;109(1):61–71. Review. German.

Weimann A, Wolfert A, Zantop T, Eggers AK, Raschke M, Petersen W. Reducing the "killer turn" in posterior cruciate ligament reconstruction by fixation level and smoothing the tibial aperture. *Arthroscopy.* 2007;23(10):1104–1111.

Wiley WB, Owen JR, Pearson SE, Wayne JS, Goradia VK. Medial femoral condyle strength after tunnel placement for single- and double-bundle posterior cruciate ligament reconstruction. *J Knee Surg.* 2007;20(3):223–227.

Wind WM Jr, Bergfeld JA, Parker RD. Evaluation and treatment of posterior cruciate ligament injuries: Revisited. *Am J Sports Med.* 2004;32(7):1765–1775. Review.

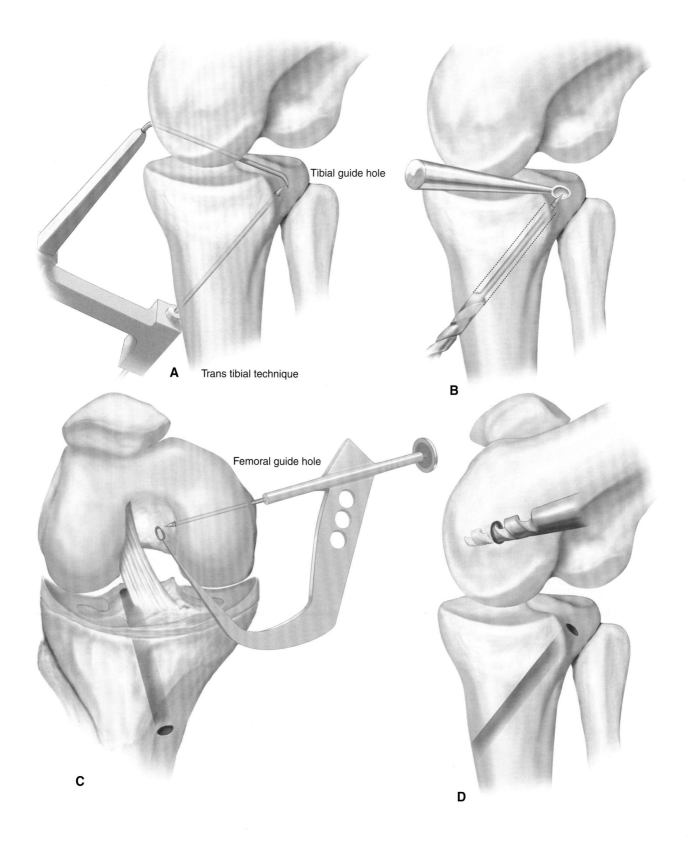

Figure 81. PCL Reconstruction. A. A Transtibial drill guide is used to place the tibial tunnel
B. The Drill tip is protected to avoid injury to the posterior structures **C, D.** The
Femoral footprint is noted and femoral tunnel is drilled. **E, F.** Graft with bone block
is prepared and fixed. **G.** Alternatively, a tibial inlay technique may be used. (*continued*)

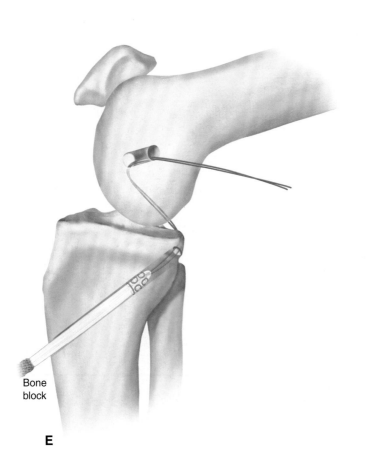

Bone
block

E

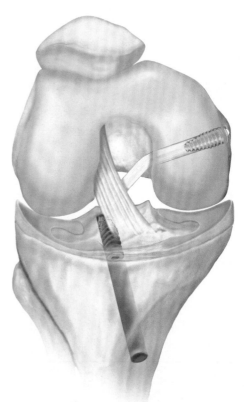

F Trans tibial technique completed

Figure 81. (*continued*)

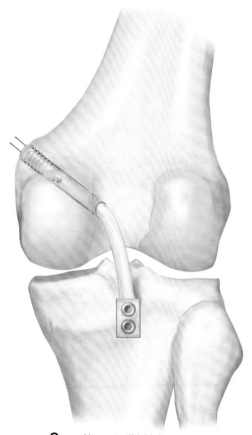

G   Alternate tibial inlay

Figure 81. (*continued*)

LCL/PLC Reconstruction

Indications and Goals: Injuries to the lateral collateral ligament (LCL) and the posterolateral corner (PLC) are rarely isolated. Injuries commonly include a rotational force and commonly include knee dislocations. Examination includes external rotation asymmetry (dial test) and may include a posterolateral drawer. Complete LCL and PLC injuries mandate surgical intervention.

Procedure and Technique: Primary repair of PLC injuries involve restoring normal anatomy. Avulsion injuries are repaired back to their origin with suture anchors or drill holes. These are typically backed-up with static grafts that limit external rotation. Chronic reconstruction involves using static grafts in a variety of techniques. The Larson Figure 8 technique involves passing a graft across the fibular neck and securing it anterior to the lateral femoral epicondyle. The Muller popliteal bypass technique includes passing a graft across the tibia from anterior to posterior and securing it anterior to a point anterior to the lateral femoral epicondyle. These procedures can be combined. Other procedures attempt to produce a more anatomical reconstruction using two fixation points on the femur.

Post-surgical Precautions/Rehabilitation: The early post-operative phase should focus on pain reduction, minimizing knee joint effusion, and initiating gentle range of motion exercises. A knee brace is applied locked at full extension for approximately 6 weeks, during which time minimal to no weight bearing is allowed. Straight-leg-raise exercises may be initiated immediately post-operative with the exception of hip extension, waiting until 4 months post-operative to begin these. Three months after surgery weight-bearing strengthening exercises can begin with a focus on regaining neuromuscular control. Running in a single plane should not begin until approximately 4 to 6 months post-operatively and should be based on patient's goals, leg strength, proprioceptive control, neuromuscular control, range of motion, and confidence level.

Expected Outcomes: Reconstruction of the posterior lateral corner via an allograft of the popliteus, popliteofibular, and fibulocollateral ligaments yield stable reconstructions with excellent functional results. Post-operatively, individuals with isolated PCL injuries demonstrated greater range of motion and reduced incidence of failure versus those with multiligamentous knees.

Return to Play: With major multiple ligament injuries (which usually include PLC injury), return to play at the previously performed level may never be possible. Return to play in general may be possible, but not any earlier than 1 year post-operatively.

Recommended Readings

Arciero RA. Anatomic posterolateral corner knee reconstruction. *Arthroscopy.* 2005;21(9):1147.

Bicos J, Arciero RA. Novel approach for reconstruction of the posterolateral corner using a free tendon graft technique. *Sports Med Arthrosc.* 2006;14(1):28–36.

Cooper JM, McAndrews PT, LaPrade RF. Posterolateral corner injuries of the knee: Anatomy, diagnosis, and treatment. *Sports Med Arthrosc.* 2006;14(4):213–220.

Markolf KL, Graves BR, Sigward SM, Jackson SR, McAllister DR. How well do anatomical reconstructions of the posterolateral corner restore varus stability to the posterior cruciate ligament-reconstructed knee? *Am J Sports Med.* 2007;35(7):1117–1122.

Sanchez AR II, Sugalski MT, LaPrade RF. Anatomy and biomechanics of the lateral side of the knee. *Sports Med Arthrosc.* 2006; 14(1):2–11.

Stannard JP, Brown SL, Robinson JT, et al. Reconstruction of the posterolateral corner of the knee. *Arthroscopy.* 2005;21(9):1051–1059.

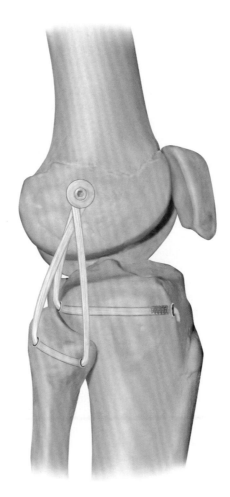

Figure 82. Lateral collateral ligament and Posteriorolateral corner reconstruction

MCL/Posteromedial Corner Reconstruction

Indications and Goals: Medial collateral ligament (MCL) injuries are common, but rarely require surgical treatment. These injuries are a result of a valgus contact force. The knee should be examined in both 30 degrees of flexion and in full extension. Valgus opening in flexion only is typical of an isolated MCL injury, which is treated non-operatively with a hinged brace for 6 to 8 weeks. Valgus opening in full extension is a more ominous sign and may represent a combined MCL and ACL/PCL injury. Treatment of MCL injuries is usually only indicated in knee dislocations or with chronic MCL laxity.

Procedure and Technique: Primary repair or advancement should be attempted, especially with acute injuries. Suture anchor, staples, or screw-washer constructs can be used. The posterior oblique ligament (capsular thickening posterior to the MCL) should be imbricated/advanced anteriorly if there is laxity in this structure. The repair can be supplemented with a tendon using the modified Bosworth technique. This involves stripping the semitendinosus tendon after leaving it intact at its distal insertion. Muscle fibers are removed from the tendon and a whip stitch is placed in its free end. The tendon is then looped over a screw and soft tissue washer that is placed at the medial femoral epicondyle and then secured distally with a screw and/or staple. It is important to check for isometric positioning of the femoral screw before securing the graft. This can be accomplished by provisionally selecting a location for the screw, wrapping the graft over this location and then flexing and extending the knee to ensure that there is not excessive graft movement.

Post-surgical Precautions/Rehabilitation: The key for early post-operative rehabilitation is to avoid excessive valgus forces while encouraging controlled sagittal plane range of motion to facilitate mobilization. Immediate post-operative phases will include wearing a long leg brace, oftentimes locked during ambulation at 30 degrees of flexion. However, active and passive range of motion should occur outside of the brace in a controlled manner beginning day one. Gentle cross-friction massage to the incisional region will reduce localized sensitivity, and regular ice, compression and elevation will assist with controlling post-operative effusion. The patient should regain full extension and 90 degrees of knee flexion within 4 to 6 weeks post-operative, with ambulation using crutches weaned off in a similar timeframe based upon progression level. Quadricep and hamstring strength can be assessed between 12 and 16 weeks, and straight line jogging can begin when range of motion, strength, and proprioception return to acceptable functional levels. Lateral movements are the last functional activity to be restored, as these movements place added and isolated stress on the medial and lateral compartments of the knee.

Expected Outcomes: Though some residual valgus joint laxity may persist for quite some time, post-operative joint stability fairs very well. Localized tenderness may persist, and the greatest complication concern is arthrofibrosis for a lack of early controlled mobilization.

Return to Play: Return to participation depends upon the degree of injury. In some cases, complete tears of the medical collateral ligament are not surgically repaired. For operative cases, 6 months or more may be required prior to an athlete having regained full function, especially if the sport requires large amounts of lateral movement (volleyball, ice hockey, basketball, soccer). For multiple ligament injuries, return to participation will be more challenging and may not be possible at the preinjury level.

Recommended Readings

Azar FM. Evaluation and treatment of chronic medial collateral ligament injuries of the knee. *Sports Med Arthros.* 2006;14(2):84–90.

Edson CJ. Conservative and postoperative rehabilitation of isolated and combined injuries of the medial collateral ligament. *Sports Med Arthrosc.* 2006;14(2):105–110.

Indelicato PA. Nonoperative management of complete tears of the medial collateral ligament. *Orthop Rev.* 1989;18(9):947–952.

Pressman A, Johnson DH. A review of ski injuries resulting in combined injury to the anterior cruciate ligament and medial collateral ligaments. *Arthroscopy.* 2003;19(2):194–202.

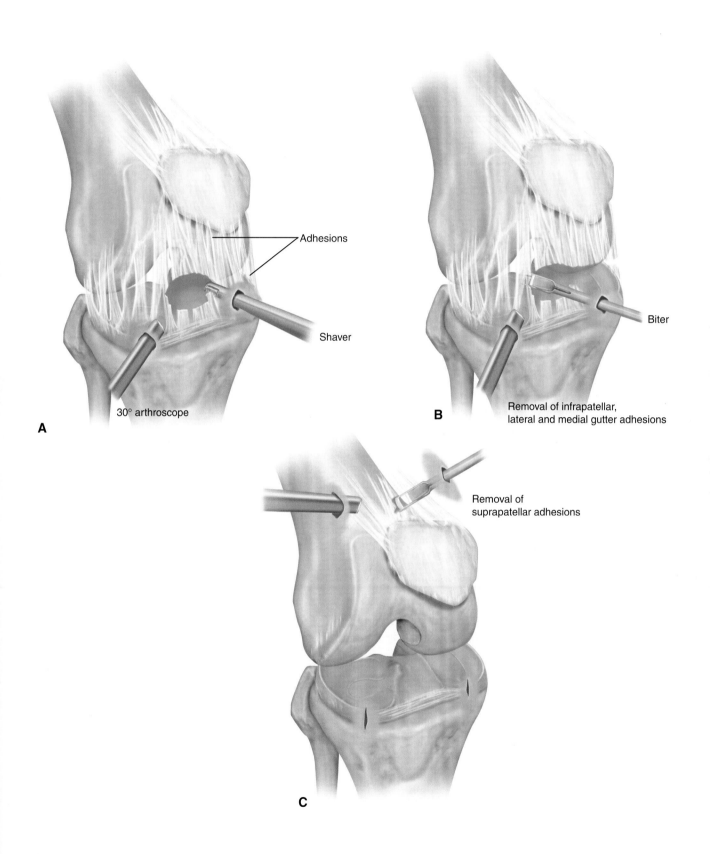

Figure 85. Arthroscopic lysis of adhesions with an arthroscopic shaver (A), and biter (B). Suprapatellar portals can be used to resect superior adhesions (C)

Osteotomy

Indications and Goals: Osteotomies are required to restore an altered mechanical axis and/or unload a portion of the joint in conjunction with meniscal or articular cartilage procedures. The normal mechanical axis falls just medial to midline in the knee. The goal is to unload the joint by moving the mechanical axis 62% of the way across the knee to the opposite compartment to unload the affected compartment.

Procedure and Technique: Most osteotomies are performed for varus knees and the idea is to shift the mechanical axis into the lateral compartment. This can be done with a closing or opening wedge osteotomy on the tibia. In a closing wedge osteotomy, a wedge of bone is removed and a plate and screws are fixed to the lateral aspect of the tibia to hold the reduction. For an opening wedge osteotomy, a cut is made in the tibia and this is opened so that a wedge of bone can be placed into the osteotomy to hold the gap open while it heals. Special plates and instruments are available for both techniques. For the opening wedge osteotomy, special plates with a block of metal in the middle allows precise control of the amount of opening. Occasionally, it is necessary to shift the axis medially for lateral compartment problems. This is typically done on the femur. The closing wedge technique is done medially with a blade plate. The opening wedge technique is done laterally with an extended plate with a metal block in the middle.

Post-surgical Precautions/Rehabilitation: Oftentimes post-operative rehabilitation involves a few days in the hospital under direct supervised care. A continuous passive motion device may be utilized to facilitate passive range of motion. Goals also consist of reducing pain and knee joint swelling, while establishing isometric quadriceps muscle volitional control. Upon hospital discharge, a knee brace will be worn to promote stability of the joint for partial weight bearing, though crutches or a walker will likely be used for up to 6 weeks post-operatively. One of the primary focuses is to allow for adequate bone healing, which may take up to 6 months. Careful attention not to increase joint forces too soon is critical. Non–weight-bearing muscular strengthening exercises are beneficial and usually begin 4 to 6 weeks after the surgery, emphasizing quadriceps and hamstrings.

Expected Outcomes: High tibial osteotomies have been shown to improve knee function and reduce joint related pain, with good results obtained in patients for up to almost 9 years post-operatively.

Return to Play: Return to participation in sports is limited as an option for those who undergo osteotomies. This procedure is often indicated for advanced deformities and arthrosis, whereby a return to functional activities of daily living with less pain and discomfort is more of a realistic goal.

Recommended Readings

Brouwer RW, Raaij van TM, Bierma-Zeinstra SM, Verhagen AP, Jakma TS, Verhaar JA. Osteotomy for treating knee osteoarthritis. *Cochrane Database Syst Rev.* 2007;18(3):CD004019. Review.

Giffin JR, Shannon FJ. The role of the high tibial osteotomy in the unstable knee. *Sports Med Arthrosc.* 2007;15(1):23–31. Review.

Jackson DW, Warkentine B. Technical aspects of computer-assisted opening wedge high tibial osteotomy. *J Knee Surg.* 2007;20(2):134–141. Review.

Preston CF, Fulkerson EW, Meislin R, Di Cesare PE. Osteotomy about the knee: Applications, techniques, and results. *J Knee Surg.* 2005;18(4):258–272. Review.

Puddu G, Cipolla M, Cerullo G, Franco V, Giannì E. Osteotomies: The surgical treatment of the valgus knee. *Sports Med Arthrosc.* 2007;15(1):15–22. Review.

Wright JM, Crockett HC, Slawski DP, Madsen MW, Windsor RE. High tibial osteotomy. *J Am Acad Orthop Surg.* 2005;13(4):279–289. Review.

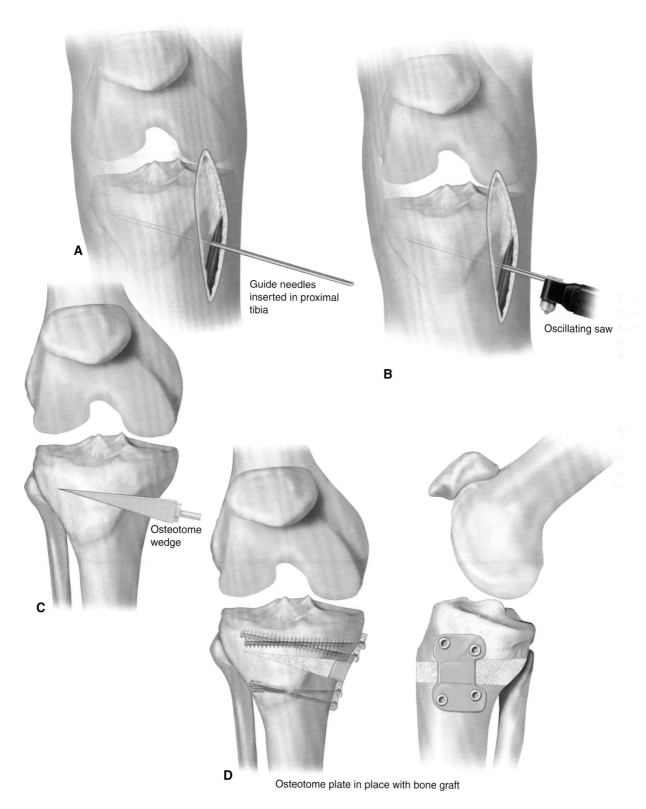

A Guide needles inserted in proximal tibia

B Oscillating saw

C Osteotome wedge

D Osteotome plate in place with bone graft

Figure 86. Opening wedge high tibial osteotomy. A Guide pin is inserted (**A**) followed by proximal tibial cut (**B**) and wedge insertion for calculated correction (**C**). A special plate is then placed to maintain the new angle.

Arthroplasty (Knee Replacement)

Indications and Goals: Knee arthroplasty is actually a "resurfacing" rather than a total replacement of the articular surfaces of the knee. It is indicated for arthritis that is refractory to non-operative management. Unicompartmental arthroplasty is used to replace one compartment, typically the medial compartment. Total knee arthroplasty replace all compartments (medial, lateral, and patellofemoral). A total knee is actually a resurfacing procedure that covers the affected surfaces with metal and high tech plastic.

Procedure and Technique: A series of cutting guides and sizing instruments are used to make the appropriate cuts on all articular surfaces of the knee. Trial components are placed and the knee is checked to ensure that appropriate sizes of all components are selected. Soft tissue "balancing" is an important part of this procedure. The final components are then cemented in place using methyl methacrylate cement.

Post-surgical Precautions/Rehabilitation: Immediate post-operative goals should focus on wound healing and prevention of arthrofibrosis. Some patients spend a few days in the hospital, and others will be discharged on the same day, pending health status. Crutches, a cane, or even a walker or wheelchair in some circumstances (bilateral replacement performed simultaneously) may be needed for up to 6 weeks, depending on one's functional ambulatory status and pain tolerance. The first few weeks of rehabilitation will emphasize knee joint mobilization and quadriceps strengthening. Weight-bearing exercises can begin immediately with supervision, and once the surgical incision closes aquatic exercises may be performed. Patients can usually resume their normal activities within 3 to 6 weeks following the total knee joint replacement. It is important to avoid overworking or straining the knee during this recovery period.

Expected Outcomes: Patients undergoing total knee arthroplasties demonstrate improvements in functional performance measures. Gait becomes more symmetric and quadriceps strength becomes stronger. Many are able to return to premorbid levels of healthy activity. High-impact sports such as running should be avoided, yet other activities such as walking, cycling, and swimming are highly encouraged.

Return to Play: Total knee joint arthroplasty procedures are not performed with the goal of returning to competitive sport. However, some can return to limited recreational activities typically after a timeframe of at least 6 months or more post-operatively.

Recommended Readings

Dorr LD, Chao L. The emotional state of the patient after total hip and knee arthroplasty. *Clin Orthop Relat Res.* 2007;463:7–12. Review.

Griffin T, Rowden N, Morgan D, Atkinson R, Woodruff P, Maddern G. Unicompartmental knee arthroplasty for the treatment of unicompartmental osteoarthritis: A systematic study. *ANZ J Surg.* 2007;77(4):214–221. Review.

Kane RL, Wilt T, Suarez-Almazor ME, Fu SS. Disparities in total knee replacements: A review. *Arthritis Rheum.* 2007;57(4):562–567. Review.

McClelland JA, Webster KE, Feller JA. Gait analysis of patients following total knee replacement: A systematic review. *Knee.* 2007; 14(4):253–263. Epub 2007 May 24. Review.

Minns Lowe CJ, Barker KL, Dewey M, Sackley CM. Effectiveness of physiotherapy exercise after knee arthroplasty for osteoarthritis: Systematic review and meta-analysis of randomised controlled trials. *BMJ.* 2007;335(7624):812. Epub 2007 Sep 20. Review.

Widuchowski W, Widuchowski J, Reszka P. Postoperative treatment and rehabilitation after total knee arthroplasty. *Ortop Traumatol Rehabil.* 2002;4(6):766–772.

Yoshida Y, Mizner RL, Ramsey DK, Snyder-Mackler L. Examining outcomes from total knee arthroplasty and the relationship between quadriceps strength and knee function over time. *Clin Biomech (Bristol, Avon).* 2008 Mar;23(3):320–328.

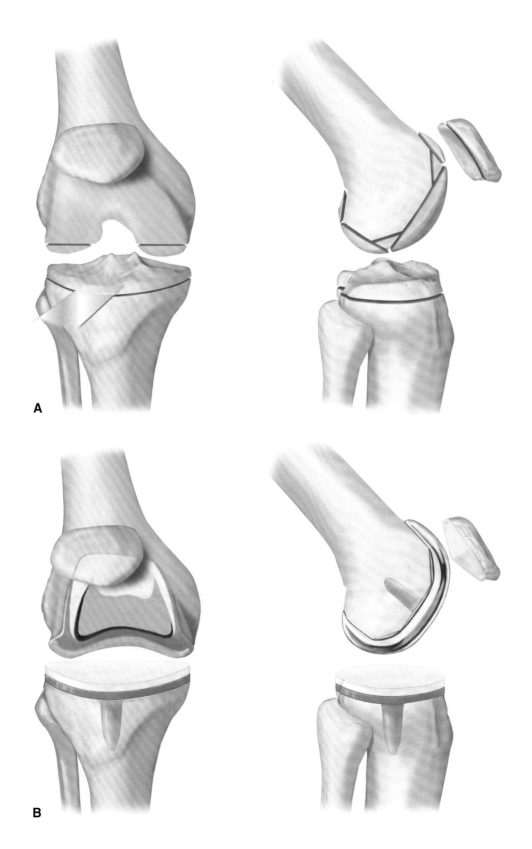

Figure 87. Typical bone cuts in total knee arthroplasty demonstrated (A). Total knee arthroplasty with cruciate retaining design (B).

Proximal Patellar Realignment

Indications and Goals: This procedure is indicated for patellar instability without an abnormal quadriceps/patellar tendon insertion axis (Q Angle) in patients who have failed non-operative treatment (quadriceps and VMO strengthening).

Procedure and Technique: Two general techniques are available: Primary repair and graft placement. Both techniques are designed to repair or replace the medial patellofemoral ligament (MPFL) which is the primary restraint to lateral displacement of the patella. Repair is usually done at the femoral insertion of the ligament, just anterior to the medial epicondyle and just below the adductor tubercle. Suture anchors are typically used and the repair is tensioned with the knee in approximately 40 degrees of flexion. Reconstruction uses a free graft (semitendinosus autograft or tibialis anterior allograft) or primary repair. If a free graft is used, the graft is passed through drill hole(s) in the upper half of the patella and secured at the femoral attachment site of the MPFL. Prior to final fixation, isometry is checked by holding both ends of the graft while cycling the knee.

Post-surgical Precautions/Rehabilitation: Immediate attention is placed upon the healing of the realigned tissue. One's leg is locked in an immobilizing brace for the first 3 weeks allowing only 0 to 30 degrees of knee flexion, using crutches with non–weight-bearing status. Supervised passive patella mobilization and gentle knee joint passive range of motion can be performed within the brace, and submaximal isometrics for the surrounding knee muscles are allowed. Each subsequent 2 weeks, the brace can be opened an additional 30 degrees of movement toward knee flexion, and partial weight bearing can progress about 25% each 2 weeks. At approximately 6 to 8 weeks post-operative, the brace can be discarded, and weaning off crutches toward full weight-bearing status is a goal. Strengthening exercises should continue for up to 6 months to assure neuromuscular control of the knee and increased emphasis on weight-bearing proprioception.

Expected Outcomes: Proximal patellar realignments appear to significantly improve congruence angles and lateral patellofemoral angles. Post-operative reports of episodes of patellar dislocation are low. Arthroscopic realignment of the patella yields less morbidity and faster rehabilitation versus established open procedures; however, MPFL imbrication or reconstruction with a free graft has been a more popular procedure.

Return to Play: Proximal patellar realignments are intensive procedures that require high levels of post-operative compliance. The timeframe to return to sport participation under optimal circumstances is 6 months or more post-operatively. It is not uncommon for minor residual discomfort to exist, and continued quadriceps muscle strengthening to be restored even after 6 months time.

Recommended Readings

Ali S, Bhatti A. Arthroscopic proximal realignment of the patella for recurrent instability: Report of a new surgical technique with 1 to 7 years of follow-up. *Arthroscopy*. 2007;23(3):305–311.

Halbrecht JL. Arthroscopic patella realignment: An all-inside technique. *Arthroscopy*. 2001;17(9):940–945.

Shen HC, Chao KH, Huang GS, Pan RY, Lee CH. Combined proximal and distal realignment procedures to treat the habitual dislocation of the patella in adults. *Am J Sports Med*. 2007;35(12):2101–2108. Epub 2007 Aug 27.

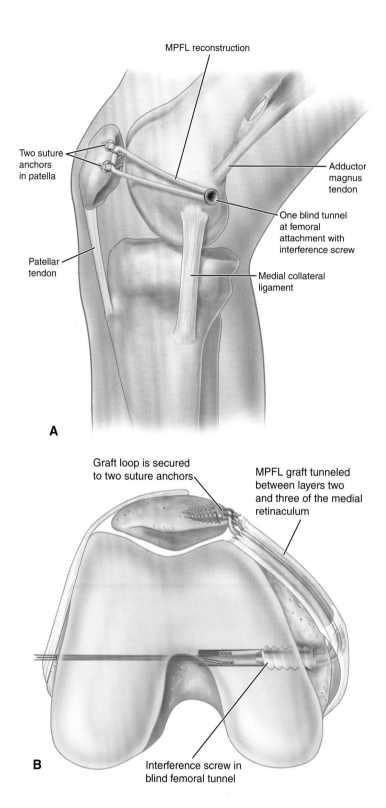

MPFL reconstruction

Two suture
anchors
in patella

Adductor
magnus
tendon

One blind tunnel
at femoral
attachment with
interference screw

Patellar
tendon

Medial collateral
ligament

A

Graft loop is secured
to two suture anchors

MPFL graft tunneled
between layers two
and three of the medial
retinaculum

Interference screw in
blind femoral tunnel

B

**Figure 88. A. Proximal patella realignment with MPFL reconstruction. B. An interference screw
and suture anchors are used to secure the graft.**

Distal Patellar Realignment

Indications and Goals: This procedure is indicated for patients with recurrent patellar instability and abnormal quadriceps-patellar tendon alignment (High Q-angles). Because this surgery increased contact pressures in the superomedial patella, chondrosis of this area is a contraindication to this procedure. There remains some controversy regarding whether a proximal or a distal realignment (or both) is required in an individual patient, and it largely remains a matter of surgeon's choice.

Procedure and Technique: Although a variety of procedures have been described, the most popular technique is anteromedialization of the tibial tubercle as popularized by Fulkerson. An oblique cut is made in the tibia at the patellar tendon insertion and the tubercle is shifted anterior and medially. It is fixed in its new location with anterior to posterior screws.

Post-surgical Precautions/Rehabilitation: Rehabilitation for a distal patellar realignment is very similar to that of the proximal patella realignment, with one of the major differences being a slightly sooner increased range of motion allowed within the brace. Immediate attention is placed upon the healing of the realigned tissue. One's leg is locked in an immobilizing brace for the first 3 weeks allowing only 0 to 30 degrees of knee flexion, using crutches with non–weight-bearing status. Supervised passive patella mobilization and gentle knee joint passive range of motion can be performed within the brace, and submaximal isometrics for the surrounding knee muscles are allowed. At approximately 4 weeks post-operative, the brace may be unlocked from 0 to 90 degrees of flexion and partial weight bearing can progress about 25% each 2 weeks, based upon evidence of bone healing through radiographs. At approximately 6 to 8 weeks post-operative, the brace can be discarded, and weaning off crutches toward full weight-bearing status is a goal. Strengthening exercises should continue for up to 6 months to assure neuromuscular control of the knee.

Expected Outcomes: Overall results are reported to be satisfactory. Studies have been unable to identify any correlations between clinical results and age, sex, body weight, body height, preoperative pain scores or Lysholm scores. Clinical outcomes do however, correlate with the severity of articular damage and the increased amount of patellar realignment required.

Return to Play: Typical return to participation may take 4 to 6 months post-operatively, following the complete healing of the osteotomy and restoration of full range of motion and muscle control. It is not uncommon for minor residual discomfort to exist, and continued quadriceps muscle strengthening to be restored even after 6 months time.

Recommended Readings

Gibson WK, Dugdale TW. A trigonometric analysis of distal patellofemoral realignment. *Orthop.* 1995;18(5):457–460.

Mangine RE, Eifert-Mangine M, Burch D, Becker BL, Farag L. Postoperative management of the patellofemoral patient. *J Orthop Sports Phys Ther.* 1998;28(5):323–335.

Post WR, Fulkerson JP. Distal realignment of the patellofemoral joint. Indications, effects, results, and recommendations. *Orthop Clin North Am.* 1992;23(4):631–643. Review.

Wang CJ, Chan YS, Chen HH, Wu ST. Factors affecting the outcome of distal realignment for patellofemoral disorders of the knee. *Knee.* 2005;12(3):195–200. Epub 2004 Oct 19.

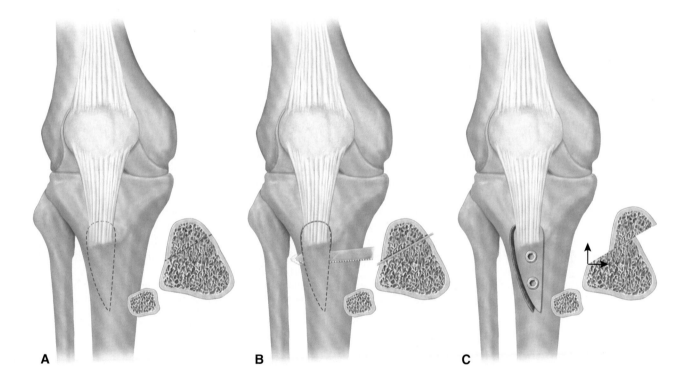

Figure 89. Knee distal patella realignment (A-C). Note that the tubercle is cut obliquely and shifted anterior and medial.

Quadriceps and Patellar Tendon Debridement/Repair

Indications and Goals: Patellar, or less commonly, quadriceps tendon debridement is indicated in patients with refractory tendinosis that has failed extended non-operative treatment. Tendon ruptures may or may not have antecedent tendinosis. Patellar tendon ruptures classically occur in patients under 40 years old and quadriceps tendon ruptures occur in patients over 40. Repair is indicated for all ruptures unless there are other mitigating factors (health, ambulatory status, etc.).

Procedure and Technique: Tendon debridement involves excising an ellipse of tissue from the tendon. The area of tendinosis is typically immediately adjacent to the patella. Recently, debridement of the inferior pole of the patella with an arthroscopic burr has been described. Patellar and quadriceps tendon ruptures are repaired by placing heavy running/locking sutures (Bunnell or Krackow) into the ends of the tunnel and then pulling these sutures through drill holes to the opposite side of the patella where they are tied.

Post-surgical Precautions/Rehabilitation: Rehabilitation depends upon the amount of surgical work performed, and the relationship between tissue removal and tissue repair. With tissue debridement, mildly conservative care is approached with the use of a long leg brace as needed, and weight bearing determined by the surgeon. Emphasis is placed upon reestablishing functional range of motion and neuromuscular control without over-stressing the debrided tissue. With repaired procedures, post-operative rehabilitation takes a much more cautious approach. Long leg brace is applied immediate post-operative, with no weight bearing allowed for up to 4 weeks, based upon the type of structural tissue repair performed. Range of motion within the brace is limited, and supervised rehabilitation is required to assist with passive range of motion. Once adequate healing of the repaired tissue has occurred and tissue tensile strength has improved, controlled active exercises, increased passive and active range of motion, increased progressive weight bearing, and discarding of the brace may occur.

Expected Outcomes: Outcomes vary based upon the procedure performed and the amount of tissue debrided/repaired. Most patients, regardless of procedure performed, will reach their preinjury levels of activity 6 months post-operative. It is not uncommon to lack a few degrees of knee extension, thus this should be emphasized during the rehabilitation process, through not too early or aggressively for fear of over-stressing the tissue.

Return to Play: Typically, return to sport participation may take up to 4 to 6 months post-operatively. However, this is a significant injury and procedure, and some athletes may not be able to return to play, particularly at the same level.

Recommended Readings

Greis PE, Holmstrom MC, Lahav A. Surgical treatment options for patella tendon rupture, Part I: Acute. *Orthop.* 2005;28(7):672–679; quiz 680–1. Review.

Greis PE, Lahav A, Holmstrom MC. Surgical treatment options for patella tendon rupture, part II: Chronic. *Orthop.* 2005;28(8):765–769; quiz 770–1. Review.

Hardy JR, Chimutengwende-Gordon M, Bakar I. Rupture of the quadriceps tendon: An association with a patellar spur. *J Bone Joint Surg Br.* 2005;87(10):1361–1363. Erratum in: *J Bone Joint Surg Br.* 2006;88(6):837.

Kaeding CC, Pedroza AD, Powers BC. Surgical treatment of chronic patellar tendinosis: A systematic review. *Clin Orthop Relat Res.* 2007;455:102–106. Review.

Moonot P, Fazal MA. Traumatic patella tendon rupture: Early mobilisation following surgical repair. *Inj.* 2005;36(11):1385. Epub 2005 Sep 26.

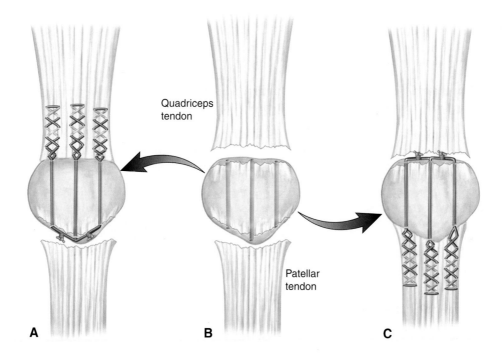

Figure 90. Quadriceps (A) and patella (B) tendon repair using longitudinal drill holes through the patella for passage of suture (C).

Nerve Decompression

Indications and Goals: Lower extremity nerves can be compressed at a variety of locations. Below are some of the more common:

Nerve	Site of Entrapment
Saphenous	Adductor canal
Common peroneal	Neck of fibula
Superficial peroneal	Fascia 10–12 cm proximal to the tip of the lateral malleolus
Posterior tibial	Tarsal tunnel behind medial malleolus
Medial plantar	Distal to medial malleolus (Jogger's Foot)
Lateral plantar (ADQ)	Abductor Hallucis fascia (Baxter's nerve)
Digital	Web space (Morton's neuroma)

Symptoms typically include numbness, tingling, and/or weakness in the distribution of the affected nerve. Electro-diagnostic studies (EMG/NCS) can be helpful in confirming the diagnosis.

Procedure and Technique: Surgical treatment involves exploring the affected nerve and releasing any areas of entrapment. Neurolysis is commonly performed after the nerve is released.

Post-surgical Precautions/Rehabilitation: Rehabilitation following a nerve decompression requires careful attention to wound closure, then a short time of reduced activity prior to any stressful muscular activity that would lead to increased lower extremity swelling. No formal supervised rehabilitation is necessary as long as patient education occurs in a meaningful way early on.

Expected Outcomes: Nerve decompressions are relatively safe and effective procedures, with outcomes yielding improvements with restored sensation, increased muscular strength, and decreased pain.

Return to Play: Return to participation in sport typically requires 2 to 4 months depending upon the extent of surgery required for the release.

Recommended Readings

Humphreys DB, Novak CB, Mackinnon SE. Patient outcome after common peroneal nerve decompression. *J Neurosurg.* 2007;107(2): 314–318.

Malavolta M, Malavolta L. Surgery for superficial peroneal nerve entrapment syndrome. *Oper Orthop Traumatol.* 2007;19(5–6):502–510.

Morganti CM, McFarland EG, Cosgarea AJ. Saphenous neuritis: A poorly understood cause of medial knee pain. *J Am Acad Orthop Surg.* 2002;10(2):130–137. Review.

Oh SJ, Meyer RD. Entrapment neuropathies of the tibial (posterior tibial) nerve. *Neurol Clin.* 1999;17(3):593–615, vii. Review.

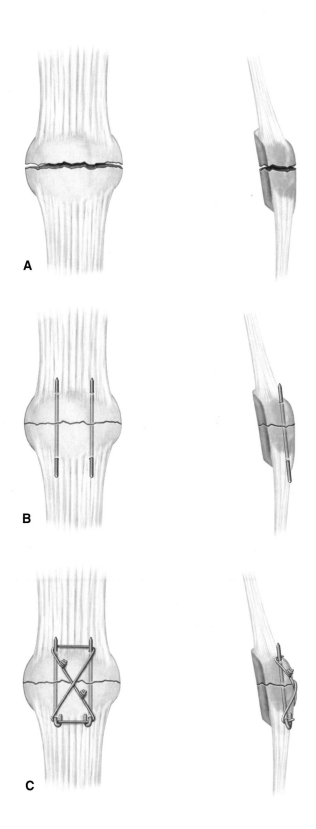

Figure 93. A. Transverse patella fracture. B. K-wires are placed to hold the reduction. C. Tension wiring is applied for compression

ORIF Distal Femoral Fractures

Indications and Goals: Distal femoral fractures typically occur in two populations—young men with high energy trauma, and the elderly population (typically female). These fractures are classified regarding their location (extra- versus intra-articular [whether or not the extend into the knee joint]) and degree of comminution (how many pieces there are).

Procedure and Technique: Treatment typically consists of open reduction and internal fixation. Major pieces may need to be put back together (like a jigsaw puzzle) and then connected with plate(s) and screws. Newer implants with locking capability (locks the screws into the plate) have improved fixation of these difficult fractures.

Post-surgical Precautions/Rehabilitation: There is no single established protocol to follow for open reduction internal fixation procedures for distal femur fractures. The specific type and location of the fracture, the procedure performed, and the healing rate of the bone will all determine the speed to which one can return to ambulation, function, and ultimately work or sports participation.

Expected Outcomes: The treatment methods may influence the final outcomes. A higher incidence rate of complications has been reported when the physis is violated by hardware. Salter Harris classifications and displacement of the fracture have been identified as predictors of the final outcome, though the degree and the direction of displacement do not statistically correlate with outcome.

Return to Play: After complete fracture union and restoration of muscle function return to sport participation is likely 4 to 6 months post-operatively.

Recommended Readings

Haidukewych GJ, Berry DJ, Jacofsky DJ, Torchia ME. Treatment of supracondylar femur nonunions with open reduction and internal fixation. *Am J Orthop.* 2003;32(11):564–567.

Rademakers MV, Kerkhoffs GM, Sierevelt IN, Raaymakers EL, Marti RK. Intra-articular fractures of the distal femur: A long-term follow-up study of surgically treated patients. *J Orthop Trauma.* 2004;18(4):213–219.

Zlowodzki M, Bhandari M, Marek DJ, Cole PA, Kregor PJ. Operative treatment of acute distal femur fractures: Systematic review of 2 comparative studies and 45 case series (1989 to 2005). *J Orthop Trauma.* 2006;20(5):366–371. Review.

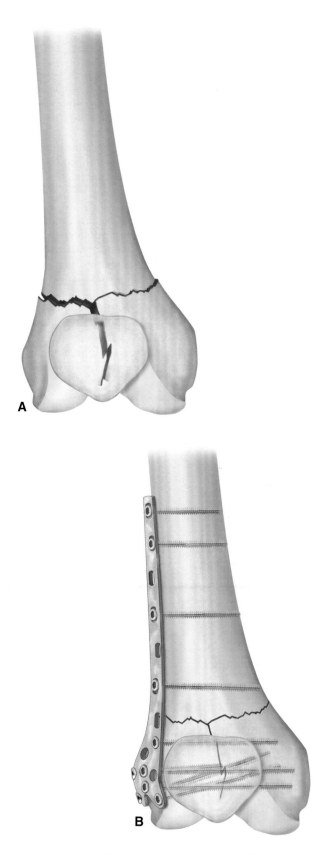

Figure 94. Open reduction and internal fixation distal femur fracture with intercondylar component (A) with lateral plate (B).

ORIF Tibial Plateau Fractures

Indications and Goals: These fractures are typically a result of a blow from the side or an axial (compressive) force on the knee (or both). Classification is based upon the compartment(s) involved (medial or lateral, with lateral the most common, by far), the degree of compression/comminution (number of pieces), and whether it involves the cortex of the injured compartment.

Procedure and Technique: Treatment involves open reduction and internal fixation of the fracture. It is often necessary to elevate the articular surface of the affected tibial plateau and add bone graft to support these fragments. A plate and screws are typically used to stabilize the fracture. Again, locking plates have improved the fixation of these sometimes difficult fractures.

Post-surgical Precautions/Rehabilitation: The main focus of rehabilitative intervention following open reduction internal fixation is to protect the forces at the tibiofemoral joint. Patients will be non-weight bearing for an extended period of time, with the application of a knee brace and assistive device for ambulation. CPM may be helpful in the early post-operative period. Gradual weight bearing and resistive quadriceps exercises that place added stress to the joint will be initiated once radiographs show signs of bone healing.

Expected Outcomes: Open reduction and internal fixation tibial plateau fractures typically unite, though cases of delayed and non-unions have been reported (requiring additional procedures and bone grafting). Functional results are oftentimes good as reported up to 3 years post-operative, with not as good outcomes possibly related to abnormal mechanical axes and multiple comorbid injuries. Long-term follow-up radiographs have demonstrated degenerative changes in the lateral compartment. Patients can expect to refrain from a weight-bearing occupation for up to 8 weeks.

Return to Play: Assuming that complete restoration of articular congruity is achieved, return to sport participation can occur anywhere from 3 to 6 months post-operatively. However, post-traumatic arthrosis is common and athletes may not be able to return to play in some cases.

Recommended Readings

Canadian Orthopaedic Trauma Society. Open reduction and internal fixation compared with circular fixator application for bicondylar tibial plateau fractures. Results of a multicenter, prospective, randomized clinical trial. *J Bone Joint Surg Am.* 2006; 88(12):2613–2623.

Chin TY, Bardana D, Bailey M, Williamson OD, Miller R, Edwards ER, Esser MP. Functional outcome of tibial plateau fractures treated with the fine-wire fixator. *Inj.* 2005;36(12):1467–1475. Epub 2005 Oct 21.

Ebraheim NA, Sabry FF, Haman SP. Open reduction and internal fixation of 117 tibial plateau fractures. *Orthop.* 2004;27(12): 1281–1287.

Rademakers MV, Kerkhoffs GM, Sierevelt IN, Raaymakers EL, Marti RK. Operative treatment of 109 tibial plateau fractures: Five- to 27-year follow-up results. *J Orthop Trauma.* 2007;21(1):5–10. Erratum in: *J Orthop Trauma.* 2007;21(3):218.

Toro-Arbelaez JB, Gardner MJ, Shindle MK, Cabas JM, Lorich DG, Helfet DL. Open reduction and internal fixation of intraarticular tibial plateau nonunions. *Inj.* 2007;38(3):378–383.

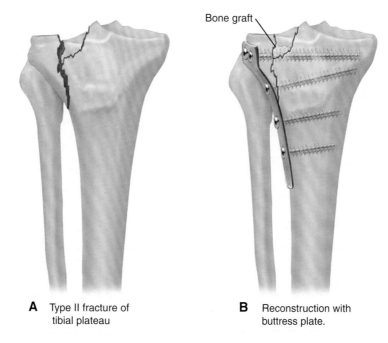

A Type II fracture of tibial plateau

B Reconstruction with buttress plate.

Bone graft

Figure 95. Open reduction internal fixation of a tibial plateau fracture (A). B. Reconstruction with buttress plate and elevation of articular depression with bone graft.

ORIF Tibial Shaft Fractures

Indications and Goals: Fractures of the tibia are relatively common and slow to heal. They can occur as a result of a fall with a twisting force or a direct force. They need to be monitored early to ensure that the patient does not develop a compartment syndrome (bleeding into the soft tissues can elevate the pressure and require emergent decompression). Fractures are classified on the basis of their location, displacement, fracture pattern, and degree of comminution (number of pieces).

Procedure and Technique: Although some fractures can be treated with casting and then fracture braces, the mainstay of treatment for tibial shaft fractures has become intramedullary nailing. An incision is made next to the patella tendon which is retracted, and a starting hole is made in the proximal tibia. A long guide wire is inserted into the starting hole and down the shaft of the tibia. Flexible reamers are then introduced and the canal is dilated to the appropriate size. A titanium rod with a hollow center is then tapped down into the canal to stabilize the fracture. Locking screws are typically used to stabilize the rod.

Post-surgical Precautions/Rehabilitation: Range of motion of the knee and ankle should begin in the early post-operative phase. Weight bearing is restricted for the initial period, usually 4 to 6 weeks, until there is early radiographic evidence of healing. After that point, weight bearing may be progressed as tolerated by the patient. If there is only minimal or no evidence of healing at 12 weeks, dynamization (removal of the distal interlocking screws) should be considered.

Expected Outcomes: Tibial shaft fractures treated with intramedullary nailing have excellent outcomes reported in the literature with healing rates as high as 98%. Compared with closed fixation and casting, the rate of non-union, malunion, and shortening are remarkably low. The hardware is tolerated well and rarely requires additional surgery for removal.

Return to Play: After complete healing and restoration of muscle tone, return to sport participation may be around 4 months post-operatively.

Recommended Readings

Bhandari M, Guyatt GH, Tornetta P 3rd, Swiontkowski MF, Hanson B, Sprague S, Syed A, Schemitsch EH. Current practice in the intramedullary nailing of tibial shaft fractures: An international survey. *J Trauma.* 2002;53(4):725–732.

Littenberg B, Weinstein LP, McCarren M, Mead T, Swiontkowski MF, Rudicel SA, Heck D. Closed fractures of the tibial shaft. A meta-analysis of three methods of treatment. *J Bone Joint Surg Am.* 1998;80(2):174–183.

Reuss BL, Cole JD. Effect of delayed treatment on open tibial shaft fractures. *Am J Orthop.* 2007;36(4):215–220.

Tang P, Gates C, Hawes J, Vogt M, Prayson MJ. Does open reduction increase the chance of infection during intramedullary nailing of closed tibial shaft fractures? *J Orthop Trauma.* 2006;20(5):317–322.

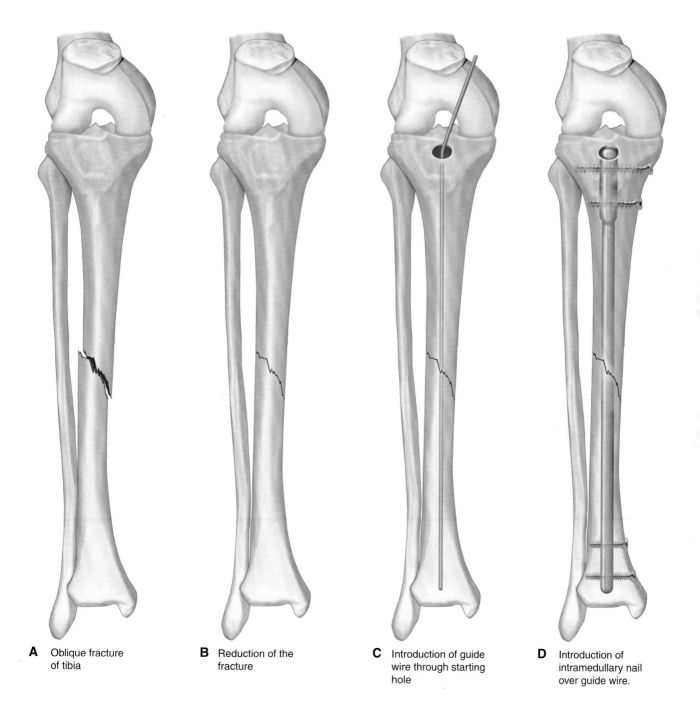

A Oblique fracture of tibia

B Reduction of the fracture

C Introduction of guide wire through starting hole

D Introduction of intramedullary nail over guide wire.

Figure 96. **Tibial shaft fracture stabilized with a locked intramedullary nail. A,** Oblique tibial fracture. **B,** Reduction of fracture. **C,** Introduction of guide wire. **D,** Introduction of medullary nail over guide wire.

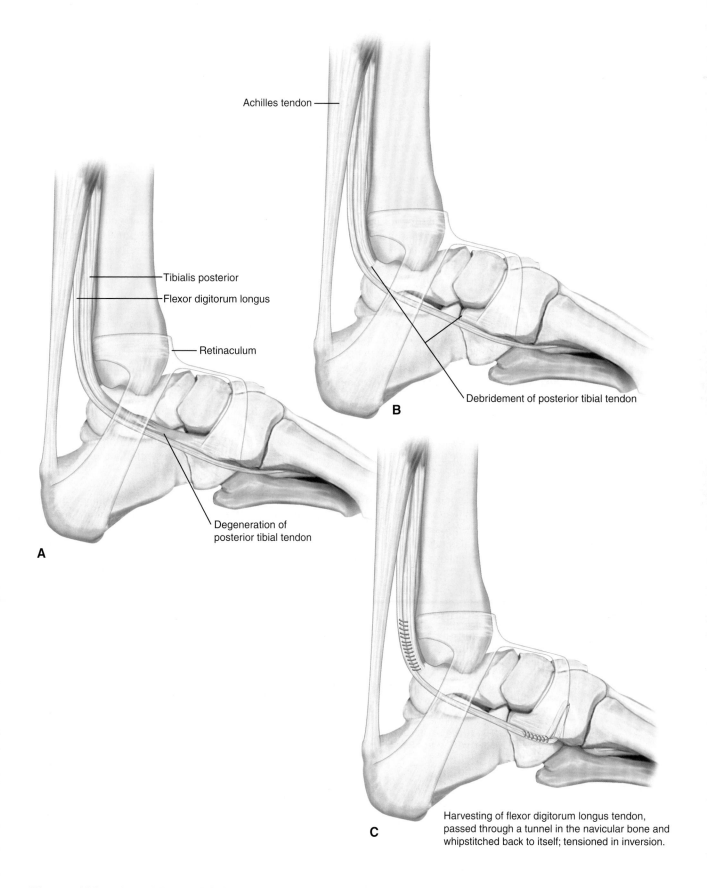

Achilles tendon

Tibialis posterior

Flexor digitorum longus

Retinaculum

Debridement of posterior tibial tendon

B

Degeneration of
posterior tibial tendon

A

Harvesting of flexor digitorum longus tendon,
passed through a tunnel in the navicular bone and
whipstitched back to itself; tensioned in inversion.

C

Figure 102. FDL (Flexor Digitorum Longus Transfer) for Posterior Tibial Tendon Dysfunction

Peroneal Tendon Surgery

Indications and Goals: Rupture of the peroneal tendons is extremely rare. Tendinosis and subluxation/dislocation of these tendons are more common. Tendinosis is a result of overuse and is treated conservatively with rest, ice, NSAIDs, and arch supports. Subluxation or dislocation is a result of a violent contraction of these muscles in an everted, dorsiflexed foot. This results in tearing or attenuation of the superior peroneal retinaculum. It most commonly occurs in skiers and football players. Tenderness and visualization of the tendon subluxing with active eversion confirms the diagnosis. Conservative treatment includes a short leg non–weight-bearing cast in slight plantarflexion and eversion for 5 to 6 weeks. Failing this, stabilization may be required.

Procedure and Technique: Tenolysis should be performed by opening the tendon sheath at the location of tenderness. In some cases, normal superior peroneal retinacular anatomy can be restored by repairing the avulsed fibrocartilaginous rim to the fibula. Peroneal groove deepening may also be required if the posterior fibula is flat or convex. Associated longitudinal tears in the peroneus brevis are common and should be repaired with running sutures. Tears involving greater than 50% of the tendon may require tenodesis to the remaining peroneal tendon or allograft reconstruction. Low-lying brevis muscle belly or peroneus quartus should be excised if present.

Post-surgical Precautions/Rehabilitation: Most repairs are immobilized in a cast for 4 to 6 weeks before beginning any range of motion. Once the cast is removed, active, active-assisted, and passive range of motion can be initiated with extra caution placed upon active and passive inversions, and active eversion movements. Weight bearing is gradually increased as tolerated, with crutches utilized during the casting period and immediately after the cast is removed. Resistive ankle exercises can progress emphasizing low weight and early repetitions to restore ankle musculature endurance. Balance and proprioceptive exercises can also begin once the cast is removed and slowly progress to more difficult activities.

Expected Outcomes: Surgical intervention of peroneal tendon tears are reported to yield successful and predictable results with few clinically significant complications. However, patients with previous steroid injections and those with symptoms for more than 12 months had poorer outcomes. Prevention of recurrent subluxation is critical to ensure maximal chance of recovery.

Return to Play: The anatomic structures involved play a critical role with nearly all ankle movements in sport activities, thus a safe return to participation will likely take 6 months or more following surgical repair. If a repair of the longitudinal split is performed, one should protect the repair for approximately 3 months with early ROM to minimize scarring. For an allograft reconstruction or tenodesis, patients will often require 6 months to return. After groove deepening, patients may return at ~5 months, similar to a Broström procedure, which is often performed in tandem.

Recommended Readings

Adachi N, Fukuhara K, Tanaka H, Nakasa T, Ochi M. Superior retinaculoplasty for recurrent dislocation of peroneal tendons. *Foot Ankle Int.* 2006;27(12):1074–1078.

Dombek MF, Lamm BM, Saltrick K, Mendicino RW, Catanzariti AR. Peroneal tendon tears: A retrospective review. *J Foot Ankle Surg.* 2003;42(5):250–258.

Krause JO, Brodsky JW. Peroneus brevis tendon tears: Pathophysiology, surgical reconstruction, and clinical results. *Foot Ankle Int.* 1998;19(5):271–279.

Ogawa BK, Thordarson DB, Zalavras C. Peroneal tendon subluxation repair with an indirect fibular groove deepening technique. *Foot Ankle Int.* 2007;28(11):1194–1197.

Safran MR, O'Malley D Jr, Fu FH. Peroneal tendon subluxation in athletes: New exam technique, case reports, and review. *Med Sci Sports Exerc.* 1999;31(7 suppl):S487–S492. Review.

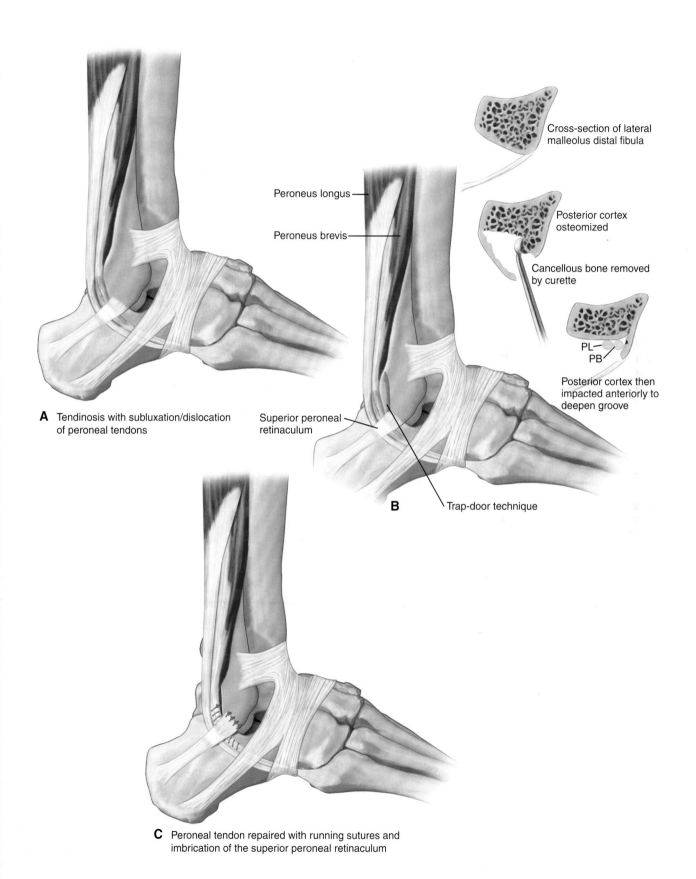

Cross-section of lateral malleolus distal fibula

Posterior cortex osteomized

Cancellous bone removed by curette

PL
PB

Posterior cortex then impacted anteriorly to deepen groove

Peroneus longus

Peroneus brevis

A Tendinosis with subluxation/dislocation of peroneal tendons

Superior peroneal retinaculum

B Trap-door technique

C Peroneal tendon repaired with running sutures and imbrication of the superior peroneal retinaculum

Figure 103. Peroneal Groove Deepening, with Retinacular Repair and Peroneus Brevis Repair

Plantar Plate Injuries/Turf Toe

Indications and Goals: Extreme dorsiflexion of the great toe can result in significant injuries to the plantar plate. This injury is most commonly seen in offensive linemen and occurs during push off from their stance. A similar injury (sand toe) can occur in beach volleyball players with extreme plantarflexion. Examination will reveal tenderness and swelling in the metatarsophalangeal (MTP) joint and pain with passive flexion. Patients may also have instability (varus/valgus and "Lachmans" test) and weakness of flexion and extension against resistance. Significant injury can result in traumatic bunion deformities or MTP arthritis. Radiographs can be helpful (especially a forced dorsiflexion lateral view) because the sesamoids may be retracted proximally on the injured side. MRI can be helpful. Initial treatment is conservative with rest, ice, NSAIDs, taping, and rehabilitation. Shoe modifications (rigid metatarsal bar) may help prevent reinjury. A cast or walking boot may be helpful in the management of acute cases. The plantar plate of the second toe may also be ruptured with similar mechanisms.

Procedure and Technique: Surgery involves restoration of normal anatomy, usually primary repair of the plantar plate complex, sesamoids, and sometimes the flexor hallucis brevis. A medial "J" incision is made, and care is taken not to injure the plantar medial cutaneous nerve. Working lateral to medial, the capsule and plantar plate is repaired anatomically to the base of the proximal phalanx. Suture anchors are sometimes required.

Post-surgical Precautions/Rehabilitation: The foot is initially immobilized for 7 to 10 days postoperative (including the ankle joint) in a non–weight-bearing splint. Wound management and control of distal swelling are key elements early post-operatively.

Active dorsiflexion is restricted to neutral for 3 to 4 weeks to avoid stress on the plantar plate, and gradual weight bearing can begin after a few weeks based upon surgeon preference, with limited push off during the gait phase to prevent against excessive dorsiflexion of the first metatarsophalangeal joint. A Morton's extension splint can be used post-operatively to restrict dorsiflexion

Expected Outcomes: Results of plantar-plate repairs often yield good outcomes. Patient's age, activity level, joint status prior to surgery, and compliance post-operatively will contribute to the functional level of activity after the repair. Complete healing may take up to 1 year. Late recognition may lead to hallux rigidus. Delayed diagnosis or advanced disease has led to the early termination of the careers of many elite athletes.

Return to Play: Despite the small area being addressed, the majority of one's push-off weight bearing occurs at this joint. As such, a safe return to sports participation may take between 6 months to a year.

Recommended Readings

Blitz NM, Ford LA, Christensen JC. Plantar plate repair of the second metatarsophalangeal joint: Technique and tips. *J Foot Ankle Surg.* 2004;43(4):266–270.

Ford LA, Collins KB, Christensen JC. Stabilization of the subluxed second metatarsophalangeal joint: Flexor tendon transfer versus primary repair of the plantar plate. *J Foot Ankle Surg.* 1998;37(3):217–222.

Good JJ, Weinfeld GD, Yu GV. Fracture-dislocation of the first metatarsophalangeal joint: Open reduction through a medial incisional approach. *J Foot Ankle Surg.* 2001;40(5):311–317.

Watson TS, Anderson RB, Davis WH. Periarticular injuries to the hallux metatarsophalangeal joint in athletes. *Foot Ankle Clin.* 2000;5(3):687–713. Review.

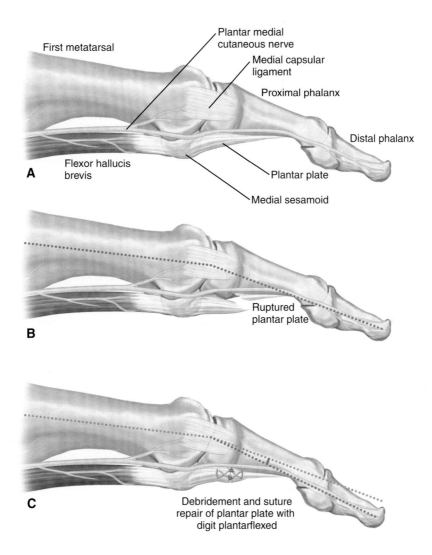

First metatarsal

Plantar medial
cutaneous nerve

Medial capsular
ligament

Proximal phalanx

Distal phalanx

Flexor hallucis
brevis

A

Plantar plate

Medial sesamoid

Ruptured
plantar plate

B

Debridement and suture
repair of plantar plate with
digit plantarflexed

C

Figure 104. **Anatomy of Plantar Plate and Repair**

Bunion/Bunionette Surgery

Indications and Goals: Hallux valgus (bunion) is caused by shoewear that compresses the forefoot in predisposed individuals. Vallux varus (bunionette), also known as tailor's bunion, occurs from excessive pressure on the lateral foot. Both problems result in a painful prominence on the border of the foot (bunion medial, bunionette lateral); and both likely have a hereditary component. Over half of patients complain of pain over the prominence and conservative measures (wider shoes, pads, etc) may have some benefit early. Radiographic measurements of the hallux valgus/varus (HV) angle (at the metatarsophalangeal joint) and the intermetatarsal (IM) angle help to plan treatment.

Procedure and Technique: Both distal and proximal procedures have been described. Most require an osteotomy of the metatarsal or proximal phalanx. For smaller bunions/bunionettes, distal procedures (chevron with soft tissue releases/imbrications) may be all that is required. With large intermetatarsal angles, proximal procedures are typically necessary.

Post-surgical Precautions/Rehabilitation: Post-operative protocol after hallux valgus surgery depends on the location of metatarsal osteotomy, with goals of pain management and swelling reduction. Heel weight bearing is permitted after a distal chevron. Following a proximal osteotomy, the patient may not bear weight for 6 weeks with up to 8 weeks non–weight-bearing following a Lapidus procedure. Soon thereafter, ankle- and foot-strengthening exercises can be implemented in all directional planes, with additional weight-bearing activity to improve proprioception. Individuals should be able to perform activities of daily living unrestricted and begin more progressive return to sporting-type activities between 8 and 10 weeks post-operatively.

Expected Outcomes: Bunionectomy surgery yields good or excellent results with high patient satisfaction and a low complication rate. Recurrence rates can be reduced with successful reduction of inter-metatarsal angle and narrowing of the forefoot. Return to activity levels depend upon the patient's general health status and goals, and many times are improved from pre-operative levels of function. Results are less predictable in adolescent athletes.

Return to Play: Following complete bony union and painless running, a return to sports participation may take 3 months or more post-operatively.

Recommended Readings

Barouk LS, Barouk P, Baudet B, Toullec E. The great toe proximal phalanx osteotomy: The final step of the bunionectomy. *Foot Ankle Clin.* 2005;10(1):141–155. Review.

Coughlin MJ, Shurnas PS. Hallux valgus in men. Part II: First ray mobility after bunionectomy and factors associated with hallux valgus deformity. *Foot Ankle Int.* 2003;24(1):73–78.

Dayton P, Glynn A, Rogers WS. Use of the Z osteotomy for Tailor bunionectomy. *J Foot Ankle Surg.* 2003;42(3):167–169.

Gill LH. Distal osteotomy for bunionectomy and hallux valgus correction. *Foot Ankle Clin.* 2001;6(3):433–453. Review.

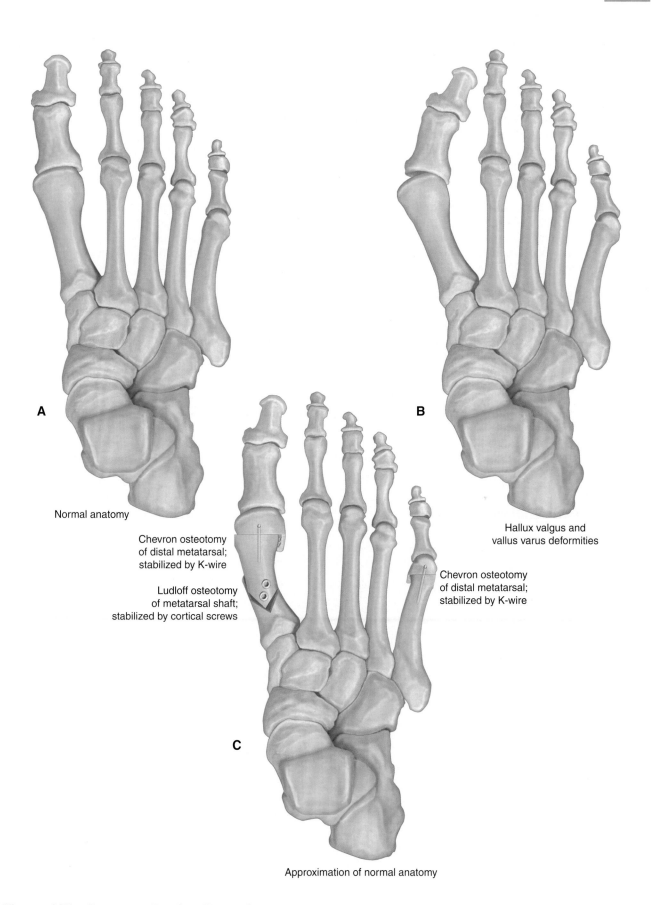

A

Normal anatomy

B

Hallux valgus and
vallus varus deformities

Chevron osteotomy
of distal metatarsal;
stabilized by K-wire

Ludloff osteotomy
of metatarsal shaft;
stabilized by cortical screws

Chevron osteotomy
of distal metatarsal;
stabilized by K-wire

C

Approximation of normal anatomy

Figure 105. Common Bunion Procedures

Cheilectomy (for Hallux Rigidus)

Indications and Goals: Hallux rigidus (proliferative bone formation at the dorsum of top of the first toe proximal phalanx) is a disabling painful condition of the first MTP joint. In athletes, it can be a result of a chronic turf toe or osteochondritis dissecans. Clinical findings typically include loss of great toe dorsiflexion, a palpable, painful ridge dorsally, and an osteophyte best seen on lateral radiographs. Conservative management includes NSAIDs, padding, and a stiff shoe insert. Failing this, a cheilectomy may be required. For more severe arthrosis, other techniques to include MTP fusion may be necessary.

Procedure and Technique: A longitudinal incision is made over the MTP joint and the extensor hood and capsule is opened. A synovectomy is completed, loose bodies removed, and the joint is inspected. Using a saw or osteotome, the dorsal 20% to 30% of the metatarsal head is removed. Additional osteophytes are removed, irregularities are smoothed, and the capsule and skin is closed. Full restoration of full dorsiflexion should be confirmed on lateral C-arm imaging.

Post-surgical Precautions/Rehabilitation: Patients are typically placed in a rigid post-operative shoe to reduce forces with early weight-bearing activity. Controlled range of motion may begin immediately, or a few days post-operative, based upon surgeon preference. Post-operative pain is a common complaint, and can be addressed with medication and therapeutic modalities as needed. Most surgeons utilize 2 weeks heel weight bearing with advance to as tolerated with aggressive range of motion.

Expected Outcomes: Cheilectomy typically results in good pain relief and improvement in function. Complications can include injury to the medial branch of the dorsal cutaneous nerve and wound complications. Cheilectomy has been reported to have predictable success when treating isolated osteophytes without advanced cartilage loss. More severe cases may require an arthrodesis.

Return to Play: While a return to sports participation is typically 2 to 3 months post-operatively, some individuals with advanced arthritis may not be able to return to play.

Recommended Readings

Beertema W, Draijer WF, van Os JJ, Pilot P. A retrospective analysis of surgical treatment in patients with symptomatic hallux rigidus: Long-term follow-up. *J Foot Ankle Surg.* 2006;45(4):244–251.

Coughlin MJ, Shurnas PS. Hallux rigidus. Grading and long-term results of operative treatment. *J Bone Joint Surg Am.* 2003;85-A(11):2072–2088.

Debnath UK, Hemmady MV, Hariharan K. Indications for and technique of first metatarsophalangeal joint arthroscopy. *Foot Ankle Int.* 2006;27(12):1049–1054.

Dereymaeker G. Surgical treatment of hallux rigidus. *Orthopade.* 2005;34(8):742–744, 746–747. Review.

Keiserman LS, Sammarco VJ, Sammarco GJ. Surgical treatment of the hallux rigidus. *Foot Ankle Clin.* 2005;10(1):75–96. Review.

Lau JT, Daniels TR. Outcomes following cheilectomy and interpositional arthroplasty in hallux rigidus. *Foot Ankle Int.* 2001;22(6): 462–470.

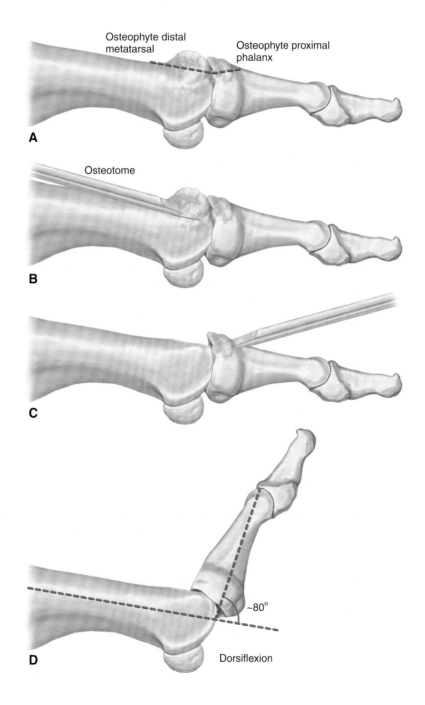

Figure 106. Cheilectomy

Os Trigonum Excision

Indications and Goals: An unfused os trigonum, on the posterior aspect of the talus, can sometimes be a problem in dancers, especially with extreme ankle plantarflexion (such as a ballerina in the "en pointe" position). The os can impact the distal tibia in this position and it can be painful. In patients who fail conservative management, excision may be necessary. The os is located just lateral to the flexor hallucis longus tendon in the posterior ankle.

Procedure and Technique: Excision can be completed from a posterolateral or posteromedial approach. Posterolateral approaches avoid dissection of the medial neurovascular bundle. Alternatively, arthroscopic excision, using portals that are immediately adjacent to the medial and lateral border of the Achilles tendon and with the patient in the prone position, has been successful.

Post-surgical Precautions/Rehabilitation: Post-operative rehabilitation following an excision begins immediately. Emphasis is placed on pain reduction, swelling reduction, and enhancing range of motion. Weight-bearing status will depend upon the surgeon's preference, as it is not uncommon to initiate immediate weight bearing. Progression to full weight-bearing status, increased proprioception, and strengthening exercises can be implemented as tolerated.

Expected Outcomes: A symptomatic os trigonum that does not respond favorably to non-operative treatment for 3 months can be treated with surgical excision. Results of excision have been good, with most athletes returning to previous levels of competition. Possible complications from surgery include sural nerve injury, superficial wound infections, and reflex sympathetic dystrophy.

Return to Play: Return to full sports participation is usually within 6 to 8 weeks post-operatively.

Recommended Readings

Abramowitz Y, Wollstein R, Barzilay Y, London E, Matan Y, Shabat S, Nyska M. Outcome of resection of a symptomatic os trigonum. *J Bone Joint Surg Am.* 2003;85-A(6):1051–1057.

Chao W. Os trigonum. *Foot Ankle Clin.* 2004;9(4):787–796, vii. Review.

Mouhsine E, Crevoisier X, Leyvraz PF, Akiki A, Dutoit M, Garofalo R. Post-traumatic overload or acute syndrome of the os trigonum: A possible cause of posterior ankle impingement. *Knee Surg Sports Traumatol Arthrosc.* 2004;12(3):250–253. Epub 2004 Jan 28.

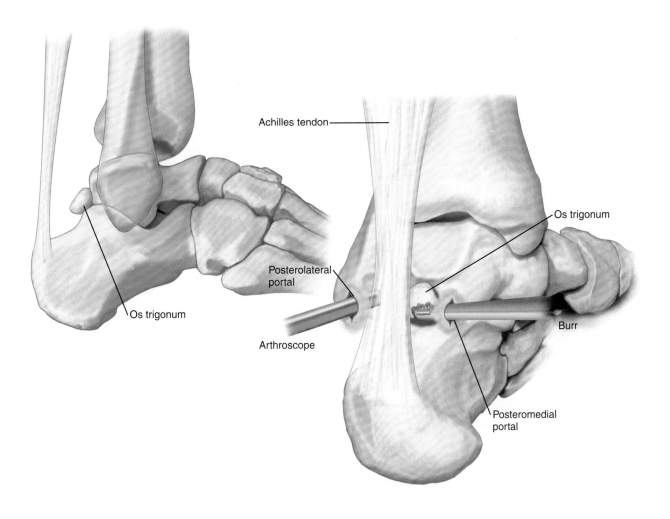

Figure 107. Arthroscopic Excision of Os Trigonum

Plantar Fascia Release

Indications and Goals: Plantar fasciitis is a result of inflammation of the plantar fascia in the central to medial subcalcaneal region. It commonly occurs in runners. It is exacerbated by excessive pronation. Initial treatment includes rest, orthotics, NSAIDs, and stretching. Heel cord stretching several times per day can be helpful. Release of the fascia and nerve can be helpful for intractable symptoms, but should be considered only after failure of conservative measures. Resolution of symptoms can take greater than 10 months in some cases. Repetitive steroid injections should be avoided, as they can result in plantar fascia rupture, as well as skin/fat pad atrophy.

Procedure and Technique: An oblique incision is made medially, at the level of the insertion of the plantar fascia in the heel. The lateral plantar nerve, which is often entrapped in this process, is released and protected. The superficial fascia of the abductor hallucis muscle is released. Then the abductor hallucis muscle is reflected proximally and the remaining fascia is released. The procedure can also be done arthroscopically.

Post-surgical Precautions/Rehabilitation: Following a plantar fascia release, it is important to be careful with gradual increased weight bearing during early rehabilitation. Scar management and soft tissue mobilization are encouraged immediately. Cushioning under the sole of the foot may be helpful. Between 1 and 2 weeks post-operatively, weight bearing can slowly increase using pain as a relative guideline.

Expected Outcomes: Post-operative function will improve for most patients, with those who presented with preoperative symptoms for longer than 2 years before surgery having lower post-operative scores. Individuals may return to activity approximately 3 months after surgery. Obesity has not been shown to affect outcomes except for in athletes who possess a body mass index greater than 27. A partial release of less than 40% of the fascia is recommended to minimize the effect on arch instability and maintain normal foot biomechanics. Residual pain, flattening of the medial longitudinal arch, and wound issues can be possible complications.

Return to Play: Although a seemingly minor operation, results and ability to return to play are mixed. Return to play may be within 8 to 12 weeks following successful surgery.

Recommended Readings

Bazaz R, Ferkel RD. Results of endoscopic plantar fascia release. *Foot Ankle Int.* 2007;28(5):549–556.

Brugh AM, Fallat LM, Savoy-Moore RT. Lateral column symptomatology following plantar fascial release: A prospective study. *J Foot Ankle Surg.* 2002;41(6):365–371.

Cheung JT, An KN, Zhang M. Consequences of partial and total plantar fascia release: A finite element study. *Foot Ankle Int.* 2006;27(2):125–132.

Hogan KA, Webb D, Shereff M. Endoscopic plantar fascia release. *Foot Ankle Int.* 2004;25(12):875–881.

Jerosch J, Schunck J, Liebsch D, Filler T. Indication, surgical technique and results of endoscopic fascial release in plantar fasciitis (E FRPF). *Knee Surg Sports Traumatol Arthrosc.* 2004;12(5):471–477. Epub 2004 Apr 14.

Saxena A. Uniportal endoscopic plantar fasciotomy: A prospective study on athletic patients. *Foot Ankle Int.* 2004;25(12):882–889.

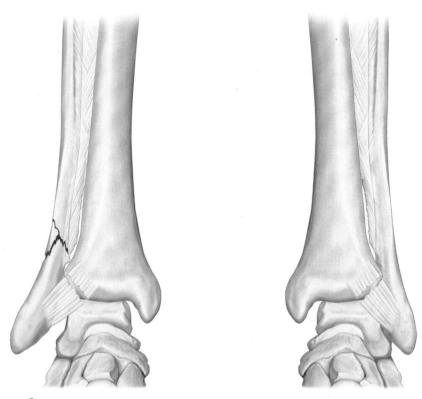

A Syndesmotic injury, with and without fracture, resulting in incongruity of mortise

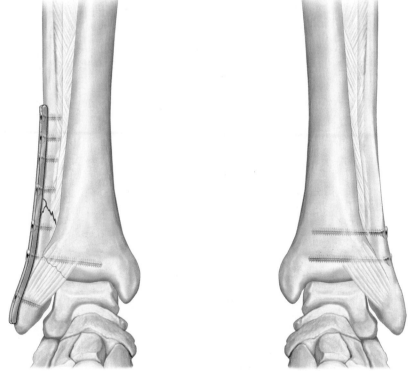

B Internal fixation of fracture with stabilization and return to functional mortise.

Figure 110. Open Reduction Internal Fixation (ORIF) of Syndesmosis

ORIF Ankle Fractures

Indications and Goals: Ankle fractures are typically the result of a rotational injury with the foot fixed. The classification is typically based on the location of the fibular fracture. Any talar displacement in the mortise is an indication for ORIF because of the effect on altered contact pressures. Displaced fractures require ORIF.

Procedure and Technique: A vertical incision is made to approach the distal fibula. Care is taken to look for and protect the superficial peroneal nerve. The fibula is exposed subperiosteally and the fracture is reduced with a clamp. If there is an associated medial malleolus fracture, this is reduced and provisionally fixed with K-wires. Definitive fixation of the fibula is carried out with interfragmentary screw(s) for oblique fractures and with a plate and screws for most fractures. Definitive fixation of the medial malleolus fracture is typically two screws. Cannulated screws can be used by taking advantage of the K-wires placed after reduction of the medial side. The posterior malleolus fracture, if present, typically does not need to be fixed unless it involves more than 25% of the joint or has more than 2 mm of step-off. Syndesmotic screws may need to be placed if diastasis is demonstrated on stress views.

Post-surgical Precautions/Rehabilitation: Patients will be placed in a cast/walking boot with non–weight-bearing status for 6 to 8 weeks. Once bony healing has occurred, supervised range of motion, strengthening, and proprioception exercises can be initiated and progressed as tolerated. Adjacent joint mobilization is highly encouraged to restore ankle and foot biomechanics.

Expected Outcomes: Patients who had early mobilization in a removable cast had higher functional scores and were able to return to work sooner.

Return to Play: Return to sports participation must follow a complete bony union, control of swelling, functional range of motion, and proprioception. The typical timeframe for this is usually 4 to 6 months post-operatively.

Recommended Readings

Honigmann P, Goldhahn S, Rosenkranz J, Audigé L, Geissmann D, Babst R. Aftertreatment of malleolar fractures following ORIF—functional compared to protected functional in a vacuum-stabilized orthesis: A randomized controlled trial. *Arch Orthop Trauma Surg.* 2007;127(3):195–203. Epub 2006 Dec 30.

Vioreanu M, Dudeney S, Hurson B, Kelly E, O'Rourke K, Quinlan W. Early mobilization in a removable cast compared with immobilization in a cast after operative treatment of ankle fractures: A prospective randomized study. *Foot Ankle Int.* 2007;28(1):13–19.

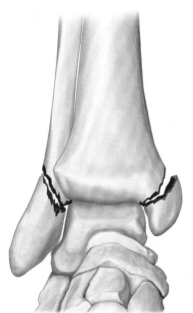

A Bimalleolar ankle fracture

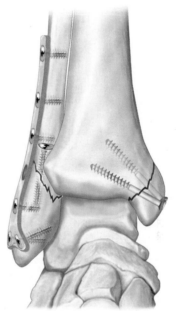

B ORIF of fibula with lag screw/neutralization plate, ORIF of medial malleolus with partially threaded cancellous screws

Figure 111. Open Reduction Internal Fixation (ORIF) of Bimalleolar Ankle Fracture

ORIF Talar Fractures

Indications and Goals: Talar neck fractures are the most common fracture of the talus. Displaced fractures have a high risk of avascular necrosis, even with fixation, because of the tenuous blood supply of the talus. Treatment requires ORIF with an anatomic reduction. Talar body fractures and talar process fractures (lateral > medial) require fixation only if they are significantly displaced. Lateral talar process fractures are commonly referred to as the snowboarder's ankle. Subtalar dislocations (basketball foot) are usually medial, and are quite stable following closed reduction.

Procedure and Technique: For talar neck fractures, treatment requires ORIF with an anatomic reduction. Dual incisions (medial and lateral) are usually required and two posterior to anterior cannulated screws (one medial and one lateral) are usually used. Plate fixation is sometimes required for fractures with significant comminution.

Post-surgical Precautions/Rehabilitation: Patients are non–weight-bearing until evidence of healing exists. The Hawkins sign (subchondral lucency) is a positive finding as it represents subchondral reabsorption consistent with maintained vascularity/perfusion. The alternative may signify osteonecrosis which is common in these injuries. Cast or boot is surgeon preference. Range of motion, strengthening, and proprioceptive exercises can be initiated as tolerated post-operatively and progressed accordingly.

Expected Outcomes: Urgent open reduction and internal fixation is recommended for the treatment of displaced talar neck and/or body fractures, although some have reported that a delay in surgical fixation does not appear to affect the outcome, union, or prevalence of osteonecrosis. Post-traumatic arthritis and avascular necrosis are complications associated with displaced fractures even after anatomic reduction and stable fixation.

Return to Play: Return to sports participation depends upon the location and extent of the fracture and the quality of the reduction and fixation. Some displaced talar neck fracture progress to avascular necrosis and return to play may not be possible.

Recommended Readings

Cronier P, Talha A, Massin P. Central talar fractures–therapeutic considerations. *Injury.* 2004;35(suppl 2):SB10–SB22. Review.

Frawley PA, Hart JA, Young DA. Treatment outcome of major fractures of the talus. *Foot Ankle Int.* 1995;16(6):339–345.

Lindvall E, Haidukewych G, DiPasquale T, Herscovici D Jr, Sanders R. Open reduction and stable fixation of isolated, displaced talar neck and body fractures. *J Bone Joint Surg Am.* 2004;86-A(10):2229–2234.

Tezval M, Dumont C, Stürmer KM. Prognostic reliability of the Hawkins sign in fractures of the talus. *J Orthop Trauma.* 2007;21(8):538–543.

Vallier HA, Nork SE, Benirschke SK, Sangeorzan BJ. Surgical treatment of talar body fractures. *J Bone Joint Surg Am.* 2004;86-A(suppl 1 pt 2):180–192.

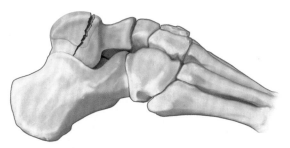

A Talar fracture; lateral view

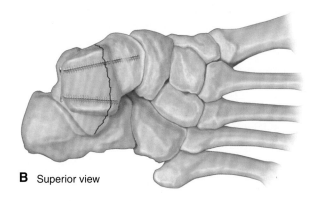

B Superior view

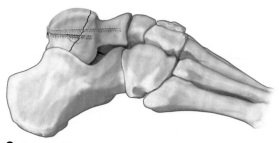

C Lateral view

Figure 112. ORIF of Talar Body Fracture

ORIF Calcaneal Fractures

Indications and Goals: Calcaneus fractures are usually a result of a significant axial load. They are sometimes associated with other lower extremity and lumbar fractures. The heel is typically shortened, widened, and in varus following these fractures. CT scanning is helpful in the classification and treatment of these fractures. Displaced fractures usually require ORIF. Complications (wound complications, compartment syndrome, post-traumatic arthritis, etc.) are unfortunately common, even with optimum treatment.

Procedure and Technique: For most calcaneal fractures, treatment involves ORIF through an extensile lateral approach. Deep flaps are created and the skin is protected. K-wires are helpful in obtaining initial fixation prior to definitive fixation with specially contoured plates. The joint surfaces are restored, and a perimeter plate is utilized to connect the tuberosity to the posterior facet and anterior process.

Post-surgical Precautions/Rehabilitation: Patients are non–weight-bearing until evidence of healing exists. Cast or boot treatment depends on surgeon preference. Range of motion, strengthening, and proprioceptive exercises can be initiated as tolerated post-operatively and progress accordingly. Weight bearing is typically started at 6 to 8 weeks post-operatively.

Expected Outcomes: Open reduction internal fixation for calcaneal fractures tends to yield good results only for minimally displaced, simple fracture patterns. Most result in decreased subtalar ROM, regardless of healing. Healing has been reported to occur within 4 months in most cases. Functional outcomes and anatomic axis alignment is reported to be excellent nearly 5 years post-operative. Complications may include non-union, malunion, infection, and arthritic changes. Advanced arthritis can be treated with delayed subtalar arthrodesis. The most common complication remains wound problems including dehiscence. Limited subtalar range of motion can effect ambulation, especially on uneven surfaces.

Return to Play: Return to sports participation is entirely dependent upon the extent of the fracture and the quality of the reduction. Fractures that heal in a near-anatomic fashion may allow return to play within 6 months. More advanced fractures may preclude return to play.

Recommended Readings

Bajammal S, Tornetta P 3rd, Sanders D, Bhandari M. Displaced intra-articular calcaneal fractures. *J Orthop Trauma*. 2005;19(5):360–364. Review.

Carr JB. Surgical treatment of the intra-articular calcaneus fracture. *Orthop Clin North Am*. 1994;25(4):665–675. Review.

Germann CA, Perron AD, Miller MD, Powell SM, Brady WJ. Orthopedic pitfalls in the ED: Calcaneal fractures. *Am J Emerg Med*. 2004;22(7):607–611. Review.

Harvey EJ, Grujic L, Early JS, Benirschke SK, Sangeorzan BJ. Morbidity associated with ORIF of intra-articular calcaneus fractures using a lateral approach. *Foot Ankle Int*. 2001;22(11):868–873.

Howard JL, Buckley R, McCormack R, Pate G, Leighton R, Petrie D, Galpin R. Complications following management of displaced intra-articular calcaneal fractures: A prospective randomized trial comparing open reduction internal fixation with nonoperative management. *J Orthop Trauma*. 2003;17(4):241–249.

Hüfner T, Geerling J, Gerich T, Zeichen J, Richter M, Krettek C. [Open reduction and internal fixation by primary subtalar arthrodesis for intraarticular calcaneal fractures] *Oper Orthop Traumatol*. 2007;19(2):155–169. Review.

Rammelt S, Zwipp H. Calcaneus fractures: Facts, controversies and recent developments. *Injury*. 2004;35(5):443–461. Review.

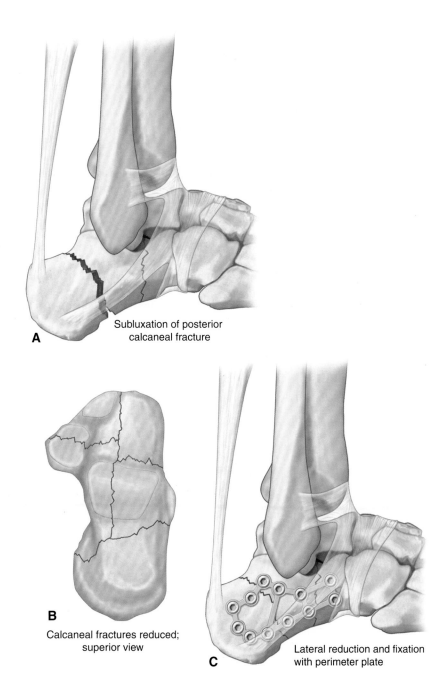

Subluxation of posterior
calcaneal fracture

A

B

Calcaneal fractures reduced;
superior view

Lateral reduction and fixation
with perimeter plate

C

Figure 113. Open Reduction Internal Fixation (ORIF) of Calcaneus Fracture

ORIF Fifth Metatarsal (Jones) Fractures

Indications and Goals: Jones fractures are located at the junction of the metaphysis and diaphysis of the fifth metatarsal. This should be distinguished from "Pseudo-Jones" fractures that are more proximal. The distinction is important because the true Jones fracture has a poor healing rate and, at least in the competitive athlete, ORIF should be considered. This allows for earlier return to training. Initial treatment for non-operatively treated Jones fractures is non–weight-bearing.

Procedure and Technique: Treatment of Jones fractures within specific indications can be accomplished with an intramedullary screw placed through a percutaneous incision. This procedure is done under fluoroscopic guidance. It is helpful to use the cannulated screw system, at least for canal preparation, even if a conventional screw is placed. In general, the larger the screw, the better, and non-cannulated screws are preferred. This is because hardware failure (screw breakage) has been reported. Newer headless compression screws are also popular

Post-surgical Precautions/Rehabilitation: Patients will be placed non–weight-bearing in a Cam walker for 3 to 4 weeks. Progression to full weight bearing as tolerated will be guided by surgeon preference though early return to activity has been shown to predispose to recurrent fracture. The initiation of proprioceptive exercises can also be progressed coinciding with weight bearing.

Expected Outcomes: Expect return to full activity 6 to 8 weeks post surgery. Recurrent fractures, or incomplete healing is often the result of varus hindfoot malalignment leading to lateral column overload. This can be addressed with orthotics, first MT dorsiflexion osteotomy or sometimes a Dwyer calcaneal osteotomy.

Return to Play: Ideally, a return to sports participation should follow radiographic evidence of bony healing, pain-free activity, and the ability to run and cut without apprehension or difficulty. Radiographic healing can occur as early as 6 to 8 weeks post-operatively. CT scans can be performed to document full healing of the metatarsal.

Recommended Readings

Johnson JT, Labib SA, Fowler R. Intramedullary screw fixation of the fifth metatarsal: An anatomic study and improved technique. *Foot Ankle Int.* 2004;25(4):274–277.

Mologne TS, Lundeen JM, Clapper MF, O'Brien TJ. Early screw fixation versus casting in the treatment of acute Jones fractures. *Am J Sports Med.* 2005;33(7):970–975. Epub 2005 May 11.

Porter DA, Duncan M, Meyer SJ. Fifth metatarsal Jones fracture fixation with a 4.5-mm cannulated stainless steel screw in the competitive and recreational athlete: A clinical and radiographic evaluation. *Am J Sports Med.* 2005;33(5):726–733. Epub 2005 Feb 16.

Reese K, Litsky A, Kaeding C, Pedroza A, Shah N. Cannulated screw fixation of Jones fractures: A clinical and biomechanical study. *Am J Sports Med.* 2004;32:1736–1742.

Rehman S, Kashyap S. Proximal fifth metatarsal stress fracture treated by early open reduction and internal fixation. *Orthopedics.* 2004 Nov;27(11):1196–1198.

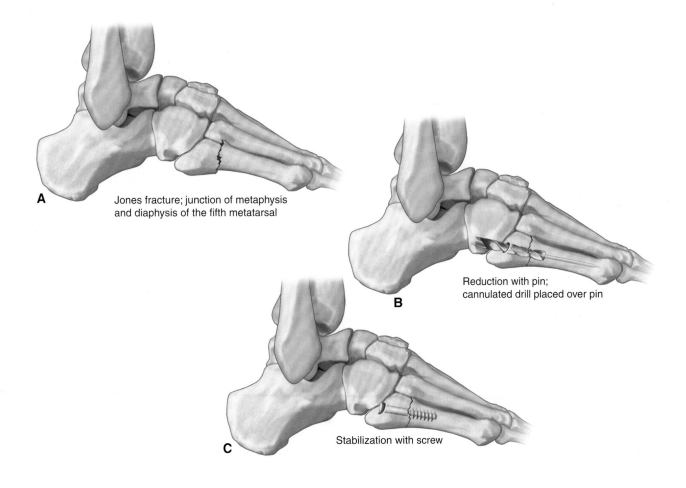

A   Jones fracture; junction of metaphysis
    and diaphysis of the fifth metatarsal

B   Reduction with pin;
    cannulated drill placed over pin

C   Stabilization with screw

Figure 114. Open Reduction Internal Fixation of Jones Fracture

ORIF Lisfranc Injuries

Indications and Goals: Tarsometatarsal fracture dislocations (Lisfranc injuries) are typically a result of a twisting injury with a fixed forefoot. Injury to the Lisfranc's ligament (which runs from the base of the second metatarsal to the medial cuneiform) is common. There is a loss of congruity of the tarsometatarsal alignment, which is best demonstrated with standing radiographs. These injuries can be classified as homolateral (to the same side), isolated (only one joint is injured), or divergent (in different directions). Treatment of displaced injuries requires ORIF.

Procedure and Technique: Anatomic reduction is achieved with open reduction. Cannulated screws and K-wires are used to fix the tarsometatarsal joints. Arthrodesis can also be considered for significant joint displacement or high-energy injuries.

Post-surgical Precautions/Rehabilitation: Open reduction internal fixation to this area is challenging. Anatomic reduction is necessary but not sufficient to reduce the risk of arthritic changes. Early ankle range of motion may begin shortly after surgery in a supervised manner. Gradual progressive resistive strengthening exercises can be prescribed for rehabilitation and post-operative swelling should be kept to a minimum for facilitation of restoration of normal joint mechanics. Once weight bearing, progression from partial to full weight bearing will occur, with proprioceptive exercises implemented.

Expected Outcomes: Temporary rigid screw fixation of Lisfranc injury maintains anatomic reduction and maximizes functional outcomes for the patients. Those injuries with significant displacement have yielded worse outcomes as compared to others. Poorer outcomes have also been associated with pre-operative high-energy trauma and additional associated injuries on the ipsilateral limb. Complications can include post-traumatic arthritis, painful hardware, malreduction, and injuries to nerves.

Return to Play: Return to participation depends upon the restoration of the normal alignment of the foot. With near-anatomic restoration, return to play may be within 4 to 6 months. In competitive athletes, screws may be taken out at 4 months post-operatively to avoid breakage and midfoot pain.

Recommended Readings

Aronow MS. Treatment of the missed Lisfranc injury. *Foot Ankle Clin.* 2006;11(1):127–142, ix. Review.

Desmond EA, Chou LB. Current concepts review: Lisfranc injuries. *Foot Ankle Int.* 2006;27(8):653–660. Review.

Hatch RL, Alsobrook JA, Clugston JR. Diagnosis and management of metatarsal fractures. *Am Fam Physician.* 2007;76(6):817–826. Review.

Owens BD, Wixted JJ, Cook J, Teebagy AK. Intramedullary transmetatarsal Kirschner wire fixation of Lisfranc fracture-dislocations. *Am J Orthop.* 2003;32(8):389–391. Review.

Perron AD, Brady WJ, Keats TE. Orthopedic pitfalls in the ED: Lisfranc fracture-dislocation. *Am J Emerg Med.* 2001;19(1):71–75.

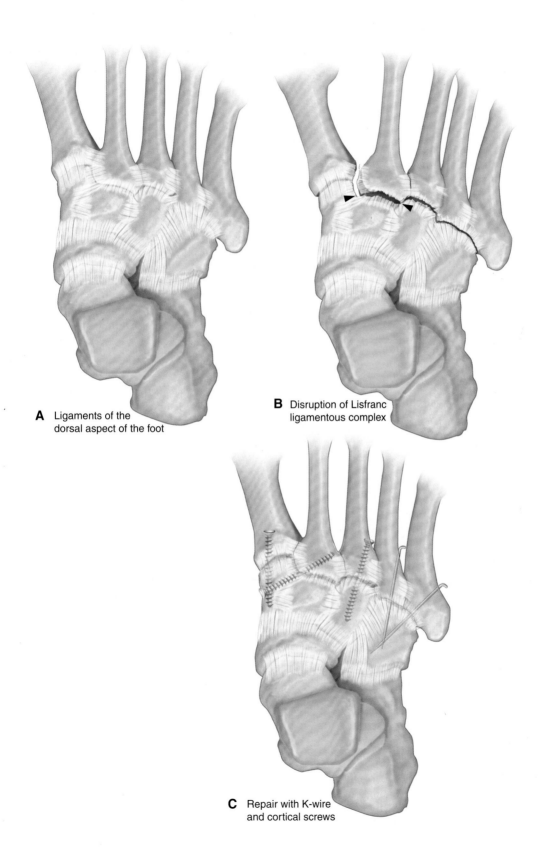

A Ligaments of the
dorsal aspect of the foot

B Disruption of Lisfranc
ligamentous complex

C Repair with K-wire
and cortical screws

Figure 115. Screw and K-wire Fixation of Lisfranc Injury

ORIF Metatarsal and Phalangeal Fractures

Indications and Goals: Most of these fractures can be treated non-operatively. Open fractures, border metatarsal fractures (first and fifth), multiple metatarsal fractures, intra-articular fractures of the great toe, and all open fractures require operative intervention.

Procedure and Technique: The advent of smaller screw and plate systems has made anatomic fixation of metatarsal and phalangeal fractures easier both in the hand and the foot. A vertical incision is made over the injured bone and the fracture is reduced and fixed. Some fractures can be treated with intramedullary K-wires or K-wires placed horizontally to achieve an internal splint.

Post-surgical Precautions/Rehabilitation: Immobilization in a boot or cast occurs for 4 to 8 weeks based upon the severity of the injury and the type of fixation. Once removed, local range of motion can begin. Lower-leg strengthening, cardiovascular activity, and general balance activity performed during the rehabilitation. phase early can assist with return to overall function.

Expected Outcomes: Patients tend to do well overall if length and rotation can be restored with stable fixation. Individuals returning to repetitive running or jumping activities will require additional time for rehabilitation.

Return to Play: Following complete fracture healing and progressive weight bearing, running, and functional return. Typically 3 to 4 months post-operatively.

Recommended Readings

Galuppo LD, Stover SM, Willits NH. A biomechanical comparison of double-plate and Y-plate fixation for comminuted equine second phalangeal fractures. *Vet Surg.* 2000;29(2):152–162.

Mereddy PK, Molloy A, Hennessy MS. Osteochondral fracture of the fourth metatarsal head treated by open reduction and internal fixation. *J Foot Ankle Surg.* 2007;46(4):320–322.

Bacterial External Otitis

Introduction (Definitions/Classification): Bacterial infection of the external auditory canal is the most common form of external otitis. Common pathogens include *Pseudomonas aeruginosa* and *Staphylococcus aureus.* Predisposing factors include the following.

- Excess wetness—alters protective skin–cerumen barrier and increased pH of the ear canal that favors bacterial growth.
- Aggressive cleaning of the external ear canal—reduces amount of protective cerumen and induces abrasions, which allows bacteria to ingress into deeper tissues.

History and Physical Examination: Individuals typically have a history of recurrent external otitis, and may present with a history of either tympanic membrane perforation or ear surgery. Common symptoms include discharge, earache, pruritus, and change in hearing acuity. Tinnitus or vertigo may be present in more severe cases. Physical examination typically reveals the following.

- Erythematous external canal impacted to varying degrees (depending on severity) with discolored debris that varies in color (white, gray, or brown).
- Tympanic membrane maybe erythematous and "boggy," yet should be intact and mobile.
- Increased pain with superior distraction of the auricle.
- Fever, periauricular lymphadenopathy, or periauricular erythema in more severe cases.

Diagnosis:

- Signs/symptoms on physical examination.
- Cultures are typically unnecessary. Consider cultures, complete blood count (CBC) with differential, erythrocyte sedimentation rate (ESR), and imaging (CT or MRI) in individuals with increased ear discharge, fever, periauricular lymphadenopathy, periauricular erythema, or earache out of proportion to clinical examination findings to rule out necrotizing otitis externa.

Treatment:

- Examine all patients before commencing treatment.
- Remove debris with gentle irrigation using 3% hydrogen peroxide only *if* tympanic membrane is visible and intact.
- Topical preparations containing acetic acid reduce pH and inhibit growth of common pathogens.
- Topical preparations that contain corticosteroids and either acetic acid or antibiotics have a higher cure rate.
- Compared to topical preparations, there is no difference in clinical response with systemic antibiotics.
- Various combinations of topical antibiotics polymyxin and neomycin are available and effective.
- Neomycin can be ototoxic if the tympanic membrane is perforated and is a common cause of contact dermatitis following treatment for bacterial external otitis.
- Topical fluoroquinolones (FQs), including ciprofloxacin and ofloxacin used once to twice daily may improve compliance because of reduced dosing; as compared to topical preparations containing polymyxin and neomycin that need to be used at least three times daily.
- Duration of treatment is typically from 2 to 7 days and varies with disease severity and individual compliance and response to therapy.
- Patient education to prevent recurrence should include "dry ear" precautions, regular use of acidifying ear drops, the avoidance of ear phones and hearing aids, and the use of ear plugs for swimming practice.

Other Considerations:

- Consider fungal (candida) infections in individuals who frequently use hearing aids and headphones, and those who do not respond to antibiotic therapy.
- Refer to otolaryngology if the tympanic membrane is not intact.
- Refer all individuals to otolaryngology who have severe ear discharge, fever, periauricular lymphadenopathy, periauricular erythema, or earache out of proportion to clinical examination findings to rule out necrotizing otitis externa—a potential life-threatening complication of bacterial external otitis.

Return to Play Criteria:

- Improving symptoms and normal hearing acuity.
- Absence of fever, severe ear discharge, fever, periauricular lymphadenopathy, periauricular erythema, or earache out of proportion to clinical examination findings.

Recommended Readings

Clark WB, Brook I, Bianki D, Thompson DH. Microbiology of otitis externa. *Otolaryngol Head Neck Surg.* 1997;116:23–25.

Cohen D, Friedman P. The diagnostic criteria of malignant external otitis. *J Laryngol Otol.* 1987;101:216–221.

Goffin FB. pH as a factor in external otitis. *N Engl J Med.* 1963;268:287–289.

Kaushik V, Malik T, Saeed SR. Interventions for acute otitis externa. *Cochrane Database Syst Rev.* 2010;(1):CD004740.

Rosenfeld RM, Brown L, Cannon CR, et al. Clinical practice guideline: acute otitis externa. *Otolaryngol Head Neck Surg.* 2006;134:S4–S23.

Russell JD, Donnelly M, McShane DP, Alun-Jones T, Walsh M. What causes acute otitis externa? *J Laryngol Otol.* 1993;107:898–901.

van Balen FA, Smit WM, Zuithoff NP, Verheij TJ. Clinical efficacy of three common treatments in acute otitis externa in primary care: Randomised controlled trial. *BMJ.* 2003;327:1201–1205.

Van Ginkel CJ, Bruintjes TD, Huizing EH. Allergy due to topical medications in chronic otitis externa and chronic otitis media. *Clin Otolaryngol.* 1995;20:326–328.

Yelland MJ. The efficacy of oral cotrimoxazole in the treatment of otitis externa in general practice. *Med J Aust.* 1993;158:697–699.

Otitis Media

Introduction (Definitions/Classification): Mucosal infection or inflammation of the middle ear. Eustachian tube obstruction or dysfunction leads to accumulation of fluid in the middle ear which is a precursor for infection or inflammation. *Streptococcus pneumoniae* is the most common bacteria implicated in adults. Several viruses may induce otitis media in children. Various pathologic variants include the following.

- Acute otitis media with or without effusion.
  - "With effusion."
    - Usually associated with allergies or barotraumas.
    - Associated with conductive hearing loss.
- Chronic otitis media.
  - Serous.
  - Purulent.

History and Physical Examination: Individuals typically have a history of seasonal allergies or an upper respiratory infection preceding the following symptoms and signs.

- Otalgia.
- Otorrhea—serous or purulent associated with tympanic membrane perforation.
- Conductive hearing loss.
- Tympanic membrane fluid level.
- Fever is usually absent.

Diagnosis:

- Signs/symptoms on physical examination.
- Otoscopic examination of tympanic membrane may reveal bulging, erythema, blisters (bullous myringitis), opacities, or decreased mobility.
- Lack of inflammation, an immobile tympanic membrane with retraction, or an air–fluid level usually signifies otitis media with effusion.
- Either serous or purulent fluid in the external ear canal signifies tympanic membrane perforation.
- Weber tuning fork test lateralizes to affected ear secondary to conductive hearing loss.
- Rinne tuning fork test (512 Hz) may reveal bone conduction greater than air conduction secondary to conductive hearing loss.

Treatment:

- Treat all adults with antibiotics.
- Intact tympanic membrane.
  - First-line antibiotic—amoxicillin for 7 to 10 days.
  - Individuals with penicillin allergy—macrolide (azithromycin or clarithromycin).
  - Failure to respond to first-line antibiotics—amoxicillin–clavulanate or second-generation cephalosporin (PO cefdinir or IM ceftriaxone).
- Ruptured tympanic membrane.
  - Topical ofloxacin otic drops.
  - Avoid acidic, antiseptic, and otic drops containing neomycin that can be ototoxic if used in the presence of a perforated tympanic membrane.
  - Patient education to prevent recurrence should include "dry ear" precautions.
- Supportive care with antihistamines, decongestants, or nasal steroids may be beneficial in otitis media with effusion.

Other Considerations:

- Consider mastoiditis in individuals with swelling or pain behind the auricle.
- Refer all individuals to otolaryngology who have the following.
  - Swelling or pain behind the auricle.
  - Hearing loss that persists after resolution of infection.
  - Persistent or recurrent tympanic membrane perforation.
  - Fever.
  - Persistent, painful effusion.
  - Forthcoming airline travel (for consideration of myringotomy and placement of pressure equalization tubes).

Return to Play Criteria:

- Improving symptoms and intact tympanic membrane without hearing loss.
- No fever or symptoms or signs concerning for mastoiditis.

Recommended Readings

Chole RA, Cook GB. The Rinne test for conductive deafness. A critical reappraisal. *Arch Otolaryngol Head Neck Surg.* 1988;114:399–403.
Chonmaitree T, Revai K, Grady JJ, et al. Viral upper respiratory tract infection and otitis media complication in young children. *Clin Infect Dis.* 2008;46:815–823.
Ginsburg CM, Rudoy R, Nelson JD. Acute mastoiditis in infants and children. *Clin Pediatr.* 1980;19:549–553.
Gray BM, Converse GM 3rd, Dillon HC Jr. Serotypes of Streptococcus pneumoniae causing disease. *J Infect Dis.* 1979;140:979–983.
Luxford WM, Sheehy JL. Myringotomy and ventilation tubes: A report of 1,568 ears. *Laryngoscope.* 1982;92:1293–1297.

Vertigo

Introduction (Definitions/Classification): A type of dizziness, with a sense of "spinning," "swaying," or "tilting" "movement" while stationary. It is not a disease but a symptom of numerous underlying disorders that affect vestibular function (balance and equilibrium). It is two to three times more common in women. Common causes in "otherwise healthy individuals" include the following.

- Benign paroxysmal positional vertigo (BPPV)—most common cause, secondary to canalithiasis.
- Ménière disease—idiopathic, endolymphatic hydrops (excessive fluid in inner ear).
- Vestibular neuritis—viral-induced inflammation of vestibular nerve.
- Labyrinthitis—inflammation of the inner ear labyrinth induced by either infection, stress, trauma, medications, or autoimmune diseases.
- Other causes—posttraumatic, motion sickness, otitis media, acoustic neuroma, multiple sclerosis, vertebrobasilar stroke.

History and Physical Examination: All except BPPV, usually associated with nausea and vomiting.

- BPPV—**RECURRENT** and **BRIEF** (<1 minute) with change in position.
- Ménière disease—**THERE** (**T**innitus, **H**earing loss, **E**pisodic vertigo, **R**ecurrent, **E**ar fullness) that lasts several hours to days, progressive, usually **UNILATERAL**.
- Vestibular neuritis—**SAW** (**S**ingle or **S**udden, **A**cute vertigo, **W**ithout hearing loss) that last days to weeks.
- Labyrinthitis—**US** (**U**nilateral, **S**udden) hearing loss *and* vestibular function.

Diagnosis:

- In addition to history and physical evaluation:
  - BPPV—Dix–Hallpike maneuver.
  - Ménière disease—Weber test (sound localizes to normal ear).
  - Vestibular neuritis—check hearing acuity (usually normal).
  - Labyrinthitis—consider temporal bone CT or MRI in selected cases.

Treatment:

- Examples of common medications used to suppress vestibular symptoms include antihistamines (diphenhydramine, meclizine), antiemetics (promethazine, ondansetron), and benzodiazepines (diazepam).
- BPPV.
  - Epley maneuver (canalith repositioning).
  - Vestibular rehabilitation (recommend early).
- Ménière disease.
  - Low sodium diet.
  - Intratympanic dexamethasone or gentamicin.
- Vestibular neuritis.
  - Steroids may be superior than antivirals (valacyclovir).
- Labyrinthitis.
  - First-line management—bed rest and hydration.
  - Short course of steroids in refractory cases.
  - No clear role for antivirals.

Other Considerations:

- If associated with vertigo, consider brain MRI/MRA.
  - Acoustic neuroma—ipsilateral sensorineural loss, deafness, and/or tinnitus.
  - Multiple sclerosis—episodic neurologic symptoms.
  - Vertebrobasilar stroke—diplopia, dysphagia, dysarthria, and/or weakness.
- Refer athletes to ENT or neurologist if common measures fail to resolve symptoms.
- Caution with medications includes the following.
  - Use medications for the shortest duration possible.
  - Promethazine can potentially prolong QT interval and induce fatal arrhythmia.
  - Drugs used to treat vertigo can have undesirable side effects including dry mouth and urinary retention.

Return to Play Criteria:

- Normal balance, hearing, vision with sport-specific tasks.
- No nausea or vomiting.

Recommended Readings

Furman JM, Barton J. Approach to the patient with vertigo. *UpToDate,* Accessed September 1, 2010.

Herraiz C, Plaza G, Aparicio JM, Gallego I, Marcos S, Ruiz C. Transtympanic steroids for Ménière's disease. *Otol Neurotol.* 2010;31(1): 162–167.

Mark AS, Seltzer S, Nelson-Drake J, Chapman JC, Fitzgerald DC, Gulya AJ. Labyrinthine enhancement on gadolinium-enhanced magnetic resonance imaging in sudden deafness and vertigo: Correlation with audiologic and electronystagmographic studies. *Ann Otol Rhinol Laryngol.* 1992;101(6):459–464.

Neuhauser HK, Lempert T. Vertigo: Epidemiologic aspects. *Semin Neurol.* 2009;29(5):473–481.

Schuknecht HF, Kitamura K. Second Louis H. Clerf Lecture. Vestibular neuritis. *Ann Otol Rhinol Laryngol Suppl.* 1981;90(1 Pt 2):1–19.

Strupp M, Zingler VC, Arbusow V, et al. Methylprednisolone, valacyclovir, or the combination for vestibular neuritis. *N Engl J Med.* 2004;351(4):354–361.

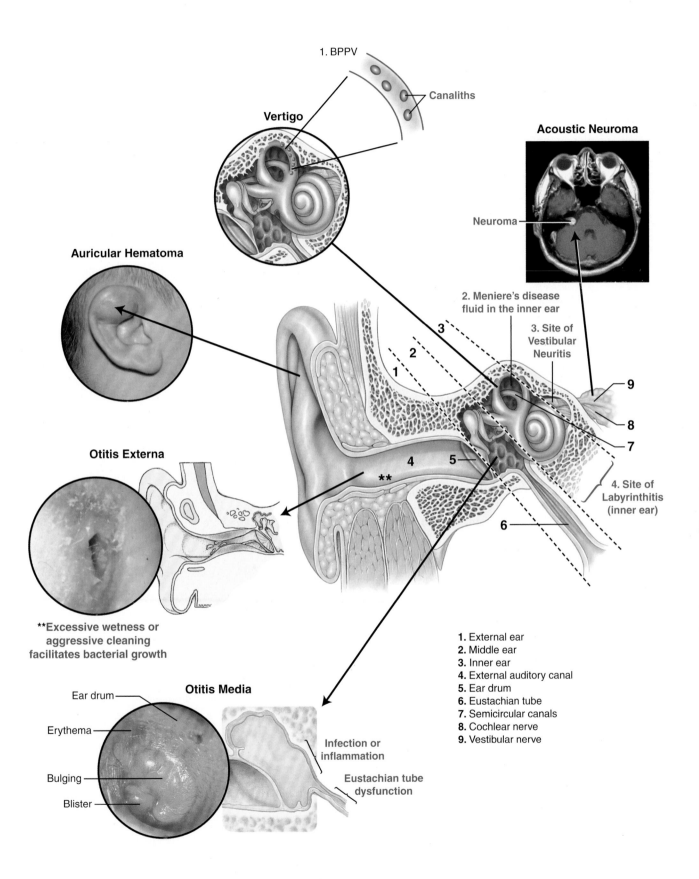

1. BPPV

Canaliths

Vertigo

Acoustic Neuroma

Neuroma

Auricular Hematoma

2. Meniere's disease
fluid in the inner ear

3. Site of
Vestibular
Neuritis

3

2

1

9

8

7

Otitis Externa

4

5

4. Site of
Labyrinthitis
(inner ear)

6

****Excessive wetness or
aggressive cleaning
facilitates bacterial growth**

1. External ear
2. Middle ear
3. Inner ear
4. External auditory canal
5. Ear drum
6. Eustachian tube
7. Semicircular canals
8. Cochlear nerve
9. Vestibular nerve

Ear drum

Erythema

Bulging

Blister

Otitis Media

Infection or
inflammation

Eustachian tube
dysfunction

Figure 117. Ears

Section 2: Eyes

Conjunctivitis

Introduction (Definitions/Classification): Commonly known as "pink or red eye;" caused by inflammation of the "conjunctiva," which covers the eyeball and lines the inner portion of eyelids. Etiologic factors include the following.

- Noninfectious—allergic, chemical exposure, mechanical.
- Infectious—viruses (more common) and bacteria.

History and Physical Examination: Chemosis (conjunctival edema), erythema, discharge, morning "eyes stuck," and "lid crusting" are typical features, yet not useful in distinguishing different types of conjunctivitis. Other differentiating features may include the following.

- Bilateral itching and watery discharge with a history of seasonal or environmental allergies—**allergic**.
- Unilateral or bilateral pain and thick purulent discharge—especially at the lid margins—**bacterial**.
- Unilateral, bilateral involvement over 2 days, "sandy, gritty, or burning" feeling, or watery discharge with mucus during an ongoing upper respiratory infection—**viral**.

Diagnosis:

- Signs/symptoms on physical examination.
- Cultures are usually unnecessary.
- Consider gram stain of discharge to rule out gonococcal conjunctivitis.
- Consider rapid 10-minute test (RPS Adeno Detector) for adenovirus.
  - Can save costs and reduce bacterial resistance by eliminating need for empiric topical antibiotic therapy.
- Visual acuity testing as needed on an individual basis.

Treatment:

- Examine all patients before commencing treatment.
- Allergic and viral conjunctivitis are usually self-limited.
  - Over-the-counter antihistamine and decongestant eye drops provide symptomatic relief but do not treat disease.
  - Extended use of drops can be toxic and irritating.
  - Preservative-free eye drops are effective for refractory symptoms and may reduce toxicity and irritation noted with prolonged use of antihistamine and decongestant eye drops.
- Various drops and ointments for bacterial conjunctivitis.
  - Sulfacetamide, azithromycin, or FQ drops—latter highly effective against pseudomonas.
  - Bacitracin, polymyxin–bacitracin, or sulfacetamide ointment.
  - Counsel individuals regarding blurring of vision following the application of ointments.
- Discontinue contact lens use.
- No role for glucocorticoids for conjunctivitis. Can be extremely toxic and may cause various complications.
- Educate on contagiosity. Avoid sharing linens, towels, cups, and silverware.
- Obtain ophthalmology consult for all individuals with failure to respond to antibiotic therapy, change in visual acuity, inability to keep the eye open, persistent and severe foreign body sensation, nausea, headache, refractory photophobia, pupil dysfunction, or corneal opacities.

Other Considerations:

- Consider gonococcal conjunctivitis in individual with a purulent discharge that develops hyperacutely within 12 hours, eyelid swelling, marked chemosis, with or without preauricular lymphadenopathy and concomitant urethritis. Gonococcal conjunctivitis is severe and can cause blindness if treatment is delayed.
- Consider keratoconjunctivitis (adenovirus) in individuals with "foreign body" sensation, acute vision changes, and corneal infiltrates that may not be readily visible on penlight corneal examination. May be severe and cause blindness if treatment is delayed.
- Consider chlamydia-induced inclusion conjunctivitis in individuals with chronic symptoms refractory to topical antibiotic therapy.

- Consider keratitis (corneal inflammation) in individuals who use contact lenses. Empiric treatment of conjunctivitis without ruling out keratitis can potentially cause eye perforation.
- Consider "pterygium" in individuals with a localized, triangular area of conjunctival thickening or redness extending from the inner canthus to the medial corneal margin.

Return to Play Criteria:

- Improving symptoms and normal visual acuity.
- At least 24 hours on antibiotics for bacterial conjunctivitis.
- Address vision needs for individuals who use contact lenses and are unable to use during recovery from conjunctivitis.

Recommended Readings

Cheng KH, Leung SL, Hoekman HW, et al. Incidence of contact-lens-associated microbial keratitis and its related morbidity. *Lancet.* 1999;354:181–185.

Jernigan JA, Lowry BS, Hayden FG, et al. Adenovirus type 8 epidemic keratoconjunctivitis in an eye clinic: Risk factors and control. *J Infect Dis.* 1993;167:1307–1313.

Rietveld RP, ter Riet G, Bindels PJ, Sloos JH, van Weert HC. Predicting bacterial cause in infectious conjunctivitis: Cohort study on informativeness of combinations of signs and symptoms. *BMJ.* 2004;329:206–210.

Udeh BL, Schneider JE, Ohsfeldt RL. Cost effectiveness of a point-of-care test for adenoviral conjunctivitis. *Am J Med Sci.* 2008;336:254–264.

Ullman S, Roussel TJ, Culbertson WW, et al. Neisseria gonorrhoeae keratoconjunctivitis. *Ophthalmology.* 1987;94:525–531.

Wan WL, Farkas GC, May WN, Robin JB. The clinical characteristics and course of adult gonococcal conjunctivitis. *Am J Ophthalmol.* 1986;102:575–583.

Eyelid Diseases

Introduction (Definitions/Classification): Common eyelid diseases encountered in athletes include the following.

- Hordeolum.
  - **External**—commonly known as a "*stye.*" Caused by bacterial infection of the eyelid sebaceous (Zeis) or sweat glands. *S. aureus* is the most common bacteria. May be associated with eyelid (*periorbital, preseptal*) cellulitis.
  - **Internal**—inflammation of meibomian glands.
- Chalazion.
  - Chronic noninfectious, inflammatory lesion following obstruction of either the Zeis sebaceous glands or meibomian glands.

History and Physical Examination:

- Eyelid pain with foreign body sensation in eyelid.
- Increased tearing (*epiphora*).
- Blurring of vision.
- **Stye**—focal swelling noted on inner lid, best noted following eversion of lid.
- **Chalazion**—focal pustule or papule at lid margin (external or internal).
- Medial, lower eyelid swelling—concerning for infection of either lacrimal sac (*dacryocystitis*) or lacrimal gland (*dacryoadenitis*).
- In individuals with preseptal cellulitis look for
  - diffuse eyelid erythema and edema.
  - lack of pustule or papule at lid margin.
  - preauricular, submandibular, or cervical lymphadenopathy.
- Impaired eyeball motility, change in vision, bulging eyeballs (*proptosis*), altered pupillary reflexes, or optic nerve swelling and retinal vein engorgement on fundus examination—concerning for orbital cellulitis.

Diagnosis:

- Signs/symptoms on physical examination.
- Cultures of tissue fluid for styes that fail to respond to common therapies.
- CBC with differential in selected cases.
- CT scan of orbit for all individuals with symptoms or signs concerning for
  - dacryocystitis.
  - dacryoadenitis.
  - orbital cellulitis.

Treatment:

- Examine all patients before commencing treatment.
- Warm compresses for 10 to 15 minutes, up to four times per day.
- For stye and chalazion, gentle massage for 5 minutes, up to four times per day. *NO massage for diffuse eyelid erythema or edema.*
- Topical antibiotic ophthalmic drops containing bacitracin or erythromycin.
- Consider oral antibiotics for concomitant periorbital cellulitis.
  - First-line antibiotic—amoxicillin–clavulanate or first-generation cephalosporin.
  - Failure to respond to first-line antibiotics—IM ceftriaxone or oxacillin.
  - Consider IV antibiotics (oxacillin or nafcillin) if symptoms fail to improve in 48 to 72 hours.
- Consider clindamycin or Bactrim for methicillin-resistant *S. aureus* (MRSA) as directed by cultures.
- Counsel treated individuals on eyelid hygiene—to keep eyelid margins clean by regular, gentle washing with a few drops of baby shampoo.

Other Considerations:

- When to refer to ophthalmologist?
  - Refractory or recurrent chalazion for biopsy to rule out malignancy, and treatment with either corticosteroid injection and/or curettage.
  - Individuals being considered for IV antibiotics.
  - *To rule out orbital cellulitis*—individuals with impaired eyeball motility, change in vision, proptosis, altered papillary reflexes, or optic nerve swelling and retinal vein engorgement on fundus examination.
  - Consider infection with MRSA in individuals who fail to respond to common therapeutic interventions.

Return to Play Criteria:

- Improving symptoms and normal vision.
- No fever or symptoms or signs concerning for orbital cellulitis.

Recommended Readings

Goawalla A, Lee V. A prospective randomized treatment study comparing three treatment options for chalazia: Triamcinolone acetonide injections, incision and curettage and treatment with hot compresses. *Clin Experiment Ophthalmol.* 2007;35:706–712.

Mueller JB, McStay CM. Ocular infection and inflammation. *Emerg Med Clin North Am.* 2008;26:57–72.

Wald ER. Periorbital and orbital infections. *Pediatr Rev.* 2004;25:312–320.

Corneal Abrasion

Introduction (Definitions/Classification): Defect of the corneal epithelium. Common causes in athletes include the following.

- Trauma.
- Prolonged use of contact lenses.
- Foreign body.

History and Physical Examination:

- Severe eye pain.
- Foreign body sensation.
- Inability to open eyelids that precludes activities of daily living.
- Increased tearing (*epiphora*), blurring of vision, corneal edema (*grayish appearance*).
- Recurrent corneal abrasions induce "nocturnal" and "early morning" pain.
- Perform thorough eye examination to rule out penetrating trauma.
  - Check for foreign body with penlight examination.
  - Check for discharge, opacities, or infiltrate—corneal abrasions induce *only tearing*.
  - Check pupils.
    - Small (corneal abrasion).
    - *Large and nonreactive* (*consider penetrating trauma*).
  - Check eyelids for foreign bodies.

- Check anterior chamber for blood or pus.
- Visual acuity may be completely normal.
- Funduscopic examination to confirm *red reflex* (*absent in retinal detachment*).

Diagnosis:

- Signs/symptoms on physical examination.
- Fluorescein examination should be performed *only to confirm diagnosis after* physical examination has been completed (*presumptive diagnosis*). Visualization of cornea under cobalt blue light reveals *green discoloration* of the affected area.
- Stained abrasion appears yellow to the naked eye.

Treatment:

- As needed, remove foreign body using gentle irrigation with saline.
- May benefit from eye lubrication with hourly application of "over-the-counter lubricant" (e.g., preservative-free artificial tears).
- Pain relief with systemic narcotics or nonsteroidal anti-inflammatory medications.
- Choice of topical antibiotics (sulfacetamide, erythromycin, ciprofloxacin, ofloxacin, polymyxin/trimethoprim).
  - Optimal dosing—QID for 3 to 5 days.
  - Ointment facilitates lubrication of cornea and is preferred.
- Eye patch for 24 hours may help healing of corneal epithelium and relief of symptoms.
  - No data to prove that patching reduces symptoms or improves healing.
  - Noninfected corneal abrasions, those secondary to trauma (*with the exception of abrasions induced by contact lens*), and abrasions following removal of foreign bodies can be treated without an eye patch.
  - Properly placed eye patch will prevent athlete from blinking.
  - *Contraindicated*, if abrasion induced by contact lenses. Using an eye patch for corneal abrasions induced by contact lenses can lead to "*sight-threatening infections.*"
- Avoid topical steroids or anesthetics (*delays corneal healing*).

Other Considerations:

- When to refer to ophthalmologist?
  - Corneal abrasions >3 mm.
  - Lack of improvement within 24 hours following use of common therapies, even if the abrasion is <3 mm in size.
  - Clinical features of penetrating trauma (large, nonreactive pupil; blood in anterior chamber [*hyphema*]; pus in anterior chamber [*hypopyon*]; extrusion of ocular contents).
  - Change in acuity *and/or* questionable corneal infection (*altered color and infiltrate of cornea*), especially following prolonged use of contact lenses while sleeping.
    - Contact lenses can induce infectious pseudomonas keratitis complicated by corneal perforation.
  - With foreign body that cannot be removed by gentle irrigation with saline.
- Consider a short course of cycloplegic eye drops that can alleviate pain induced by pupil miosis.
  - Cyclopentolate or homatropine.
  - Avoid use before consulting with an ophthalmologist.
- Consider tetanus prophylaxis for penetrating eye injuries.
- Educate athletes to avoid driving with an eye patch secondary to "*altered depth perception.*"

Return to Play Criteria:

- Improving symptoms and normal vision.
- Off narcotics for pain relief.

Recommended Readings

Benson WH, Snyder IS, Granus V, Odom JV, Macsai MS. Tetanus prophylaxis following ocular injuries. *J Emerg Med*. 1993;11:677–683.

Clemons CS, Cohen EJ, Arentsen JJ, Donnenfeld ED, Laibson PR. Pseudomonas ulcers following patching of corneal abrasions associated with contact lens wear. *CLAO J*. 1987;13:161–164.

Jacobs DS. Corneal abrasions and corneal foreign bodies. *UpToDate*. Accessed October 10, 2010 and October 27, 2012.

Kaiser PK. A comparison of pressure patching versus no patching for corneal abrasions due to trauma or foreign body removal. Corneal abrasion patching study group. *Ophthalmology*. 1995;102:1936–1942.

www.ncemi.org. Accessed October 27, 2012.

Pterygium

Introduction (Definitions/Classification): Wing or triangular shaped, proliferation of conjunctival tissue of unclear etiology. Pathogenic factors include genetic predisposition, viral (human papilloma virus), ultraviolet light (UV), and immunologic alterations. Commonly in athletes exposed to sun and wind for prolonged durations.

History and Physical Examination:

- Growth (over months to years) arises from limbus and progresses to cornea.
  - As opposed to "pinguecula"—arise from *and* stay confined to the conjunctiva.
- Most common symptoms are irritation and redness.
- If growth extends to cornea:
  - Mild to moderate—can cause blurring of vision (induced by astigmatism).
  - Severe—can reduce visual acuity.

Diagnosis:

- Clinical, based on characteristic appearance.

Treatment:

- Symptomatic measures:
  - Sunglasses with good UV protection.
  - Avoid excess sun and wind exposure, when possible.
  - Topical over the counter decongestants, nonsteroidal anti-inflammatory drugs (NSAIDs), and steroids may be effective.
    - *Only* ophthalmologists should prescribe steroids (which can raise intraocular tension).
    - All may induce side effects when used on a chronic basis, especially "*rebound*."
    - No data to show that any of these treatments can either arrest growth or cure.
- Routine, scheduled checks to document growth or stability of lesion.
- Surgical excision of large, refractory, problematic pterygia are associated with the following.
  - Astigmatism.
  - Changes in visual acuity.

Other Considerations:

- Educate—"prevention better than cure."
  - Encourage prophylactic use of sunglasses in athletes exposed to elements (wind and sun).
  - UV protection after development of pterygium, does not guarantee growth limitation.
- Usually benign, yet can be problematic and cause vision changes if growth extends to corneal visual axis.
- Refer to ophthalmologist/optometrist for
  - rapid growth.
  - untreatable irritation.
  - restricted eye movement.
  - blurring of vision—to rule out astigmatism.
  - change in visual acuity.
  - cosmetic reasons.
- Educate athletes regarding
  - high recurrence rate after surgery.
  - decreased risk of recurrence after surgery with advancing age. Therefore, the best is to delay surgical excision.

Return to Play Criteria:

- Corrected astigmatism.
- Normal visual acuity.
- Postsurgical cases—off narcotics for pain relief.

Recommended Readings

Bradley JC, Yang W, Bradley RH, Reid TW, Schwab IR. The science of pterygia. *Br J Ophthalmol.* 2010;94:815–820.
en.wikipedia.org. Accessed October 10, 2010 and October 27, 2012.
Hirst LW. The treatment of pterygium. *Surv Ophthalmol.* 2003;48:145–180.
Jacobs DS. Pterygium. *UpToDate.* Accessed October 10, 2010 and October 27, 2012.
Threlfall TJ, English DR. Sun exposure and pterygium of the eye: A dose-response curve. *Am J Ophthalmol.* 1999;128:280–287.

Traumatic Hyphema

Introduction (Definitions/Classification): Blood in the anterior chamber of the eyeball induced by trauma.

History and Physical Examination:

- History of blunt trauma to orbit or head.
- **First** evaluate for open globe.
  - **BEET: B**lood + **E**ccentric pupil + **E**xtrusion of ocular contents + **T**enting of sclera, **with**
- **PEA: P**hotophobia secondary to miosis (pupillary constriction; direct and consensual) to bright light, **E**ye pain, Decreased Visual **A**cuity, **with**
- **Blood** in anterior chamber, which may be
  - *visible, or*
  - *invisible* (seen only on slit examination; *microhyphema*).
- Other symptoms and signs.
  - Worsening vision while lying flat.
  - Pupil dilation (*mydriasis*).
- Check for other complications.
  - Tearing of iris at its root (*iridodialysis*).
  - Lens subluxation or dislocation.
  - Retinal tear.
- Physical examination of orbit.
  - "*Step-off*"—infraorbital ridge.
  - Crepitus.
  - Decreased and painful extraocular movements.
  - Orbital swelling.
  - Check for foreign body.

Diagnosis:

- Signs/symptoms on physical examination (characteristic appearance).
- Other blood tests.
  - Sickle cell solubility (screening test for sickle cell trait).
  - Hemoglobin electrophoresis (confirmatory test for sickle cell trait; especially in athletes for higher risk—based on ethnicity).
  - CBC, PT, PTT, INR—to evaluate for bleeding disorders.
- Fine-cut (1- to 2-mm cuts) CT without contrast to rule out
  - intraocular foreign body.
  - ruptured globe.
  - facial (orbital) fractures.
- Defer fluorescein examination (if corneal abrasion is suspected) until an open (ruptured) globe has been excluded.
- Funduscopy may be limited secondary to miosis.

Treatment:

- *Refer to ophthalmologist early!* Early recognition and expeditious referral is pivotal for preservation of vision (even if blood is not readily visible and high index of clinical suspicion).
- All decisions regarding activity modification and treatment should be made by ophthalmologist.
- Activity limitation is of pivotal importance.
- Bed rest and elevation of the head of the bed to 30 degrees not shown to be advantageous over infrequent movement.

- Consider sedation and hospitalization for highly active, young athletes.
- Restrict reading.
- *On-field management.*
  - Place an eye shield without compressing underlying globe.
  - Avoid eye patches.
  - Pain relief with Tylenol and/or opioids.
  - *Do not administer NSAIDs*—to prevent further bleeding.
  - *Do not instill any eye drops.*
  - Control nausea and vomiting with ondansetron expeditiously—to prevent rise in intraocular pressure.

Other Considerations:

- Prognosis based on grading of hyphema.
  - Microhyphema and grade I (<33%) have a 90% prognosis for 20/50 vision or better.
  - Grade II (33% to 50%) hyphema has a 70% prognosis for 20/50 vision or better.
  - Grade III (>50%) and grade IV (100%) hyphemas have a 50% prognosis for 20/50 vision or better.
- Consider "orbital hemorrhage" or "orbital compartment syndrome" in athletes with proptosis following blunt force orbital trauma.
  - These conditions can cause permanent blindness very rapidly.
- Test for "sickle cell trait," "bleeding disorders," or diabetes mellitus in athletes with spontaneous hyphema.
- Hospitalization for the following.
  - Grade III and IV hyphemas.
  - Bleeding disorders and sickle hemoglobinopathy.

Return to Play Criteria:

- After full clearance by ophthalmologist.
- Normal visual acuity.
- Postsurgical cases—off narcotics for pain relief.

Recommended Readings

Andreoli CM, Gardiner MF. Traumatic hyphema: Clinical features and management. *UpToDate*, Accessed September 1, 2010 and October 27, 2012.
Brandt MT, Haug RH. Traumatic hyphema: A comprehensive review. *J Oral Maxillofac Surg*. 2001;59:1462–1470.
Walton W, Von Hagen S, Grigorian R, Zarbin M. Management of traumatic hyphema. *Surv Ophthalmol*. 2002;47:297–334.
Wright KW, Sunalp M, Urrea P. Bed rest versus activity ad lib in the treatment of small hyphemas. *Ann Ophthalmol*. 1988;20:143–145.

Retinal Detachment

Introduction (Definitions/Classification): Parting of the retinal pigment epithelium and choroid from the neurosensory retinal layer with resultant ischemia of the retina, progressive degeneration of photoreceptors, and loss of vision. Caused by either

- a tear or a hole in the retina which allows vitreous fluid to leak into the subretinal space that causes detachment.
  - Spontaneous: More common; 1 in 10,000 individuals per year.
  - Traumatic: Less common.
- traction of vitreous on retina.
  - In athletes with sickle cell or diabetic retinopathy.
  - Following previous "eyeball perforation" injuries.

History and Physical Examination:

- Symptoms may develop suddenly and progress from hours to days to weeks.
  - Change in vision, including "change in peripheral vision in one eye."
  - Loss of vision.
- Commonly described symptoms:
  - "Floaters" described as either "cobwebs" or "housefly."
  - "Progressive" loss of peripheral vision of affected eye.
  - Fleeting (<1 second), "light flashes" with eye movement of the affected eye.
  - A "shower of black spots."
  - "A curtain coming across my eye."

Diagnosis:

- Clinical:
  - Signs/symptoms on physical examination.
  - History (personal and family history).
- Allergen testing:
  - Percutaneous skin test—introducing controlled amounts of allergen into skin and observing for reaction (acute, delayed, none).
  - Allergen-specific IgE (radioallergosorbent testing [RAST])—blood test looking for presence of IgE to precise allergen.
- Miscellaneous:
  - Nasolaryngoscopy/nasal cytology in addition to percutaneous skin testing.

Treatment:

- Avoidance of allergens.
- Medications (most commonly used):
  - Intranasal glucocorticoids.
    - Most effective maintenance therapy.
    - Use with caution during concurrent use of topical or inhaled glucocorticoids for asthma or dermatitis.
    - *Superior to other medications.*
  - Antihistamines.
    - Variety of oral and topical (sprays) available.
    - Combination (intranasal glucocorticoid + antihistamine) is effective for refractory cases.
    - *First* generation (diphenhydramine, chlorpheniramine, hydroxyzine)—*not advised secondary to sedative effects.*
    - *Second* generation (cetirizine, loratadine) and *third* generation (fexofenadine) effective.
    - Third generation thought to have, yet unproven, fewer central nervous system side effects.
    - *Superior to cromolyn.*
  - Mast cell stabilizers (cromolyn sodium).
    - Available over-the-counter (OTC), safe, yet requires frequent dosing.
    - Choice for individuals unresponsive to antihistamines.
  - Leukotriene modifiers (montelukast).
    - May have equal efficacy to antihistamines *and* superior efficacy when combined with an antihistamine.
    - May be beneficial in those with nasal polyps and coexistent asthma.
- Refractory cases:
  - Referral to allergist for allergen testing and consideration of immunotherapy.
  - Consider evaluation for asthma.

Other Considerations:

- Educate—intranasal glucocorticoids.
  - To direct spray away from nasal septum.
  - Can potentially cause epistaxis and nasal perforation; yet, have been generally shown to be extremely safe following long-term use.
  - May be effective within hours, yet may take days to weeks to be fully effective in athletes with chronic symptoms.
- Educate—side effects.
  - Have athletes consult with medical staff before using OTCs.
  - OTC or prescription medicines containing pseudoephedrine (PSE) can induce insomnia, irritability, and hypertension, and thus should be avoided in athletes (*author opinion*).
  - Antihistamines can cause sedation, flushing, fever, and electrolyte imbalance.
  - Leukotriene modifiers can induce anaphylaxis and aggressive behaviors.
- Swimmers may find benefit from nasal clips to prevent nasal mucosa contact and irritation with chlorinated water.
- Educate athletes on national teams.
  - Systemic glucocorticoids and PSEs are banned "in-competition."
  - Inhaled corticosteroids require a "Declaration of Use," *both* on the website of United States Anti-doping Agency (USADA) *and* on the Doping Control Official Record (DCOR), at the time of drug testing.

Return to Play Criteria:

- If athlete feels well and has no difficulty breathing.
- Adequate treatment and control of concurrent respiratory illness or conditions (asthma).

Recommended Readings

Carr W, Bernstein J, Lieberman P, et al. A novel intranasal therapy of azelastine with fluticasone for the treatment of allergic rhinitis. *J Allergy Clin Immunol.* 2012;129:1282–1289.

Cingi C, Ozlugedik S. Effects of montelukast on quality of life in patients with persistent allergic rhinitis. *Otolaryngol Head Neck Surg.* 2010;142:654–658.

deShazo RD, Kemp SF. Allergic rhinitis: Clinical manifestations, epidemiology, and diagnosis. *UpToDate.* Accessed October 28, 2012.

Dykewicz MS, Fineman S, Skoner DP, et al. diagnosis and management of rhinitis: Complete guidelines of the Joint Task Force on Practice Parameters in Allergy, Asthma and Immunology. American Academy of Allergy, Asthma, and Immunology. *Ann Allergy Asthma Immunol.* 1998;81(5 pt 2):478–518.

Gelardi M, Ventura MT, Fiorella R, et al. Allergic and non-allergic rhinitis in swimmers: Clinical and cytological aspects. *Br J Sports Med.* 2012;46:54–58.

http://www.usantidoping.org/files/pdfs/wallet-card.pdf. Accessed October 28, 2012.

Nayak A, Langdon RB. Montelukast in the treatment of allergic rhinitis: An evidence-based review. *Drugs.* 2007;67:887–901.

Patel D, Garadi R, Brubaker M, et al. Onset and duration of action of nasal sprays in seasonal allergic rhinitis patients: Olopatadine hydrochloride versus mometasone furoate monohydrate. *Allergy Asthma Proc.* 2007;28:592–599.

Salib RJ, Howarth PH. Safety and tolerability profiles of intranasal antihistamines and intranasal corticosteroids in the treatment of allergic rhinitis. *Drug Saf.* 2003;26:863–893.

Settipane RA, Charnock DR. Epidemiology of rhinitis: Allergic and nonallergic. *Clin Allergy Immunol.* 2007;19:23–34.

van Bavel J, Findlay SR, Hampel FC Jr, Martin BG, Ratner P, Field E. Intranasal fluticasone propionate is more effective than terfenadine tablets for seasonal allergic rhinitis. *Arch Intern Med.* 1994;154:2699–2704.

Nasal Trauma

Introduction (Definitions/Classification): The nose is the most commonly injured area of the face. Logically, nasal trauma is more common during participations in contact sports. Injuries include the following.

- Nose bleeding (epistaxis).
- Nasal fracture.
- Nasal septum deviation.

Epistaxis

History and Physical Examination:

- History:
  - Mechanism: Usually posttraumatic, sustained during play.
  - Recurrent and difficult to control: Hereditary hemorrhagic telangiectasia, thrombocytopenia, platelet dysfunction, or coagulopathy.
  - Medications and drugs: Warfarin, aspirin, intranasal glucocorticoids (fluticasone), alcohol, and cocaine abuse.
  - Miscellaneous: Cold and dry environments, sinusitis, allergic rhinitis, septal deviation, "nose picking," and remote history of head and neck surgery.
- Physical examination:
  - Source of the bleed should be identified by direct visualization using good light source, nasal speculum, or bayonet forceps; suction may help.
  - Approximately *90%* of nosebleeds occur from the *anterior* blood vessels involving the Kiesselbach plexus; *10%* are *posterior* bleeds.
  - Yet, may be difficult to pinpoint location; persistent bleeding despite thorough anterior nasal packing suggests posterior bleed.

Treatment:

- *First rule out fracture!*
- General measures:
  - Nose blowing will help clear existing clots, which otherwise can lengthen duration of bleeding.
  - Have patient sit with head elevated (to prevent swallowing blood).
  - Squeeze nose with constant pressure for 10 minutes, while leaning forward at the waist.
  - Two sprays of intranasal oxymetazoline.
  - Cold compress.
- Specific measures:
  - Cautery.

- Administer local anesthetic (lidocaine with epinephrine) or oxymetazoline, and/or oral anxiolytic (lorazepam) prior to procedure.
- First-line management for anterior bleeds.
- Chemical (silver nitrate) or electrical—equally effective, yet thorough hemostasis prior to cautery is essential for success.
  - Nasal packing.
    - Synthetic nasal (Merocel) tampons coated with antibiotic ointment *not* vaseline (to reduce risk for toxic-shock syndrome [TSS]).
    - Compared to traditional gauze packing, use of Merocel tampons may decrease risk for infection with *S. aureus*.
    - Hemostatic agents such as oxidized cellulose or gelatin foam. Can use for 2 to 3 days.
  - Refractory bleeding.
    - Consider etiology to be a posterior bleed.
    - Refer emergently to otolaryngologist for posterior packing (balloon or Foley catheters), embolization, or surgery.
  - Miscellaneous treatment information.
    - Foams and gels for thrombogenesis—under development.

Other Considerations:

- Routine use of NSAIDs is not associated with increased risk for epistaxis.
- Counsel that use of oxymetazoline in small doses does not enhance risk for elevated blood pressure (BP).
- Posterior epistaxis can result in significant hemorrhage and it is important to rule out nasopharyngeal cancer for posterior epistaxis, especially in individuals from China and Southeast Asia.
- Routine testing for coagulopathy is unnecessary for occasional epistaxis.
- Be vigilant for the development of TSS (fever, hypotension, skin lesions) in athletes who have been treated with nasal packing.
- In healthy athletes, routine use of antibiotics to prevent TSS not studied and has no benefit in preventing secondary bacterial sinusitis.
- Hematomas can form between cartilage and overlying mucous membrane. Refer to otolaryngologist expeditiously for surgical consultation, to prevent complications including cartilage avascular necrosis, septal perforations, or irreversible nasal damage.

Return to Play Criteria:

- Bleeding controlled.
- Hemodynamically stable.
- No recurrent epistaxis with sport-specific exertion.

Nasal Fracture

- Common in athletes. The anatomy of the nose (prominence off the facial surface) increases vulnerability to injury or fracture.

History and Physical Examination:

- History:
  - Blunt facial injury.
  - Inquire regarding the mechanism of injury from available witnesses.
- Physical examination:
  - Begins with a thorough examination!
    - Complete head, eyes, ears, nose, mouth (including teeth), and throat.
    - Complete neurologic examination.
  - Dislocation, swelling, or crepitus highly suggestive of fracture.
  - During examination, remember that nasal fractures can be associated with other facial fractures.
  - Key examination points (*needing immediate specialist referral*).
    - Open fracture or septal hematoma.
    - Significantly depressed nasal dorsum, widening of palpebral fissures, and intercanthal distance—suggestive of a naso-orbito-ethmoid fracture.
    - Halo test: Clear nasal or ear discharge (that forms a halo surrounding blood on gauze)—suggestive of cerebrospinal fluid (CSF) leak. *Test maybe positive with other body fluids including saliva.*
    - Decreased facial sensation—suggestive of fifth cranial nerve injury.
    - Facial paralysis—suggestive of seventh cranial nerve injury.

- Dysphonia—suggestive of a significant hematoma surrounding the airway or an associated fracture of the maxilla or mandible.
- Postauricular ecchymosis (Battle sign)—suggestive of a basilar skull fracture. *May not develop for 2 days post injury.*

Diagnosis:

- Signs/symptoms on physical examination.
- Imaging:
  - Radiographs.
    - Unnecessary if individual can breathe comfortably, and there is no significant curvature, or septal hematoma.
    - Do not change initial management, if not needed.
  - CT scanning.
    - CT scans with three-dimensional (3D) reconstructions for concerns regarding associated facial fractures.

Treatment:

- In the acute setting:
  - Remove from activity and apply a cold pack to minimize swelling and associated bleeding.
  - If concern for CSF leak and individual is stable:
    - Elevate the head 40 to 50 degrees to decrease intracranial pressure.
    - Refer expeditiously to otolaryngologist to rule out associated fractures and consider reduction.
  - If closed fracture and no CSF leak:
    - Consider referral to otolaryngologist within 3 to 6 hours post injury.
    - After 3 to 6 hours, edema precludes adequate reduction. Thus, need to wait 5 days for reduction.
    - Most nasal fractures are responsive to elective reduction in the first 10 days following injury.

Other Considerations:

- Cover any associated lacerations with clean dressings.
- A septal hematoma can separate the nasal cartilage from the overlying perichondrium leading to pressure-induced avascular necrosis, septal perforation, or infection. It is a significant complication and should be promptly identified followed by immediate referral to otolaryngology.
- Consider tetanus prophylaxis for any contaminated wounds.
- Consider antibiotic prophylaxis for fractures complicated by exposed nasal cartilage.

Return to Play Criteria:

- Varies and should be individualized in consultation with otolaryngologist.
- Many otolaryngologists recommend customized face masks for prolonged periods following return to activity.

Nasal Septal Deviation

- May be a congenital variant, yet commonly a result of trauma from a sports injury or other facial trauma. A deviated septum may result in nasal obstruction and difficulty breathing.

History and Physical Examination:

- History: Few individuals have an entirely straight septum. Degree of deviation determines symptom severity and characteristics. Inquire regarding the following.
  - Presence of difficulty with nasal breathing.
  - Unilateral (obstruction) or bilateral (mucosal congestion) symptoms.
  - Facial pain.
  - Difficulty smelling common odors.
  - Preceding history of sinus infections or trauma.
  - Possible irritants.
    - Drug use.
    - Smoke exposure.
    - Known allergens.

- Drugs: NSAID and methotrexate use.
- Deficiencies in folic acid, iron, vitamin B-12.
- Menstrual cycle hormonal fluctuations.
- Auto-inflammatory syndromes (Behçet disease).
- Immunodeficiencies.
- Food allergies.
- Smoking cessation.
- Genetics.
- Physical examination: Lesions are limited to the oral cavity and present as the following:
  - Small (2- to 4-mm diameter) yellow or grayish circular ulcerations.
  - Circumscribed borders.
  - Surrounding erythema and edema.
  - Located mainly on the nonkeratinized tissue (labia/buccal mucosa, floor of the mouth, and lateral or under-surface of tongue).

Diagnosis: Made by clinical examination.

- In the athlete, consider basic laboratories to rule out some of the known associations listed below:
  - CBC with differential.
  - Hemoglobin.
  - Iron studies.
  - Vitamin B-12 levels.
  - Anti-endomysium antibody and transglutaminase assay to rule out celiac disease.

Treatment: Little evidence exists for medicines used to decrease rate of recurrence.

- For symptomatic treatment:
  - Topical agents:
    - Corticosteroids (hydrocortisone hemisuccinate pellets).
    - Triamcinolone acetonide in paste form.
    - Topical tetracycline.
  - Rinses:
    - Betamethasone sodium phosphate elixir rinse.
    - Chlorhexidine gluconate rinses.
- If an association exists, correct the deficiency or avoid causal agent.
- Education on avoidance of sodium sulfate (toothpaste detergent) which prolongs ulcer-healing time.

Other Considerations:

- Rule out Behçet disease, a neutrophilic inflammatory disorder that presents with recurrent oral and genital ulcerations.
- Herpes simplex virus (HSV) and aphthous ulcers have similar morphologic characteristics; differentiation is important for adequate treatment.
- Use topical corticosteroids only after excluding HSV.
- Adequate pain control necessary, especially in sports that mandate the use of mouthguards.

Return to Play Criteria:

- No restrictions.

Recommended Readings

Aphthous ulcers. In: *Kumar: Robbins and Cotran Pathologic Basis of Disease, Professional Edition*, 8th ed. Saunders; 2009. Retrieved from http://www.mdconsult.com. Accessed January 5, 2011.

Goldstein B, Goldstein A. Oral lesions. *UpToDate*. Accessed on January 13, 2011 and October 16, 2012.

Scully C. Aphthous ulcers. Retrieved from http://emedicine.medscape.com. Accessed January 5, 2011.

Tilliss T, McDowell J. Differential diagnosis: Is it herpes or aphthous? *J Contemp Dent Pract.* 2002;(3)1:1–15.

Streptococcal Pharyngitis/Tonsillitis

Introduction (Definitions/Classification): Otherwise known as "strep throat (ST)," inflammation of the pharynx and tonsils caused by primarily group A beta-hemolytic streptococcus (GAS). Less common etiologies include group C and group G streptococci. Duration of illness is 2 to 5 days in untreated patients.

History and Physical Examination: Patients will present with an array of symptoms so it is important to discern if there exists a concern for streptococcal etiology. Have a high suspicion for GAS if two or more of the following are present (think FEAT).

- **F**ever >38°C in past 24 hours.
- **E**nlarged tonsils or erythematous oropharynx; **E**xudate.
- **A**bsence of cough.
- **T**ender anterior cervical lymph nodes.

Overlapping signs and symptoms that are suggestive of a viral etiology include the following.

- Cough.
- Diarrhea.
- Conjunctival injection.
- Coryza.
- Hoarse voice.

Complications include the following.

- *Acute rheumatic fever:* Results from persistence of GAS organisms in respiratory tract leading to increased risk of acute rheumatic fever (particularly in children). Antibiotics beneficial in prevention, if initiated within the first 9 days of symptoms. Symptoms may include arthritis, carditis, chorea, subcutaneous nodules, erythema marginatum.
- *Poststreptococcal glomerulonephritis:* Inflammation of glomeruli vasculature can cause hematuria, proteinuria, and hypertension. No clear benefit with antibiotic therapy.
- *PANDAS* ("**P**ediatric **A**utoimmune **N**europsychiatric **D**isorders **A**ssociated with group A *Streptococci*"): Symptoms may include exacerbation of tic or obsessive compulsive disorder. Consider group A *Streptococcus* testing for abrupt onset of tic disorder. No good evidence for efficacy of antibiotic treatment.
- *Scarlet fever:* A desquamating, diffuse, papular, "sandpaper-like" rash accompanied by circumoral pallor and a strawberry tongue.
- *Streptococcal TSS:* Widespread infection leads to shock and organ failure.
- *Tonsillopharyngeal cellulitis or abscess:* Occurs in <1% of acute pharyngitis infections.
- *Other potential complications:* Sinusitis, otitis media, necrotizing fasciitis.

Diagnosis:

- Rapid antigen detection test for high clinical level of suspicion for GAS tonsillopharyngitis; if positive, treat.
- If negative, obtain a confirmatory throat culture for verification.
- Consider testing for infectious mononucleosis (IM).

Treatment:

- For high level of suspicion, initiate antibiotic therapy while awaiting laboratory confirmation.
- Discontinue treatment if cultures are negative.
- Antibiotics have been shown to shorten duration of symptoms by approximately 1 day and also decrease rate of infectivity.
- Antibiotic regimens for GAS include the following.
  - No penicillin (PEN) allergy: Penicillin is first-line.
  - PEN allergy but *not* anaphylactic-type reaction: narrow-spectrum cephalosporin (cephalexin, cefadroxil).
  - True PEN allergy: Macrolide (erythromycin, clarithromycin).
- Avoid sulfonamides, FQs, and tetracyclines because of high failure rate and increasing resistance.
- Treat for 10 days.
- Supportive therapy.
  - Fever, sore throat: NSAIDs and acetaminophen (use with caution in concomitant mononucleosis because of possible, mononucleosis-induced thrombocytopenia and infective hepatitis).
  - Sore throat: Consider liquids and soft foods for sore throat.
  - Miscellaneous: Hydration and rest.

- Educate.
  - Contagiosity—rate of transmission with close contacts is ~35%. Antibiotic use will lessen the rate, yet reinforce good hand hygiene, and avoidance of sharing toothbrushes, linens, and utensils.
- Currently, no vaccine available.
- Prophylaxis is only indicated in the setting of previous rheumatic fever.

Other Considerations:

- If duration of pharyngitis lasts longer than 5 days, consider alternative etiologies (viral—Epstein–Bar virus (EBV), CMV; bacterial—mycoplasma, chlamydia; fungal).
- Tests for cure (e.g., repeat rapid antigen tests or cultures) after treatment are unnecessary unless
  - personal history of rheumatic fever.
  - acute pharyngitis presents during an outbreak of poststreptococcal glomerulonephritis or acute rheumatic fever.
- Group C and G streptococcal infections warrant a course of antibiotics for only 5 days, as rheumatic fever is not a complication of these strains.

Return to Play Criteria:

- Minimum of 24 hours on antibiotics.
- Improvement of symptoms—afebrile for at least 24 hours without antipyretic.
- No concerning respiratory symptoms.

Recommended Readings

Bisno A, Lichtenberger P. Evaluation of acute pharyngitis in adults. *UpToDate*. Accessed October 16, 2012.

Bisno AL, Gerber MA, Gwaltney JM Jr, Kaplan EL, Schwartz RH. Practice guidelines for the diagnosis and management of group a streptococcal pharyngitis. *Clin Infect Dis*. 2002;35:113–125.

Catanzaro FJ, Stetson CA, Morris AJ, et al. The role of the streptococcus in the pathogenesis of rheumatic fever. *Am J Med*. 1954;17: 749–756.

Del Mar CB, Glasziou PP, Spinks AB. Antibiotics for sore throat. *Cochrane Database Syst Rev*. 2000;(4):CD000023.

Gerber MA, Baltimore RS, Eaton CB, et al. Prevention of rheumatic fever and diagnosis and treatment of acute Streptococcal pharyngitis: A scientific statement from the American Heart Association Rheumatic Fever, Endocarditis, and Kawasaki Disease Committee of the Council on Cardiovascular Disease in the Young, the Interdisciplinary Council on Functional Genomics and Translational Biology, and the Interdisciplinary Council on Quality of Care and Outcomes Research: endorsed by the American Academy of Pediatrics. *Circulation*. 2009;119(11):1541–1551.

Gerber MA. Treatment failures and carriers: Perception or problems?. *Pediatr Infect Dis J*. 1994;13:576–579.

Micromedex. Accessed February, 2011.

Webb KH, Needham CA, Kurtz SR. Use of a high-sensitivity rapid strep test without culture confirmation of negative results: 2 Years' experience. *J Fam Pract*. 2000;49:34–38.

Infectious Mononucleosis

Introduction (Definition/Classification): Known as "mono" or "the kissing disease," IM is a widespread illness spread by saliva. The most common etiology is the EBV. Peak incidence is 10 to 24 years of age. Complications may include involvement of any organ, yet more common problems include the following.

- Spleen—enlargement/rupture.
- Hematologic—neutropenia, thrombocytopenia, and rarely aplastic anemia, disseminated intravascular coagulation, or hemolytic uremic syndrome.
- Neurologic—Guillain–Barré syndrome, neuritis, meningitis.
- Cardiac—myocarditis, *risk for sudden cardiac death (SCD)*.
- Respiratory—airway compromise.

History and Physical Examination:

- Fatigue, malaise, changes in appetite, and chills are common presenting symptoms that appear between 4 and 6 weeks' postexposure. These symptoms usually last a few days prior to the onset of the characteristic triad (that can be observed in "ST" as well).
  - Fever between 102°F and 104°F.
  - Cervical lymphadenopathy.
  - Tonsillitis/pharyngitis—erythema with or without an exudate.

- Other features may include the following.
  - Fatigue.
  - Splenomegaly in 50% to 60%; *only 20% to 50% palpable on examination*.
  - Hepatomegaly—less common.
  - Rash—petechial or maculopapular rash; before or after the administration of antibiotics.
  - Palatal petechiae (*with cervical lymphadenopathy and splenomegaly, is highly suggestive of IM*).

Diagnosis: Established by a combination of clinical and laboratory data.

- Signs/symptoms on physical examination, *with the following*.
  - Positive "*monospot*" or "*heterophile antibody (Paul Bunnell)*" tests.
    - Sensitivity ~85%; specificity ~100%.
    - If positive with clinical features of IM, no further testing necessary.
    - Not as sensitive or specific in younger athletes.
  - EBV-specific antibody testing—in selected cases, to establish diagnosis and detect past illness or reactivation of EBV. Summary:
    - EBV VCA (viral capsid antigen) IgM—*suggests acute infection*.
    - EBV VCA IgG—*suggests previous infection/immunity*.
    - EBNA (Epstein–Barr nuclear antigen)—typically appears 6 weeks after onset of illness, *suggests previous infection*.
  - Miscellaneous:
    - Leukocytosis or leukopenia.
    - Lymphocytosis >50% on differential count.
    - Increased atypical lymphocytes >10%.
    - Mild, self-limited neutropenia and thrombocytopenia.
    - Liver Function Tests (LFTs).
      - Highly suggestive of mononucleosis in individuals with pharyngitis.
      - Recheck weekly if high on initial assessment (*author opinion*).
- Peripheral smear evaluation—confirm viral characteristics in those with clinical or laboratory features concerning for occult hematologic pathology.

Treatment:

- *Discontinuation from all activities for a minimum of 3 weeks.*
- Supportive therapy for symptoms.
  - Fever, malaise, sore throat—NSAIDs at the lowest effective dose.
  - Avoid acetaminophen to minimize liver dysfunction, especially in those with elevated LFTs.
  - Appropriate diet—avoidance of fatty foods.
- No effective antiviral drugs or vaccines available.
- *Conflicting data on the role of steroids.*
  - May be warranted in individuals with either airway compromise from impending obstruction or fulminant organ failure (liver). Yet, used more often than conventionally recommended.
  - May decrease overall duration and severity of disease.
  - Often used for symptom relief. However, may need more than a single dose for symptom relief.
  - Thus, need to consider potential for systemic immunosuppression during EBV infection known to be linked to malignancies.
- Educate.
  - Contagiosity.
    - Avoid intimate contact, and sharing of toothbrushes, linens, and utensils.
    - EBV is often found in the saliva of healthy people who spread the virus intermittently throughout their lives, thus transmission is almost impossible to prevent.
    - EBV transmission does not normally occur through air or blood.
    - EBV spreads from those with active disease to healthy individuals may last several weeks after clinical resolution.
  - Steroid side effects—avoidance of alcohol and NSAIDs is recommended during treatment with steroids, to reduce the possibility of gastritis.

Other Considerations:

- Approximately 10% of cases that present with features of IM are not induced by EBV (*mono-like illness*). Other pathogens that can induce a mono-like illness include cytomegalovirus, adenovirus, and toxoplasmosis.
- *Splenic rupture:*
  - *How common*—rare, 0.1% of all cases.
  - *When*—most common, 2 to 21 days after symptom onset; no reports of spleen rupture (in medical literature) after 7 weeks of symptom onset.
  - Is there a difference between traumatic and spontaneous rupture?—*no*
  - Is there a correlation between severity of illness and likelihood of spleen rupture?—*no*
  - Can the spleen rupture in a "mono-like illness"?—*yes.*
  - Should *all* athletes with IM get an ultrasound examination during illness or prior to "return to play"?—*no.* Recommendation based on:
    - limited clinical value of obtaining only one ultrasound.
    - "high cost" for serial ultrasounds. *Routine ultrasound evaluation of all individuals with IM would cost ~1 million dollars to prevent one rupture.*
    - study that showed no difference in spleen size >30 days between IM and controls.
  - Yet, consider splenic ultrasound in selected cases to establish reduction in size—particularly, individuals involved in contact sports with prolonged splenic enlargement beyond 8 weeks.
  - CT or MRI is the study of choice to diagnose splenic rupture.
- *IM and ST have several overlapping features.* Establishing the correct diagnosis is critical to prompt treatment, prevention of complications, and reducing "lost time from practice and competition." Both illnesses can occur concurrently. Clinical and laboratory features highly suggestive of IM include the following.
  - Unusual fatigue.
  - Posterior cervical lymphadenopathy.
  - Hepatosplenomegaly.
  - IM-specific tests (noted above), elevated LFTs, lymphocytosis (total and atypical), neutropenia, thrombocytopenia.
- EBV establishes a lifelong dormant infection in some cells of the body and may reactivate under certain circumstances.
- Several features of HIV acute retroviral syndrome can mimic mononucleosis. Recommend HIV testing for athletes who
  - have mucocutaneous lesions; *or*
  - develop rash within 72 hours following the onset of fever (in the absence of concurrent use of antibiotics in an illness with clinical features suggestive for IM); *and*
  - have negative heterophile antibody test.

Return to Play Criteria:

- May gradually reintegrate into "light," "noncontact" activity at 4 weeks if laboratory studies and clinical examination are "*entirely normal,*" fluid and caloric intake are optimal, and there are no complicating features.
- Reassess weekly following reintegration to light activity.
- Typically, individuals can return to full activity in 6 to 8 weeks.

Recommended Readings

Aronson MD, Auwaerter PG. Infectious mononucleosis in adults and adolescents. *UpToDate.* Accessed October 29, 2012.

Asgari MM, Begos DG. Spontaneous splenic rupture in infectious mononucleosis: A review. *Yale J Biol Med.* 1997;70:175–182.

Burroughs KE. Athletes resuming activity after infectious mononucleosis. *Arch Fam Med.* 2000;9:1122–1123.

Candy B, Hotopf M. Steroids for symptom control in infectious mononucleosis. *Cochrane Database Syst Rev.* 2006;(3):CD004402.

Dommerby H, Stangerup SE, Stangerup M, Hancke S. Hepatosplenomegaly in infectious mononucleosis assessed by ultrasonic scanning. *J Laryngol Otol.* 1986;100:573–579.

Ebell MH. Epstein-Barr virus infectious mononucleosis. *Am Fam Physician.* 2004;70:1279–1287.

Epstein-Barr Virus and Infectious Mononucleosis. Retrieved from www.cdc.gov/ncidod/diseases/ebv.htm. Accessed August 14, 2010.

Evans AS, Niederman JC, Cenabre LC, West B, Richards VA. A prospective evaluation of heterophile and Epstein-Barr virus-specific IgM antibody tests in clinical and subclinical infectious mononucleosis: Specificity and sensitivity of the tests and persistence of antibody. *J Infect Dis.* 1975;132:546–554.

Haines J Jr. When to resume sports after infectious mononucleosis. How soon is safe? *Postgrad Med.* 1987;81:331–333.

Hosey RG, Mattacola CG, Kriss V, Armsey T, Quarles JD, Jagger J. Ultrasound assessment of spleen size in collegiate athletes. *Br J Sports Med.* 2006;40:251–254.

Kinderknecht JJ. Infectious mononucleosis and the spleen. *Curr Sports Med Rep.* 2002;1:116–120.

Luzuriaga K, Sullivan JL. Infectious mononucleosis. *N Engl J Med.* 2010;362:1993–2000.

Maki D, Reich R. Infectious mononucleosis in the athlete. diagnosis , complications, and management. *Am J Sports Med.* 1982;10(3):162–173.

Niu MT, Stein DS, Schnittman SM. Primary human immunodeficiency virus type 1 infection: Review of pathogenesis and early treatment intervention in humans and animal retrovirus infections. *J Infect Dis.* 1993;168:1490–1501.

Roy M, Bailey B, Amre DK, Girodias JB, Bussières JF, Gaudreault P. Dexamethasone for the treatment of sore throat in children with suspected infectious mononucleosis: A randomized, double-blind, placebo-controlled, clinical trial. 2004;158:250–254.

Peritonsillar Cellulitis/Abscess

Introduction (Definitions/Classification): A peritonsillar abscess (PTA or "quinsy") is the most common infection of the head and neck in adults. An acute pharyngitis causes local inflammation or cellulitis which compresses nearby salivary ducts. Complete obstruction leads to an abscess. The etiology is polymicrobial with a predominance of GAS although *Fusobacterium necrophorum* is much more widespread than previously thought in adolescents and young adults.

History and Physical Examination: History of recent pharyngitis or tonsillitis is common. Inquire about recurrent infections, previous abscesses, and symptoms concerning for airway compromise.

Presenting signs and symptoms:

- Sore throat, usually unilateral.
- Muffled or "hot potato" voice.
- Trismus.
- Fever.
- Dysphagia/odynophagia.
- Otalgia (ipsilateral).
- Drooling/salivary collections.
- Contralateral uvular deviation.

Complications include the following.

- Airway constriction/obstruction.
- Aspiration pneumonitis or pulmonary abscess, if abscess ruptures.
- Bacteremia.
- Vascular complications—internal jugular thrombosis, erosion of carotid sheath, and hemorrhage.
- Poststreptococcal complications—rheumatic fever, TSS, glomerulonephritis.
- *F. necrophorum* causes **Lemmiere** syndrome (an anaerobic septicemia with higher morbidity and mortality than rheumatic fever).
- Mediastinitis.
- Necrotizing fasciitis.

Diagnosis: Consider imaging for epiglottitis, retropharyngeal abscess, or airway compromise, which assists in diagnosing cellulitis versus an abscess in setting of limited physical examination.

- Imaging:
  - Plain radiographs—lateral view to rule out epiglottitis.
  - Ultrasound—transcutaneous or intraoral.
  - CT with IV contrast (preferred)—distinguishes cellulitis from PTA, quantifies spread of infection.
  - MRI—superior to CT if complications suspected (thrombus or erosion into vasculature); disadvantageous for patients with respiratory compromise.
- Laboratory tests:
  - Leukocytosis with a left shift (polymorphonuclear predominance).
  - Electrolyte disarray if decreased oral intake secondary to dysphagia.
  - Throat culture for GAS.
  - Gram stain, aerobic and anaerobic cultures with sensitivities of any aspirate.

If individual is stable without signs of airway compromise, a 24-hour trial of antibiotics may distinguish cellulitis (improvement) from PTA (no improvement).

Treatment:

- Prompt treatment is imperative to avoid serious complications.
- Antibiotics—14-day course.
  - Parenteral antibiotics.
    - Ampicillin–sulbactam.
    - Clindamycin.
    (Add vancomycin to either regimen if rapid improvement is not noted).
  - Transition to oral regimen when clinically improved and afebrile.
    - Amoxicillin–clavulanate.
    - Clindamycin.
    (Linezolid may be added if vancomycin was required).
- *F. necrophorum*—aggressive treatment with antibiotics. Avoid macrolides.
- Supportive care.
  - Maintain hydration.
  - Pain control—acetaminophen.
- For confirmed PTA:
  - Needle aspiration.
  - Incision and drainage.
  - Quinsy tonsillectomy—less common.
- Evidence for use of steroids to shorten duration of infection is inconclusive.

Other Considerations:

- Rule out epiglottitis, retropharyngeal and parapharyngeal abscess/cellulitis, and severe tonsillopharyngitis.
- Despite drainage, recurrence is 10% to 15%.
- The presence of a PTA in children or young adults pose greater risk of airway compromise given the more compact nature of their oropharynx. Consider hospitalization.

Return to Play:

- Reintegration into activity after clinically asymptomatic, afebrile, and on a suitable oral antibiotic regimen.
- Monitor closely for airway symptoms including resolution of neck swelling, presence of new airway hyperresponsiveness or cough, which may indicate incomplete resolution or recurrence.

Recommended Readings

Brodsky L, Sobie SR, Korwin D, Stanievish JF. A clinical prospective study of peritonsillar abscess in children. *Laryngoscope*. 1988;98: 780–783.

Centor R. Expand the pharyngitis paradigm for adolescents and young adults. *Ann Intern Med*. 2009;151(11):812–815.

Galioto NJ. Peritonsillar abscess. *Am Fam Physician*. 2008;77(2):199–202.

Goldenberg D, Golz A, Joachims HZ. Retropharyngeal abscess: A clinical review. *J Laryngol Otol*. 1997;111(6):546–550.

Johnson RF, Stewart MG, Wright CC. An evidence-based review of the treatment of peritonsillar abscess. *Otolaryngol Head Neck Surg*. 2003;128(3):332–343.

Ozbek C, Aygenc E, Tuna EU, Selcuk A, Ozdem C. Use of steroids in the treatment of peritonsillar abscess. *J Laryngol Otol*. 2004; 118(6):439–442.

Page C, Biet A, Zaatar R, Strunski V. Parapharyngeal abscess: diagnosis and treatment. *Eur Arch Otorhinolaryngol*. 2008;265(6):681–686.

Steyer TE. Peritonsillar abscess diagnosis and treatment. *Am Fam Physician*. 2002;65(1):93–96.

Wald ER. Peritonsillar cellulitis and abscess. *UpToDate*. Accessed October 16, 2012.

Yellon RF. Head and neck space infections. In: Bluestone CD, Casselbrant ML, Stool SE, et al. eds. *Pediatric Otolaryngology*. 4th ed. Philadelphia, PA: Saunders; 2003:1681–1701.

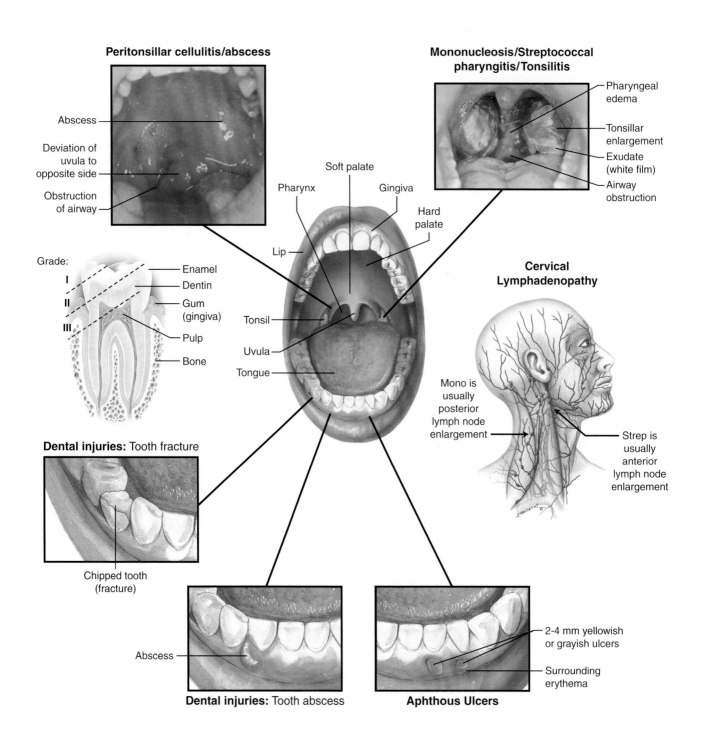

Peritonsillar cellulitis/abscess

Abscess

Deviation of uvula to opposite side

Obstruction of airway

Mononucleosis/Streptococcal pharyngitis/Tonsilitis

Pharyngeal edema

Tonsillar enlargement

Exudate (white film)

Airway obstruction

Grade:

I

II

III

Enamel

Dentin

Gum (gingiva)

Pulp

Bone

Soft palate

Pharynx

Gingiva

Hard palate

Lip

Tonsil

Uvula

Tongue

Cervical Lymphadenopathy

Mono is usually posterior lymph node enlargement

Strep is usually anterior lymph node enlargement

Dental injuries: Tooth fracture

Chipped tooth (fracture)

Abscess

Dental injuries: Tooth abscess

Aphthous Ulcers

2-4 mm yellowish or grayish ulcers

Surrounding erythema

Figure 120. Mouth

Section 5: Cardiopulmonary

Exertional Dyspnea

Introduction (Definitions/Classification):

- Breathing discomfort or difficulty with increased activity that varies in intensity.
- A common symptom that can be influenced by psychological, physiologic, environmental, and social factors.
- May be secondary to dysfunction of cardiovascular, respiratory, gastrointestinal, musculoskeletal, and/or metabolic systems.
- Two common causes of exertional dyspnea in athletes include the following:
  - Exercise-induced bronchoconstriction (EIB).
    - Airway constriction with or without underlying asthma.
    - Exercise is a trigger for EIB in those with underlying asthma.
    - More common in elite athletes participating in endurance sports, especially in winter sports (cross-country skiing, figure skaters, or ice hockey).
  - Paradoxical vocal cord motion (PVCM) or vocal cord dysfunction (VCD).
    - Inappropriate movement (paradoxical adduction) of vocal cords during inspiration or expiration resulting in airway obstruction.
    - Most frequently noted in females between 20 and 40 years old.
- Clinical distinction of these two etiologies (which may have similar clinical features) is critical for adequate management (*see figure for summary*).
- Differentiation of these two etiologies from occult, congenital, or acquired cardiac disease is critical for prevention of SCD in athletes.

Exercise-induced Bronchoconstriction

History and Physical Examination:

- History:
  - Past medical history:
    - EIB, asthma, allergic rhinitis, atopy, gastroesophageal reflux disease (GERD), smoking, second-hand smoke, irritant inhalation.
      - Athletes most affected have persistent, unidentified, or inadequately controlled asthma.
      - About 40% to 50% of athletes with allergic rhinitis also have EIB.
      - EIB can occur in 10% *without* a history of asthma or atopy.
  - Family history:
    - Inquire about congenital heart disease, pulmonary diseases, and SCD in relatives <50 years of age.
  - Symptoms:
    - Clinical manifestations are highly variable ranging from little impairment to severe bronchospasm.
    - Cough, chest tightness, shortness of breath, wheezing, activity avoidance, and diminished exercise tolerance.
    - Timing:
      - Symptoms typically commence ~3 to 8 minutes after the start of exercise, peak at 10 to 15 minutes after exercise cessation, and can last approximately 30 minutes ("locker room" cough).
    - "Refractory period":
      - For ~4 hours after exercise during which symptoms are diminished or completely absent.
- Physical examination:
  - Heart: Tachycardia.
  - Lungs: Tachypnea and expiratory wheezing, but often unremarkable at rest.
  - HEENT: Boggy and edematous nasal mucosa, especially in athletes with atopy.

Diagnosis:

- Predictive value of history and physical evaluation is poor.
  - Sixty-one percent of EIB-positive athletes and 45% of athletes with normal testing report symptoms.
  - Thus, pulmonary function tests (PFTs) for clinical suspicion of EIB is highly recommended.
- Exercise challenge (6 minutes on treadmill at 80% to 85% maximum HR).
  - FEV1 >15% drop from baseline indicative of EIB.
  - Spirometry before and after beta-agonist therapy.
  - False-negatives common with environmental stress and inadequate exercise intensity.
- Bronchoprovocation challenge tests (*for athletes with symptoms of asthma, normal PFTs and poor response to bronchodilator therapy*):
  - Pharmacologic.
    - Mannitol inhalation challenge.
    - Methacholine inhalation challenge.
  - Eucapnic voluntary hyperpnea (EVH).
    - In athletes with negative pharmacologic tests.
    - Recommended by the International Olympic Committee-Medical Commission (IOC-MC).
- Differential diagnosis pearls:
  - In the absence of an established diagnosis of EIB, exertional dyspnea may be induced by cardiovascular, pulmonary, or gastroenterologic etiologies remote from asthma.
  - Occult cardiac diseases can induce SCD (arrhythmias, cardiac shunts, and cardiomyopathy).
  - Other common mimickers include PVCM, allergic rhinitis, GERD, laryngeal dysfunction (tracheomalacia, laryngomalacia), psychological etiologies, and seeking behaviors for performance enhancement drugs (PEDs).
  - Association of EIB and GERD is debated and probably nonexistent.

Treatment:

- Nonpharmacologic.
  - Avoidance of triggers: Dry and cold air exposure, chlorine (swimming pool), pollen, animal dander, molds, house dust mites, cigarette smoke, and airborne pollutants/chemicals.
  - Breathing through a mask or loose-fitting scar in cold and dry environments.
  - Adequate warm-up prior to exercise.
  - Educate on nasal breathing and correct use of inhalers to maximize pharmacologic efficacy.
  - Diets rich in omega-3 fatty acids may have protective anti-inflammatory effects in asthmatics with EIB.
- Pharmacologic.
  - Beta-agonists.
    - Intermittent, prophylactic beta-agonists are most effective for EIB.
    - Rapid-acting beta-agonists (albuterol/formoterol) 10 minutes before exercise is effective for prophylaxis.
    - Consider long-acting beta-agonists (salmeterol/formoterol) in those who exercise on an intermittent basis daily.
      - Monotherapy may be ineffective with chronic use.
      - Thus, combine with inhaled glucocorticoid, cromolyn sodium, or anti-leukotrienes.
  - Inhaled glucocorticoids.
    - Effective for refractory EIB.
    - Do not improve EIB acutely, yet offer favorable control of EIB following several weeks to months of compliant therapy.
  - Mast cell stabilizers (cromoglycates).
    - Effective when combined with beta-agonists in high-performance athletes exercising in extreme conditions.
    - Do not independently relieve bronchoconstriction.
  - Leukotriene antagonists.
    - Once daily dose provides protection from EIB for ~12 hours.
    - Protects against EIB within 2 hours of administration.
    - Enhances postexercise recovery.
    - Superior to long-acting beta-agonists.

Other Considerations:

- Miscellaneous "key" facts:
  - EIB may lead to a severe asthma exacerbation and respiratory compromise requiring emergent care.
  - Health professionals should be prepared and equipped for intervention. Devices that monitor pulmonary function, rescue inhalers, and nebulizers should be available for emergent use.

- Rapid breathing without wheezing may be a presenting sign of exertional sickling collapse or underlying cardiac disease. Thus, not safe to assume that all rapid breathing is EIB.
- Drug interactions:
    - Beware of potential additive effects of sympathomimetic drugs.
    - Beta-agonists + stimulant medications for attention deficit hyperactivity disorder (e.g., amphetamines) + over-the-counter decongestants (e.g., PSE) can potentially induce arrhythmias.
- Doping considerations:
    - Be aware of USADA and World Anti-doping Agency (WADA) guidelines. Monitor websites for changes annually.
        - USADA: www.usada.org
        - WADA: www.wada-ama.org
    - Recommend carrying "USADA Wallet Card" in medical kit for quick reference.
        - http://www.usada.org/files/active/athletes/wallet_card.pdf
    - When in doubt, USADA resources include the following:
        - Research drugs at www.GlobalDRO.com
        - Contact "Drug Reference Department" at drugreference@usada.org
    - Current pharmacologic guidelines summary:
        - Beta-agonists.
            - Most prohibited in- and out-of-competition.
            - Albuterol (<1600 mcg per 24 hours), formoterol (<54 mcg per 24 hours), and salmeterol are permitted in- and out-of-competition.
        - Glucocorticoids.
            - Inhaled: Permitted in- and out-of-competition.
            - Oral: Prohibited in- and out-of-competition.
        - Mast cell stabilizers (cromoglycates).
            - Permitted in- and out-of-competition.
        - Leukotriene antagonists.
            - Permitted in- and out-of-competition.

Return to Play:

- Established diagnosis and stable-management protocol.
- Able to exercise without breathing difficulty or discomfort.
- Modify activity until peak expiratory flow is at least 80% of personal best.
- Recommend reporting medications to USADA and WADA to obtain therapeutic exemption (TUE), as needed, prior to competition.

Paradoxical Vocal Cord Motion or Vocal Cord Dysfunction

History and Physical Examination:

- History:
    - Past medical history:
        - Studies have shown that PVCM is associated with underlying psychosocial disorders including anxiety, childhood sexual abuse, posttraumatic stress disorder, depression, and/or personality disorders).
        - Other potential associations include GERD (LPR variant), inhalation of irritants (smoke, dust, cleaning chemicals), recent trauma, and/or surgery (postoperative phase).
        - Exercise itself, without any other underlying etiology, may be the sole precipitant of PVCM.
    - Symptoms:
        - Often normal at rest.
        - Cough (most common), choking, dyspnea, dysphagia, throat tightness, anxiety, perioral cyanosis, dysphonia, inspiratory or expiratory stridor (*as opposed to expiratory wheezing in EIB*).
    - Timing and duration varies.
        - Symptoms begin and peak during exercise.
        - Resolution of symptoms typically occurs within a few minutes after cessation of exercise.
- Physical examination:
    - Heart: Tachycardia.
    - Lungs: Tachypnea and inspiratory stridor above the cricoid cartilage which decrease over the lung fields.
    - Skin: Possible perioral cyanosis during episode.

Diagnosis:

- "Gold standard" test is fiberoptic laryngoscopy, yet typically difficult to perform during episode (*secondary to logistics*).
  - Vocal cord adduction is commonly seen only during acute episodes.
  - Yet, may be induced by asking athlete to "mimic" an attack of PVCM.
  - Methacholine challenge in conjunction with laryngoscopy:
  - To verify that inadequate airflow is secondary to PVCM.
- PFTs.
  - Normal spirometry in most individuals.
  - Flow–volume curve assessment:
    - Typically normal between episodes of PVCM.
    - May show flattening of inspiratory loop.
    - Increased proportion of forced expiratory flow to forced inspiratory flow at half the athlete's vital capacity.
- Arterial blood gas, chest x-rays (CXRs), and lung volumes are typically normal.
- Differential diagnosis pearls:
  - Asthma.
    - Typically responds to beta-agonist therapy.
  - Angioedema of the larynx induced by anaphylaxis.
    - Monitor for associated symptoms/signs of anaphylaxis.
  - Vocal cord paralysis.
    - Herpes simplex infection induced polycranial neuropathy.
    - Vagal or recurrent laryngeal nerve injury.

Treatment:

- Nonpharmacologic.
  - Reassurance and supportive care are usually sufficient.
  - "Panting" may help abort an active episode.
  - Continuous positive airway pressure (CPAP) and intermittent positive pressure ventilation (IPPV) may be helpful.
  - Prevention better than cure.
    - Speech language pathology (SLP) therapy has a 90% response rate.
      - Relaxing and breathing exercises.
    - Psychological counseling (as indicated).
- Pharmacologic.
  - Inadequate data.
  - Heliox (helium oxygen) inhalation may be beneficial.
  - Buspar may be beneficial in athletes with a psychosocial history (anecdotal evidence).
  - Prophylactic anticholinergic (ipratropium) may be beneficial (limited data).
  - Severe cases of PVCM may be amenable to intralaryngeal injection of botulinum toxin type A.

Other Considerations:

- Rarely, athletes may have respiratory distress substantial enough to require endotracheal intubation.
- PVCM can co-occur with asthma.
- A facemask that provides resistance during inspiration may be helpful in reducing inspiratory stridor and may therefore provide both physiologic and psychological benefits.

Return to Play:

- Established diagnosis and stable-management protocol.
- Cardiac etiologies that may induce SCD are excluded.
- Athlete is able to exercise without breathing difficulty or discomfort.

Recommended Readings

Anderson SD, Argyros GJ, Magnussen H, Hozer K. Provocation by eucapnic voluntary hyperpnoea to identify exercise induced bronchoconstriction. *Br J Sports Med.* 2001;35(5):344–347.

Archer GJ, Hoyle JL, Cluskey AM. Inspiratory vocal cord dysfunction, a new approach in treatment. *Eur Respir J.* 2000;15:617–618.

Corren J, Newman KB. Vocal cord dysfunction mimicking bronchial asthma. *Postgrad Med.* 1992;92:153–156.

Doshi DR, Weinberger MM. Long-term outcome of vocal cord dysfunction. *Ann Allergy Asthma Immunol.* 2006;96:794–799.

Edelman JM, Turpin JA, Bronsky EA, et al. Oral montelukast compared with inhaled salmeterol to prevent exercise-induced broncho-constriction. A randomized, double-blind trial. Exercise Study Group. *Ann Intern Med.* 2000;132:97–104.

Gavin LA, Wamboldt M, Brugman S, Roesler TA, Wamboldt F. Psychological and family characteristics of adolescents with vocal cord dysfunction. *J Asthma.* 1998;35:409–417.

Inman MD, O'Byrne PM. The effect of regular inhaled albuterol on exercise-induced bronchoconstriction. *Am J Respir Crit Care Med.* 1996;153:65–69.

Irwin CG. Bronchoprovocation testing. *UpToDate.* Accessed March 2, 2013.

Maillard I, Schweizer V, Broccard A, Duscher A, Liaudet L, Schaller M. Use of botulinum toxin type to avoid tracheal intubation or tracheostomy in severe paradoxical vocal cord movement. *Chest.* 2000;118(3):874–876.

Mickleborough TD, Lindley MR, Ionescu AA, Fly AD. Protective effect of fish oil supplementation on exercise-induced bronchoconstriction in asthma. *Chest* 2006;129:39–49.

National Asthma Education and Prevention Program: Expert panel report III: Guidelines for the diagnosis and management of asthma. Bethesda, MD: National Heart, Lung, and Blood Institute, 2007. NIH publication no. 08-4051. www.nhlbi.nih.gov/guide-lines/asthma/asthgdln.htm. Accessed on September 10, 2012.

O'Byrne PM. Exercise-induced bronchoconstriction. *UpToDate.* Accessed March 2, 2013.

Pitchenik AE. Functional laryngeal obstruction relieved by panting. *Chest.* 1991;100:1465–1467.

Powell SA, Nguyen CT, Gaziano J, Lewis V, Lockey RF, Padhya TA. Mass psychogenic illness presenting as acute stridor in an adolescent female cohort. *Ann Otol Rhinol Laryngol.* 2007;116:525–531.

Saxon KG, Shapiro J. Paradoxical vocal cord motion. *UpToDate.* Accessed March 2, 2013.

Sullivan MD, Heywood BM, Beukelman DR. A treatment for vocal cord dysfunction in female athletes: An outcome study. *Laryngoscope.* 2001;111:1751–1755.

United States Anti-doping Agency www.usada.org Accessed March 2, 2013.

Weir M. Vocal cord dysfunction mimics asthma and may respond to heliox. *Clin Pediatr (Phila).* 2002;41:37–41.

World Anti-doping Agency www.wada-ama.org Accessed March 2, 2013.

Influenza

Introduction (Definitions/Classification): An acute, typically "self-limited" viral illness caused by either Influenza A or B.

History and Physical Examination:

- Can present with either *or* both, upper *and* lower respiratory tract symptoms and signs.
- Incubation period is 1 to 4 days.
- *Abrupt* onset of symptoms including fever (>100°F), headache, malaise, myalgias (usually back and neck), sore throat, and cough (with or without sputum).
- Aside from fever, physical examination is usually benign in *uncomplicated* influenza. Physical findings may include pharyngeal erythema and/or shotty cervical lymphadenopathy.
- Symptoms after 5 to 7 days including persistent fever, cough with sputum, tachypnea, tachycardia, cyanosis, and constitutional symptoms *signify either "secondary" viral (severe) or bacterial pneumonia.*
  - Consider secondary methicillin-resistant *S. aureus* (CA-MRSA) in individuals who initially improve and then relapse with high fever, purulent sputum, and infiltrates on CXR.

Diagnosis:

- Signs/symptoms on physical examination (during the flu season).
- Laboratory testing:
  - Rapid influenza diagnostic tests (RIDTs).
    - Sensitivity = 40% to 70%; specificity = 90% to 95%; thus, false-negative rates common.
    - During the flu season, rapid tests for influenza have the same sensitivity as clinical diagnosis and are usually unnecessary in otherwise, "low-risk," healthy individuals.
- More tests:
  - Reverse transcription polymerase chain reaction (RT-PCR), viral culture, and immunofluorescence are accurate, yet take long to complete.
- Obtain CXR in all individuals with fever >100°F, respiratory rate >24, and pulse >100 *who first improve and relapse.*
- Sputum cultures are usually unnecessary except for individuals with secondary pneumonia diagnosed with a CXR.

Treatment:

- By prevention—immunize athletes (if desired by individuals).
  - On immunization: "Pros and cons" of vaccination. Information can be obtained at http://www.cdc.gov/mmwr/preview/mmwrhtml/mm6132a3.htm.
- Most cases improve with symptomatic treatment including Tylenol, NSAIDs, cough suppressants, and decongestants.

- Antiviral therapy *pearls.*
  - Do not wait for laboratory confirmation to initiate treatment.
  - Most effective when used within first 24 to 30 hours of symptoms, especially in those with fever.
  - May reduce complications and mortality.
  - Either oseltamivir (75 mg twice daily) or zanamivir (10 mg; two inhalations twice daily) for 5 days in "*high-risk*" groups.
    - Information for "high-risk" groups can be obtained at http://www.cdc.gov/flu/professionals/antivirals/summary-clinicians.htm.
  - Zanamivir not recommended in individuals with underlying asthma.
  - Due to resistance patterns, amantadine and rimantadine should not be used in the United States.
- When necessary, guided by sputum gram stain and culture, antibiotics for secondary bacterial pneumonia.
  - Options for "*non-CA-MRSA*" outpatient:
    - Azithromycin or clarithromycin: *No* recent antibiotic use, local resistance patterns, or risk for QT-interval prolongation.
    - Moxifloxacin or levofloxacin (monotherapy) or combination (beta-lactam + doxycycline): *If* nonpregnant, recent antibiotic use, local resistance patterns, or risk for QT-interval prolongation.
  - For "*CA-MRSA*" pneumonia—vancomycin.
- Educate.
  - Information regarding flu can be obtained at http://www.cdc.gov/flu/index.htm.
  - Medical providers to access weekly CDC updates on influenza activity during flu—http://www.cdc.gov/flu/weekly/fluactivitysurv.htm.
  - Treatment with either oseltamivir or zanamivir "does not cure," yet "shortens duration of symptoms" by 1 to 3 days.
  - Information on pre- and postexposure chemoprophylaxis can be obtained at http://www.cdc.gov/flu/professionals/antivirals/antiviral-use-influenza.htm. Regimens include either oseltamivir (75 mg daily) or zanamivir (10 mg; two inhalations daily).
  - Oseltamivir can induce transient neuropsychiatric symptoms including delirium and self-injury.
  - "Peak" viral shedding occurs during the first 2 days of illness.
  - Infection is transmitted by droplet contact, therefore, imperative to cover the mouth during coughing.
  - Encourage individuals to stay home until symptoms have improved and to wear a face mask for 5 days after onset of illness.
  - Avoid aspirin in children <17 years of age to prevent potential Reye syndrome.
  - Restrict use of oral decongestants in hot weather, and with other medications, including yet not limited to, stimulant medications for attention deficit-hyperactivity disorder, thyroid replacement, or bronchodilators.

Other Considerations:

- Secondary viral and bacterial (CA-MRSA) pneumonia can be life threatening even in adolescents. Yet, secondary bacterial pneumonia can be induced by non-MRSA pathogens (*S. pneumoniae* most common).
- Use CURB–65 score for decision to admit for pneumonia (*0 to 1—low severity, outpatient; 2—moderate severity, consider admission; 3 to 5—high severity, admit*).
  - **C**onfusion (*new* disorientation to person, place, or time; or based on specific mental tests).
  - **U**rea (blood urea nitrogen in the United States) >20 mg/dL.
  - **R**espiratory rate >30 breaths/minute.
  - **B**P (systolic <90 mm Hg or diastolic <60 mm Hg).
  - Age >**65** years.
- Consider myositis in younger individuals with muscular tenderness, swelling, decreased strength, and elevated creatine kinase. Obtain urinalysis for myoglobin and basic metabolic panel to assess renal function.
- Influenza can also induce complications of other systems.
  - Central nervous—aseptic meningitis, encephalitis, Guillain–Barré syndrome.
  - Cardiovascular—pericarditis, myocarditis.
  - TSS.

Return to Play Criteria:

- Improving symptoms and signs.
- No cough, fever, tachycardia, or tachypnea.
- Normal musculoskeletal examination.

Recommended Readings

Centers for Disease Control and Prevention (CDC). Severe methicillin-resistant Staphylococcus aureus community-acquired pneumonia associated with influenza—Louisiana and Georgia, December 2006–January 2007. *MMWR Morb Mortal Wkly Rep.* 2007;56: 325–329.

Dolin R. Clinical manifestations of seasonal influenza in adults. *UpToDate.* Accessed November 4, 2012.

File TM Jr. Treatment of community-acquired pneumonia in adults in the outpatient setting. *UpToDate.* Accessed August 30, 2010 and November 4, 2012.

Fiore AE, Fry A, Shay D, et al. Antiviral agents for the treatment and chemoprophylaxis of influenza—recommendations of the Advisory Committee on Immunization Practices (ACIP). *MMWR Recomm Rep.* 2011;60:1–24.

Fiore AE, Shay DK, Broder K, et al. Prevention and control of influenza: Recommendations of the Advisory Committee on Immunization Practices (ACIP), 2008. *MMWR Recomm Rep.* 2008;57:1–60.

Gamboa ET, Eastwood AB, Hays AP, Maxwell J, Penn AS. Isolation of influenza virus from muscle in myoglobinuric polymyositis. *Neurology.* 1979;29:1323–1335.

http://www.cdc.gov/flu/index.htm. Accessed November 4, 2012.

Jefferson T, Demicheli V, Rivetti D, Jones M, Di Pietrantonj C, Rivetti A. Antivirals for influenza in healthy adults: Systematic review. *Lancet.* 2006;367:303–313.

Lim WS, van der Eerden MM, Laing R, et al. Defining community acquired pneumonia severity on presentation to hospital: An international derivation and validation study. *Thorax.* 2003;58:377–382.

Zachary KC. Treatment of seasonal influenza in adults. *UpToDate.* Accessed August 30, 2010 and November 4, 2012.

Acute Bronchitis

Introduction (Definitions/Classification): Bronchial inflammation induced by infection. Classified as:

- Viral—more common.
- Bacterial and other pathogens—less common.

History and Physical Examination:

- Cough—for >5 days, usually lasts from 2 to 3 weeks.
- Purulent sputum—in ~50%; purulence does not necessarily equate to bacterial bronchitis.
- Fever—*not common*; with sputum, tachypnea, tachycardia, and constitutional symptoms *signifies either flu or pneumonia.*
- Examination:
  - Tenderness of chest wall secondary to cough.
  - *Usual—wheezing* and *rhonchi* (usually clear with coughing).
  - *Unusual*—rales, egophony, and rubs.

Diagnosis:

- Signs/symptoms on physical examination.
- Blood tests:
  - Usually mild elevation of white blood cell (WBC) count.
  - "Left shift" with higher WBC count is suggestive of bacterial pneumonia.
  - "*Procalcitonin*" test may be useful to separate bacterial and other etiologies.
- Cultures are usually unnecessary except for individuals with pneumonia diagnosed with a CXR.
- Obtain CXR in all individuals with fever >100°F, respiratory rate >24, and pulse >100.

Treatment:

- Most cases improve with symptomatic treatment including steam inhalation, Tylenol, NSAIDs, cough suppressants, and decongestants.
- Guaifenesin does not change the volume or viscosity of bronchial secretions, yet, may enhance particle clearance from airways.
- *Two key points:*
  - Beta-2 agonists (albuterol) may be effective in athletes with evidence of airway obstruction. Yet, routine use is not recommended.
  - Antibiotics are usually unnecessary, over prescribed, and not recommended in healthy athletes.
- *Current guidelines recommend specific treatment for bronchitis associated with the following.*
  - Pertussis (whooping cough).
    - Clarithromycin or azithromycin (Z-Pak).
    - *Avoid erythromycin which has been associated with acquired long QT syndrome.*
  - Influenza.
    - Either oseltamivir or zanamivir for 5 days in "high-risk" groups.
    - *Details under the section "Influenza."*

- Local outbreak of either *Chlamydophila pneumoniae* or *Mycoplasma pneumoniae.*
  - Either doxycycline, azithromycin/clarithromycin, FQs (moxifloxacin/levofloxacin).
- Educate.
  - Cover mouth during coughing.
  - Restrict use of oral decongestants in hot weather, and with other medications (including yet not limited to)—stimulant medications for attention deficit-hyperactivity disorder, thyroid replacement, and bronchodilators.

Other Considerations:

- Counsel athletes.
  - Bronchospasm can persist for 6 weeks.
  - In the absence of a history of asthma, symptoms of acute bronchitis typically resolve in 6 weeks.
- *During the flu season, exclude flu and related complications.*
- *Exclude pertussis:*
  - Nasopharyngeal swab culture and PCR.
  - Especially in individuals with prolonged cough (>2 weeks), even without "postcough emesis" or "whoop."
- Consider pulmonary function testing (and other imaging as indicated) for prolonged (>6 weeks) wheezing.
- Consider GERD as a diagnosis in athletes with chronic cough who fail to improve with treatment.

Return to Play Criteria:

- Improving symptoms and signs.
- No fever, tachycardia, or tachypnea.

Recommended Readings

Becker LA, Hom J, Villasis-Keever M, van der Wouden JC. Beta2-agonists for acute bronchitis. *Cochrane Database Syst Rev.* 2011;(7):CD001726.

Braman SS. Chronic cough due to acute bronchitis: ACCP evidence-based clinical practice guidelines. *Chest.* 2006;129:95S–103S.

File TM Jr. Acute bronchitis in adults. *UpToDate.* Accessed August 30, 2010 and November 4, 2012.

Gonzales R, Bartlett JG, Besser RE, et al. Principles of appropriate antibiotic use for treatment of uncomplicated acute bronchitis: Background. *Ann Intern Med.* 2001;134:521–529.

Gonzales R, Sande M. What will it take to stop physicians from prescribing antibiotics in acute bronchitis? *Lancet.* 1995;345:665–666.

National Quality Forum (NQF). Avoidance of antibiotic treatment in adults with acute bronchitis. Available at http://www.qualityforum.org/MeasureDetails.aspx. Accessed November 5, 2012.

Schuetz P, Chiappa V, Briel M, Greenwald JL. Procalcitonin algorithms for antibiotic therapy decisions: A systematic review of randomized controlled trials and recommendations for clinical algorithms. *Arch Intern Med.* 2011;171:1322–1331.

Snow V, Mottur-Pilson C, Gonzales R. Principles of appropriate antibiotic use for treatment of acute bronchitis in adults. *Ann Intern Med.* 2001;134(6):518–520.

Pneumothorax

Introduction (Definitions/Classification):

- A rare, yet life-threatening problem manifest by accumulation of air in the pleural space which may induce respiratory or hemodynamic compromise.
- Two categories.
  - Spontaneous.
    - Primary (PSP): Without pulmonary disease.
    - Secondary (SSP): With either pulmonary disease or systemic disease with pulmonary manifestations.
  - Traumatic (TP).
    - Iatrogenic—secondary to medical or surgical procedures.
    - Chest wall trauma.
- Tension pneumothorax.
  - Induced by blunt or penetrating trauma and the development of a "one-way valve."
  - Air enters the pleural space during inspiration and cannot escape during expiration, because pleural pressure is greater than atmospheric pressure.
- Respiratory failure may ensue from compression of the opposite, normal lung.

History and Physical Examination:

- **History:**
  - HPI.
    - PSP.
      - Age: 20's, rarely >40 and while at rest.
      - Rapid onset shortness of breath and pleuritic chest pain which may radiate to ipsilateral shoulder.
    - SSP.
      - Usually more severe secondary to compromised lung function at baseline.
    - TP.
      - Presentation similar to PSP/SSP in the presence of significant thoracic trauma (fractured ribs, stab wounds, gunshot wounds).
  - Past medical history (significant in spontaneous pneumothorax).
    - Risk factors.
      - Tobacco use.
      - PSP has been reported with cocaine and marijuana use.
      - Athletes exposed to blunt force and chest wall trauma (e.g., motocross, skiers, mountain bikers, football players, lacrosse, rugby) are at greater risk for TP.
    - PSP.
      - Substance abuse.
      - Elevated transpulmonary pressure: Power lifting and other sports that involve Valsalva maneuver, divers, pilots.
    - SSP.
      - Most common etiologies (yet infrequent in the athletic population): COPD (50% to 70%), cystic fibrosis, pneumonia, TB, pulmonary malignancy.
      - Less common: Marfan syndrome, asthma, recent pulmonary infection, thoracic endometriosis (catamenial pneumothorax), sarcoidosis, rheumatoid arthritis, ankylosing spondylitis, histiocytosis X, polymyositis, dermatomyositis, aspiration of foreign body, malignancy, homocystinuria.
  - Family history.
    - Birt–Hogg–Dubé syndrome: Characterized by skin neoplasms (benign) and renal carcinoma is a predisposition to PSP.
    - Marfan syndrome: Predisposition to SSP.

Physical Examination:

- *Athlete with either a small or uncomplicated pneumothorax may be relatively asymptomatic.*
- *Dyspnea + hypotension + tachycardia are suggestive of tension pneumothorax.*
- HEENT.
  - Lymphadenopathy, rhinorrhea, and erythematous oropharynx in infectious causes of PSP.
  - Ectopia lentis (downward dislocation of the eye lens): Marfan syndrome and homocystinuria.
  - Deviation or bifid uvula: Connective tissue disorders.
- Neck: Distended neck veins, tracheal deviation (usually a late sign).
- Pulmonary.
  - Diminished breath sounds on affected side, tachypnea, hyperressonance, diminished chest wall excursion, and absent fremitus over affected side.
  - Signs of chest wall trauma (open fractures, abrasions, flail chest).
- Cardiac: Tachycardia.
- Neurological: May be normal on initial presentation.
- Extremities: Evaluate for Marfinoid habitus (*as detailed in chapter on Marfan syndrome*).
- Skin/vascular: Cyanosis and diminished pulses with cardiovascular compromise; subcutaneous emphysema; characteristic skin lesions seen in connective tissue disorders including dermatomyositis, polymyositis, and sarcoidosis.

Diagnosis:

- Clinical suspicion and signs/symptoms on physical examination.
- Imaging.
  - Chest x-ray (standard; inspiratory).
    - Evidence of visceral-pleural line without pulmonary vasculature visible beyond edge of line, chest cavity hyperexpansion, lung wall parallel to chest wall, radiolucency, separation of ribs, deepened costophrenic angle, possible mediastinal deviation, and subcutaneous emphysema.

- **Tension pneumothorax**: Contralateral shift of mediastinum and ipsilateral flattening or inversion hemidiaphragm.
  - *Caution: As a result of trauma and possible rupture of the left hemidiaphragm, the stomach may herniate into chest and be erroneously diagnosed as a pneumothorax.*
- CT.
  - As needed to evaluate definite presence of pneumothorax, size, and location (especially in those with SSP).
  - To evaluate abnormal chest tube placement.
- Traumatic.
  - Diagnosis usually based on clinical suspicion, and mechanism of injury.
  - If athlete is stable, obtain chest radiographs and consider CT if diagnosis unclear.

Treatment:

- *All athletes with a clinical suspicion of pneumothorax should be immediately transferred to hospital.*
- First evaluate clinical "stability."

  - If **stable** place athlete in an upright position and if available, administer high-flow oxygen, pending arrival of Emergeny Medical Services (EMS), or during transfer to nearest medical facility.
  - If **unstable**, perform rapid needle decompression (*diagnosis confirmed by "hiss" of air*).
    - **When**: Diminished breath sounds on affected side, worsening shortness of breath, hypotension, distended neck veins, and/or tracheal deviation away from the affected side.
    - **How**: Insert a 14-gauge intravenous (IV) catheter into the pleural space.
    - **Where**: Either the second or third intercostal space (ICS) in the midclavicular line, or the fifth ICS in the anterior axillary line or anterior to the midaxillary line.
    - **Key point**: *Secure cannula of IV catheter to chest wall with tape until EMS arrives and chest tube has been inserted.*

Other Considerations:

- Education.
  - Athletes with either PSP or SSP can have recurrent pneumothoraces.
  - All athletes should be instructed to avoid air travel and scuba diving until complete resolution.
  - Substance use counseling for those who smoke cigarettes.
- Athletes with PSP should be evaluated for underlying pulmonary and systemic pathology (detailed above).

Return to Play:

- Incorporate "individualized approach" for return to play protocol.
- Decisions on when to return athlete to play should be made following consultation with thoracic surgeon.
- Obtain cardiac clearance if underlying connective tissue disorder suspected (e.g., Marfan syndrome).
- Recommend gradual, graded increase in exercise intensity over 3 weeks prior to full clearance for participation.
- Return athlete to full participation following complete resolution of symptoms during sports specific aerobic and anaerobic conditioning without evidence of pulmonary compromise.
- Consider use of protective taping of ribs (as needed), chest padding, or use of "flack jacket" for athletes returning to contact sport.

Recommended Readings

Legome E. Initial evaluation and management of blunt thoracic trauma in adults. *UpToDate.* Accessed March 30th, 2013.

Light RW. Secondary spontaneous pneumothorax in adults. *UpToDate.* Accessed March 18th, 2013.

Light RW. Primary spontaneous pneumothorax in adults. *UpToDate.* Accessed March 19th, 2013.

MacDuff A, Arnold A, Harvey J, BTS Pleural Disease Guideline Group. Management of spontaneous pneumothorax: British Thoracic Society Pleural Disease Guideline 2010. *Thorax.* 2010; 65 suppl 2:ii18.

Seow A, Kazerooni EA, Pernicano PG, Neary M. Comparison of upright inspiratory and expiratory chest radiographs for detecting pneumothoraces. *AJR Am J Roentgenol.* 1996;166:313.

Stark P. Imaging of pneumothorax. *UpToDate.* Accessed March 30th, 2013.

Exertional Dyspnea

Vocal cord dysfunction

Normal vocal cord abduction during exercise

Paradoxical adduction of vocal cords during exercise

- Peaks DURING exercise
- Typically resolves within a few minutes after stopping exercise
- Throat tight/choking
- Inspiratory Stridor
- No response to β agonist

Pharynx
Larynx
Trachea
Bronchus
Heart
Diaphragm

Exercise-induced bronchoconstriction

Normal bronchiole lumen
Mucosa
Smooth muscle

Constricted bronchiole lumen
Inflamed mucosa

- Peaks AFTER exercise
- Persists for 30 minutes after stopping exercise
- Cough, shortness of breath, chest pain
- Expiratory wheezing
- Good response to β agonist

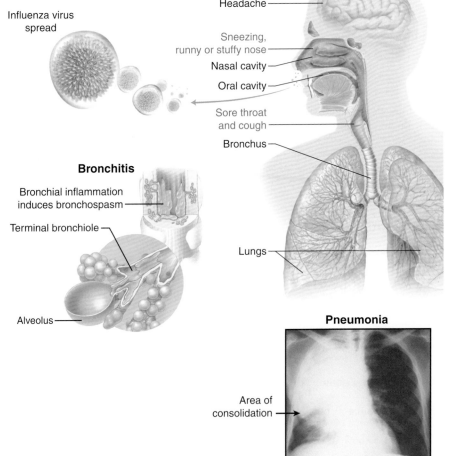

Influenza

Influenza virus spread

Headache
Sneezing, runny or stuffy nose
Nasal cavity
Oral cavity
Sore throat and cough
Bronchus
Lungs

Bronchitis

Bronchial inflammation induces bronchospasm
Terminal bronchiole
Alveolus

Pneumonia

Area of consolidation

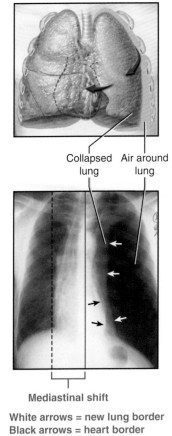

Pneumothorax

Collapsed lung   Air around lung

Mediastinal shift

White arrows = new lung border
Black arrows = heart border

Figure 121. Cardiopulmonary

Syncope

Definition: Multifactorial, unforeseen, temporary loss of consciousness followed by quick, spontaneous recovery induced by either decreased cerebral perfusion (oxygen delivery) or impaired metabolism.

- Recurrence rate ~30%.
- Ten to fifteen percent of children have syncope from various causes.
- No clear cause in 40% to 50% of cases.
- Most frequently identified causes: Unknown > vasovagal > cardiac > orthostatic.

Classification:

- Cardiac.
  - Structural (**"MVA"**).
    - **M**uscle and **m**iscellaneous—hypertrophic obstructive cardiomyopathy, arrhythmogenic right ventricular dysplasia, left ventricle dysfunction, cardiac tamponade, ventricular/atrial septal defects, myocarditis, atrial myxoma.
    - **V**alvular—bicuspid aortic valve, aortic or pulmonary stenosis.
    - **A**rterial—aortic coarctation, anomalous coronary arteries, aortic dissection pulmonary embolism or hypertension, myocardial infarction.
  - Nonstructural (**"HVCC/MAO"**).
    - **H**eat.
    - **V**asovagal (cardioinhibitory/vasodepressor).
    - **S**ituational (following bodily functions—e.g., cough, sneeze, micturition, defecation, postprandial).
    - **C**lassical (following emotional distress, pain, fear, prolonged periods of standing).
    - **C**arotid sinus syncope/hypersensitivity—rarely caused by mechanical stimulation (collared shirts or protective padding), but most often without direct stimulation.
    - **C**onduction abnormalities–Wolff–Parkinson–White syndrome, long QT syndrome, Brugada syndrome, congenital short QT syndrome, commotio cordis, idiopathic ventricular fibrillation, catecholamine-induced polymorphic ventricular tachycardia (CPVT).
    - **M**edications **"AID"** (**a**ntidepressants, **a**ntiemetics [phenothiazines], **a**ntihypertensives, **a**ntiarrhythmics, **i**nsulin, **d**iuretics, **d**rugs of abuse).
    - **O**rthostatic hypotension.
- Noncardiac (**"M, N, or P"**).
  - **M**etabolic dysfunction.
    - Hypovolemia—recent volume-depleting illness (diarrhea, vomiting), adrenocortical insufficiency (Addison disease), hemorrhage, hypoglycemia, hypoxia, or hyperventilation.
  - **N**eurologic abnormalities (**"VPN"**).
    - **V**ascular (insufficiency, subclavian steal), **P**ressure (normal pressure hydrocephalus, increased intracranial pressure), **N**erves (autonomic dysfunction, diabetic neuropathy, seizures).
  - **P**sychiatric (**"PHD"**).
    - **P**anic attacks, **H**ysteria, **D**epression.

History and Physical Examination (Yes/No):

- History:
  - Always inquire about history of sudden death, cardiac disease, prior psychiatric illness, medication change.
  - Was syncope abrupt?
    - Yes—**first** rule out cardiac etiology (ask about palpitations, syncope while in upright/prone position).
    - No—think other causes (neural, autonomic, cerebrovascular), **yet** rule out cardiac etiology.
  - Was syncope exertional?
    - Yes—think structural cardiac ("MVA") etiology.
    - No—ask about prodromal symptoms?
  - Prodromal symptoms?
    - Yes—vasovagal (ask about prolonged standing or abrupt positional change, exposure to heat, duration after exercise).
    - No—did it occur with neck stretching or possible carotid mechanical stimulation?
      - Carotid sinus hypersensitivity.
  - Subsequently, use the classification above to rule out other causes.

- Physical examination (*is usually normal, yet evaluate*):
  - Cardiac—sounds, rhythm, rate, murmurs, orthostatic BP.
    - S3 gallop—LV dysfunction.
    - Ectopy—arrhythmia.
    - Increased by Valsalva—hypertrophic cardiomyopathy.
    - Harsh, crescendo/decrescendo—aortic stenosis.
    - Orthostasis—heat illness, hypovolemia.
    - Systolic pressure drops to 50 mm following unilateral carotid sinus massage—carotid sinus hypersensitivity.
    - Check for carotid bruits.
  - Pulmonary—tachypnea, breath splinting with chest pain and fever.
    - Pulmonary embolism.
      - Ask about recent travel, birth control medications, tobacco use, and sickle cell trait.
  - Skin—signs of hypovolemia.
    - Diminished skin turgor.
    - Dry mucous membranes.
    - Weak peripheral pulses.

Diagnosis (R = routine/A = as indicated):

- Cardiopulmonary tests:
  - Electrocardiogram (EKG) (**R**).
  - Echocardiogram (**R**).
  - Cardiac MRI (**A**).
  - Exercise stress test (**A**).
  - Holter/event monitor (**A**).
  - Electrophysiologic study (**A**).
  - Upright tilt table testing (**A**).
  - Chest CTA (**A**)—rule out pulmonary embolus.
- Blood tests:
  - CBC, CMP (**A**).
  - D-dimer (**A**)—rule out pulmonary embolus.
  - Cardiac enzymes (**A**).
- Neurologic:
  - CT/MRI–MRA (**A**).
  - EEG (**A**)—to differentiate true syncope from seizure disorder.

Treatment:

- On-field.
  - **First**, place athlete in supine position to maintain BP and brain perfusion.
  - Evaluate and monitor ABCs (**A**irway, **B**reathing, **C**irculation).
  - **Do not administer** any fluids or medications by mouth until athlete is fully recovered and has been thoroughly evaluated—to prevent risk of aspiration.
- Preventive.
  - Reassurance and education are usually sufficient first-line measures.
    - Adequate fluid and sodium intake.
    - Avoidance of triggers.
    - Assume supine position and raise legs at the onset of symptoms.
- Specific.
  - Treatment as needed—directed by etiology (*for either unexplained new-onset, recurrent, or unpredictable syncope*).

Other Considerations:

- Clinical features are usually diagnostic and further testing is recommended when etiology is questionable.
- Yet a cardiology consult is recommended to eliminate cardiac etiology.
- CPVT may not manifest on routine EKG; emotional or physical stress may show changes on EKG.
- Consider Brugada syndrome in athletes from Thailand and Laos who present with unexplained syncope.
- Routine echocardiogram may miss congenital, structural abnormalities; thus congenital echocardiogram is recommended for evaluation of syncope in athletes.
- Beta-blockers.
  - Can exacerbate vasovagal syncope.
  - On list of prohibited substances for specific sports including archery, shooting, skeleton, and darts.

Return to Play Criteria:

- Restrict athletes from participation until diagnosis has been established and therapeutic intervention has been shown to be effective.
- Cardiology clearance is highly recommended.

Recommended Readings

Battle RW, Mistry DJ, Malhotra R, Macknight JM, Saliba EN, Mahapatra S. Cardiovascular screening and the elite athlete: Advances, concepts, controversies, and a view of the future. *Clin Sports Med.* 2011;30:503–524.

Benditt DG, Lurie KG, Fabian WH. Clinical Approach to diagnosis of Syncope. *Cardiol Clin.* 1997;15(2):165–176.

Brignole M, Alboni P, Benditt D, et al. Guidelines on management (diagnosis and treatment) of syncope. *Eur Heart J.* 2001;22: 1256–1306.

Coleman B, Salerno JC. Causes of syncope in children and adolescents. *UpToDate.* Accessed January 21, 2013.

DynaMed [Internet]. Syncope evaluation. Ipswich (MA): EBSCO Publishing.]. Available from http://search.ebscohost.com direct= true&db=dme&AN=116050&anchor=How-to-cite&site=dynamed-live&scope=site. Updated March 05, 2012; cited December 2, 2012.

Gillette PC, Garson A, Jr. Sudden cardiac death in the pediatric population. *Circulation.* 1992;85:I64–I69.

Kapoor WN. Evaluation and management of the patient with syncope. *JAMA.* 1992;268:2553–2560.

Kapoor WN. Syncope. *N Engl J Med.* 2000;343:1856–1862.

Maron BJ, Mitchell JH. 26th Bethesda Conference: Recommendations for determining eligibility for competition in athletes with cardiovascular abnormalities. *J Am Coll Cardiol.* 1994;24(4):846–899.

Olshansky B. Neurocardiogenic (vasovagal) syncope. *UpToDate.* Accessed February 24, 2011.

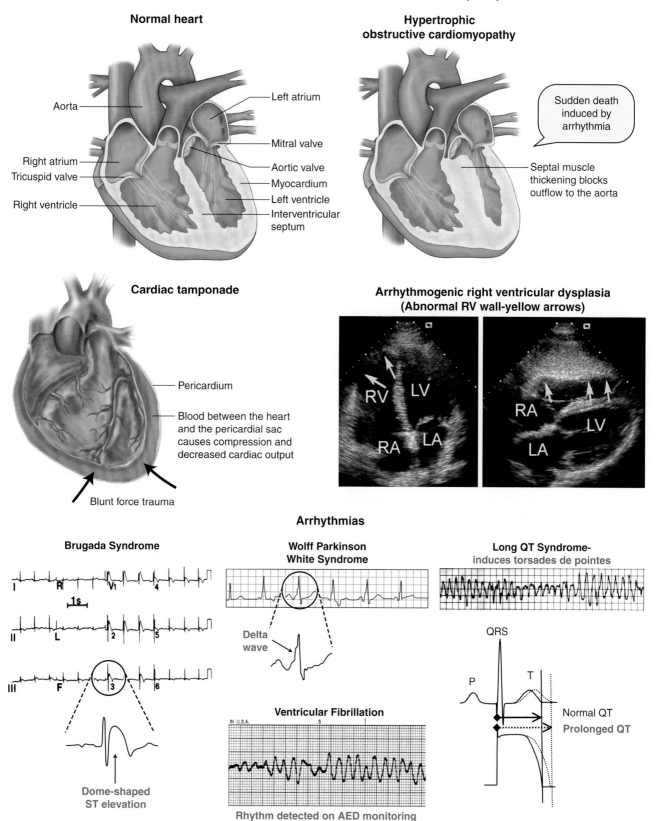

Figure 122. Syncope

Hypertension

Introduction (Definitions/Classification):

- Hypertension is the most prevalent (~25%) cardiovascular condition affecting competitive athletes.
- Defined as a persistent increase in BP >140/90 mm Hg.
- During pre-participation physical examination (PPE), 80% of athletes with BP >142/92 mm Hg will develop hypertension in 1 year.
- Conversely, athletic participation reduces incidence of hypertension by ~50%.
- Classified into two major categories:
  - Essential hypertension ("primary," "idiopathic").
    - No readily identifiable cause.
    - Combination of genetic and environmental factors.
  - Secondary hypertension.
    - Functional or structural dysfunction of a secondary system—metabolic, renal, endocrine, or cardiovascular.

History and Physical Examination:

- History:
  - Most athletes with hypertension are asymptomatic (the silent killer). Symptoms may include poor exercise tolerance, headaches, chest pain, dyspnea, orthopnea, lower extremity pain/claudication, tinnitus, visual disturbances, and changes in sexual function.
  - Past medical history:
    - Risk factors including dyslipidemia, obesity, or stress.
    - Endocrine disorders including thyroid or adrenal dysfunction.
  - Medications and drugs:
    - Prescribed stimulants for attention deficit-hyperactivity disorder.
    - Over-the-counter and other sympathomimetic agents (NSAIDs, nasal decongestants, ma huang).
    - Illicit drugs—anabolic steroids, cocaine, amphetamines.
    - Alcohol.
    - Smoking or chewing tobacco.
  - Diet:
    - Excessive fat, salt, and processed foods.
- Family history:
  - Cardiovascular disease.
    - Athletes with family history of hypertension have been shown to develop concentric hypertrophy following training.
  - Premature death, renal disease, diabetes, pheochromocytoma, gout.
- Race:
  - African Americans are affected more often than whites (2:1 ratio) with Asians being affected the least.
- Physical examination:
  - Evaluate for end-organ dysfunction.
    - HEENT: Retinopathy or papilledema.
    - Neck: Thyroid enlargement, carotid bruit.
    - Pulmonary: Rales or rhonchi on lung auscultation.
    - Cardiac: Murmur, S3 or S4 gallop, arterial bruits, point of maximal impulse (PMI) displaced laterally.
    - Neurologic: Weakness, confusion, visual changes may indicate intracranial manifestations.
    - Extremities: Edema, bounding peripheral pulses in hyperthyroidism, decreased/delayed femoral pulses with aortic coarctation, femoral bruits.
    - Abdomen: Masses, renal bruit.
    - Skin: Purple striae with Cushing syndrome.

Diagnosis:

- "White-coat hypertension" is common during PPE.
  - Record three BPs on separate occasions (out-of-office), with an appropriately sized cuff, after resting for 5 minutes on each occasion.

- Staging:
  - Pre-hypertension—120/80
  - Stage I—140/90
  - Stage II—160/100
  - Stage III—180/110
- Younger than 18 years old: average readings >95% for gender, age, and height.
- Recommended laboratory tests:
  - Comprehensive metabolic panel.
  - Fasting lipid profile.
  - CBC.
  - Urinalysis for hematuria/proteinuria.
  - EKG to rule out structural heart disease.
  - For sustained hypertension, consider further evaluation with echocardiography, to evaluate for left ventricular hypertrophy, and exercise stress testing.
  - For older athletes and in those with accelerated hypertension, consider evaluation for renal artery stenosis (fibromuscular dysplasia) and/or polycystic kidney disease.

Treatment:

- Nonpharmacologic (for those athletes with "pre-hypertension" (BP 120/80 to 139/89 mm Hg). Consider early treatment in athletes with diabetes or chronic kidney disease.
  - Dietary changes (as per DASH dietary recommendations).
    - Decrease sodium consumption, particularly processed foods (decrease 5 to 10/2 to 3 mm Hg).
    - Decrease alcohol ingestion.
    - Increase potassium intake (potatoes and bananas).
    - Weight loss (decrease of 1 mm Hg/kg lost).
  - Stress relief.
    - Muscle relaxation/meditation/yoga.
    - Stress management.
  - Regular aerobic exercise (decrease of 4 to 9 mm Hg).
- Pharmacologic.
  - Before initiating pharmacologic treatment, carefully consider side effects of antihypertensive medications to reduce potential detrimental effects on cardiovascular conditioning and exercise capacity.
  - Drugs with favorable safety profiles without significant detriments to aerobic capacity include the following.
    - *Angiotensin-converting enzyme (ACE) inhibitors.*
      - Favorable first-line agents in athletes, especially those with diabetes.
      - Decrease in ventricular remodeling (with chronic left ventricular pressure overload).
      - Short- and medium-term protective effects against cardiovascular events.
      - Most common side effect is a persistent dry cough.
    - *Calcium channel blockers (CCB).*
      - Dihydropyridines (amlodipine, nifedipine) can induce reflex tachycardia, headaches, and fluid retention.
      - Nondihydropyridines (VERAPAMIL, DILTIAZEM)—bradycardia.
    - *Beta-blockers.*
      - Cardioselective (metoprolol, atenolol) can decrease maximal cardiac output and perceived level of exertion in athletes.
    - *Angiotensin receptor blockers (ARBs):*
      - These may be a good alternative to athletes who develop a dry cough on ACE inhibitors; however, there is no data on their cardio- and renal-protective effects.
    - *Central alpha receptor antagonists.*
      - Unfavorable side effect profile includes drowsiness, dry mouth, and impotence.
      - Can cause rebound hypertension if abruptly withdrawn.
    - **Alpha-1 receptor blockers.**
      - These have very little/no effect on sports performance.
  - Drugs to be avoided in athletes:
    - *Diuretics.*
      - May predispose athletes to dehydration, electrolyte imbalance (hypokalemia), and increase risk for heat illness.
    - *Noncardioselective beta-blockers.*
      - Propranolol and nadolol which can decrease aerobic capacity.

Other Considerations:

- During PPE, athletes with elevated BP should be monitored vigilantly to confirm presence of true versus "white coat hypertension."

- Caution with ACE inhibitors in
  - ultra-endurance athletes in hot environments—can induce acute kidney damage.
  - female athletes of reproductive age—potential for birth defects.
  - athletes with renal artery stenosis.
- Beta-blockers and CCBs can blunt peak heart rate and impair performance.
- Consider CCBs versus either ACE inhibitors or ARBs in athletes of African descent (low renin).
- Beta-blockers are banned in elite (national and international) athletes competing in shooting, archery, darts, or skeleton.
- Diuretics can be used as "masking agents" and are thus banned from international competition.
- Substances which can impact BP control include the following.
  - Estrogen containing oral contraceptives (OCs).
  - NSAIDs.
  - Antidepressants.
  - Alcohol.
  - Nasal decongestants.
  - Tobacco.
  - Exogenous thyroid hormone supplementation.
- Consider evaluation for coronary artery disease as hypertension is a risk factor.

Return to Play:

- Eligibility for participation needs to be individualized if hypertension coexists with additional cardiac disease (acquired or congenital).
- During PPE, athletes with elevated BP should be monitored vigilantly to confirm presence of true versus "white coat hypertension" (described earlier).
- Recommend reporting medications to sports governing bodies to obtain TUE (as needed prior to competition).
- In athletes with diabetes and hypertension, maintain BP <130/85 mm Hg.
- Recommended guidelines according to staging:
  - Pre-hypertension—120/80
    - Lifestyle modifications; no activity restrictions.
    - Obtain echocardiogram for sustained hypertension.
  - Stage I—140/90
    - No activity restrictions if no end-organ damage or heart disease.
    - Monitor BP every 2 to 4 months; may need to monitor more frequently (if indicated).
  - Stage II—160/100 and stage III—180/110
    - Permit low-intensity dynamic exercises.
    - Restrict activity (high static sports, classes IIIA to IIIC) until hypertension is controlled.

Recommended Readings

Baggish AL, Weiner RS, Yared K, et al. Impact of family hypertension history on exercise induced cardiac remodeling. *Am J Cardiol.* 2009;104:101–106.

Basile J, Bloch M. Identifying and managing factors that interfere with or worsen blood pressure control. *Postgrad Med.* 2010;122(2): 35–48.

DynaMed [Internet]. Hypertension. Ipswich (MA): EBSCO Publishing. Available from login.aspx?direct=true&db=dme&AN=115345 &anchor&site=dynamed-live&scope=site. Updated November 26, 2012; cited December 2, 2012.

Gifford RW Jr., Kirkendall W, O'Connor DT, Weidman W. Office evaluation of hypertension. A statement for health professionals by a writing group of the Council for High Blood Pressure Research, American Heart Association. *Circulation.* 1989;79:721–731.

Lehmann M, Durr H, Merkelbach H, Schmid A. Hypertension and sports activities: Institutional experience. *Clin Cardiol.* 1990;13: 197–208.

Maron BJ, Mitchell JH. 26th Bethesda Conference: Recommendations for determining eligibility for competition in athletes with cardiovascular abnormalities. January 6–7, 1994. *J Am Coll Cardiol.* 1994;24:845–899.

Maron BJ, Zipes DP. 36th Bethesda Conference: Eligibility recommendations for Competitive athletes with cardiovascular abnormalities. *J Am Coll Cardio.* 2005;45(8).1318–1375.

Niedfeldt M. Managing hypertension in athletes and physically active patients. *Am Fam Physician.* 2002;66(3):445–453.

Petrella RJ. How effective is exercise training for the treatment of hypertension? *Clin J Sport Med.* 1998;8:224–231.

Sacks FM, Svetkey LP, Vollmer WM, et al. Effects on blood pressure of reduced dietary sodium and Dietary Approaches to Stop Hypertension (DASH) diet. DASH-Sodium Collaborative Research Group. *N Engl J Med.* 2001;344:3–10.

Seventh report of Joint National Committee on Prevention, Detection, Evaluation and Treatment of High Blood Pressure. *JAMA.* 2003;289:2560–2571.

Shafeeq A, Thompson PD. Management of hypertension in athletes. In: *Delee & Drez's Orthopedic Sports Medicine: Principles and Practice.* Elsevier; 2012.

The sixth report of the Joint National Committee on Prevention, Detection, Evaluation, and Treatment of High Blood Pressure. *Arch Intern Med.* 1997;157:2413–2446.

Tanji JL. Tracking of elevated blood pressure values in adolescent athletes at 1-year follow-up. *Am J Dis Child.* 1991;145:665–657.

Hypertension

Be aware: "White-coat hypertension" is common during preparticipation examination
- Record three blood pressures on separate occasions (out-of-office), with an appropriately sized cuff, after resting for 5 minutes on each occasion
- Staging:
  - Pre-hypertension: > 120/80
  - Stage I: > 140/90
  - Stage II: > 160/100
  - Stage III: > 180/110

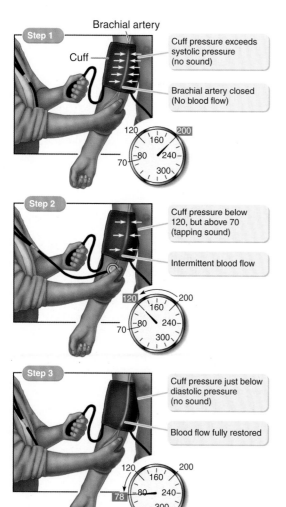

Step 1

Brachial artery

Cuff

Cuff pressure exceeds systolic pressure (no sound)

Brachial artery closed (No blood flow)

Step 2

Cuff pressure below 120, but above 70 (tapping sound)

Intermittent blood flow

Step 3

Cuff pressure just below diastolic pressure (no sound)

Blood flow fully restored

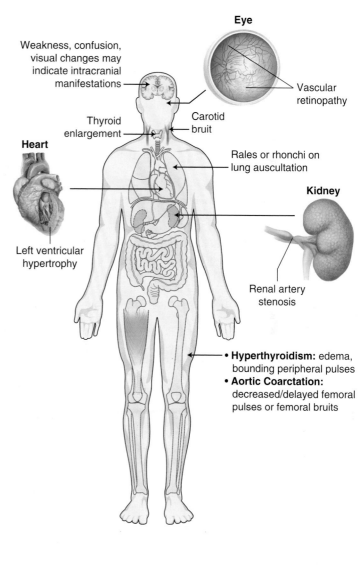

Eye

Vascular retinopathy

Weakness, confusion, visual changes may indicate intracranial manifestations

Thyroid enlargement

Carotid bruit

Heart

Rales or rhonchi on lung auscultation

Kidney

Left ventricular hypertrophy

Renal artery stenosis

- **Hyperthyroidism:** edema, bounding peripheral pulses
- **Aortic Coarctation:** decreased/delayed femoral pulses or femoral bruits

Figure 123. Hypertension

Marfan Syndrome

Introduction (Definitions/Classification):

- An autosomal dominant disorder, Marfan syndrome (MFS) results from a mutation of the fibrillin-1 gene resulting in loose ligaments and weak supporting connective tissue.
- Approximately 10% of individuals with Marfan phenotype have been linked to TGF beta receptor 2 (TGFBR2) and TGFBR1 gene mutations.
- MFS and related disorders (Ehlers–Danlos or Loeys–Dietz syndrome [LDS]) all manifest genetic deficiencies of connective tissue proteins that increase the risk of dissection of the aorta and other smaller arteries.
- Clinical manifestations may also include the ocular, musculoskeletal, respiratory, central nervous, and integumentary (skin) systems.

History and Physical Examination:

- History:
  - May have a positive family history.
  - Occasionally, may present with collapse during physical exertion.
- Physical examination:
  - "Marfanoid" features (see diagnostic criteria later).
  - Athletes are typically tall with thin body habitus, long arms and fingers, and joint hypermobility (See "screening tests" defined in Figure).
  - Wide variation of clinical presentations.

Diagnosis:

- *Based on The Revised Ghent Criteria, Updated 2010.*
- **First, check "Systemic Score" during pre-participation physical examination:** ≥ 7 *indicates systemic involvement.*
  - Wrist **and** thumb sign: 3 points (wrist OR thumb sign: 1 point)
  - Pectus carinatum deformity: 2 (pectus excavatum or chest asymmetry: 1 point)
  - Hindfoot deformity: 2 points (plain pes planus: 1 point)
  - Pneumothorax: 2 points
  - Dural ectasia: 2 points
  - Protrusio acetabuli: 2 points
  - Reduced upper segment/lower segment ratio (US/LS) **and** increased arm span/height **and** no severe scoliosis: 1 point
  - Scoliosis or thoracolumbar kyphosis: 1 point
  - Reduced elbow extension (≤ 170 degrees with full extension): 1 point
  - Facial features (at least three of the following five features: Dolichocephaly [reduced cephalic index or head width/length ratio], enophthalmos, downslanting palpebral fissures, malar hypoplasia, retrognathia): 1 point
  - Skin striae: 1 point
  - Myopia >3 D: 1 point
  - Mitral valve prolapse (all types): 1 point
- Second, ask about a family history of MFS.
  - *If negative family history of MFS, the presence of any of the following criteria is diagnostic.*
    - Aortic criterion[#] and ectopia lentis.[*]
    - Aortic criterion and a causal *FBN1* mutation.
    - Aortic criterion and a systemic score ≥ 7.
    - Ectopia lentis and a causal *FBN1* mutation found in an individual with aortic aneurysm.
  - *If positive family history of MFS, the addition of any of the following criteria is diagnostic.*
    - Ectopia lentis
    - Systemic score ≥ 7 points[*]
    - Aortic criterion (aortic diameter Z-score [Z] ≥ 2, >20 years old; $Z \geq 3$, <20 years, or aortic root dissection)[*]

---

[*]absence of discerning characteristics of either Shprintzen–Goldberg syndrome (SGS), Loeys–Dietz syndrome (LDS), or vascular Ehlers–Danlos syndrome (vEDS).
[#]Aortic diameter $Z \geq 2$ or aortic root dissection.
Note: Pay attention to body surface area when calculating Z-score for aortic dilatation; may underestimate in athletes with large BSAs.

- Medications:
  - Antispasmodic agents.
    - Dicyclomine, hyoscyamine, or enteric-coated peppermint oil capsules may be helpful to relieve gut smooth muscle contractions.
    - Use as needed, especially prophylactically for "known forthcoming stressors" (e.g., stressful competition).
  - Antidepressants (tricyclic antidepressants [TCAs] and selective serotonin reuptake inhibitors [SSRIs]).
    - Beneficial, yet, outcome data are limited.
    - Start at low dose and titrate as needed.
  - Alosetron (serotonin receptor antagonist).
    - Helpful in IBS-D.
    - Had been banned, yet is now available for a subset of patients under close monitoring.
  - Antibiotics.
    - Short-term, nonabsorbable antibiotics (neomycin, clarithromycin, metronidazole) have been suggested to be effective, yet outcome data are limited.
    - Short course of Rifaximin may help patients with IBS-D; use only after all other therapies have failed.
  - Antidiarrheal.
    - Loperamide may have a role in treatment of IBS-D; avoid in IBS-C or IBS-M.
- Probiotics.
  - Certain formulations such as *Bifidobacteria* have been shown to be effective.
  - No data available on the efficacy of *Lactobacillus*.
- Associated psychiatric disorders.
  - Cognitive behavioral therapy (CBT) may be beneficial.

Other Considerations:

- Consider diagnostic workup for celiac sprue in IBS-D.
- ESR and C-reactive protein (CRP) should be normal. If elevated, consider ulcerative colitis or Crohn disease.
- While evaluating a patient with IBS, *"alarm symptoms or signs"* that should trigger further evaluation include weight loss (>10%), family history of colon cancer, fever, anemia, hematochezia, chronic and severe diarrhea, nocturnal abdominal symptoms, guarding, or rebound tenderness on abdominal examination. If alarm symptoms are present, consider obtaining the following.
  - CBC.
  - Comprehensive metabolic panel.
  - Thyroid function tests.
  - Stool for ova and parasites.
  - Abdominal radiographs.
  - Colonoscopy.

Return to Play Criteria:

- Afebrile with normal caloric, fluid and electrolyte balance **WITHOUT** *"alarm symptoms or signs."*

Recommended Readings

American College of Gastroenterology Task Force on Irritable Bowel Syndrome, Brandt LJ, Chey WD, et al. An evidence-based position statement on the management of irritable bowel syndrome. *Am J Gastroenterol.* 2009;104 Suppl 1:S1–S35.

Catassi C, Kryszak D, Louis-Jacques O, et al. Detection of celiac disease in primary care: A multicenter case-finding study in North America. *Am J Gastroenterol.* 2007;102:1454–1460.

Drossman DA, Toner BB, Whitehead WE, et al. Cognitive-behavioral therapy versus education and desipramine versus placebo for moderate to severe functional bowel disorders. *Gastroenterology.* 2003;125:19–31.

Grundmann O, Yoon SL. Irritable bowel syndrome: Epidemiology, diagnosis and treatment: An update for health-care practitioners. *JGastroenterol Hepatol.* 2010;25(4):691–699.

Longstreth GF, Thompson WG, Chey WD, et al. Functional bowel disorders. *Gastroenterology.* 2006;130:1480–1491.

Owens DM, Nelson DK, Talley NJ. The irritable bowel syndrome: Long-term prognosis and the physician-patient interaction. *Ann Intern Med.* 1995;122:107–112.

Parisi GC, Zilli M, Miani MP, et al. High-fiber diet supplementation in patients with irritable bowel syndrome (IBS): A multicenter, randomized, open trial comparison between wheat bran diet and partially hydrolyzed guar gum (PHGG). *Dig Dis Sci.* 2002;47:1697–1704.

Pimentel M, Lembo A, Chey WD, et al. Rifaximin therapy for patients with irritable bowel syndrome without constipation. *N Engl J Med.* 2011;364:22–32.

Quartero AO, Meineche-Schmidt V, Muris J, et al. Bulking agents, antispasmodic and antidepressant medication for the treatment of irritable bowel syndrome (Cochrane Review). In: *The Cochrane Library 2007 Issue 1.* Chichester, UK: John Wiley and Sons, Ltd.

Wald AD. Treatment of irritable bowel syndrome. *UpToDate.* Accessed November 16, 2012.

Solid Organ Injury

Introduction (Definitions/Classification):

- Solid organ injuries can induce severe morbidity and can cause death in athletes.
- Failure to identify life-threatening injuries is the most common "pitfall" in the initial management of intra-abdominal trauma.
- Prompt recognition of potential solid organ injury, expeditious diagnosis, and swift management are therefore essential to prevent serious harm.
- This chapter discusses selected topics regarding solid organ injury in athletes with specific attention to the following.
  - Spleen.
  - Liver.
  - Kidney (less common).

History and Physical Examination:

- **History:**
  - History of "mechanism" of impact injury to the upper abdomen, or trunk.
    - Person-to-person contact.
    - Equipment-to-person contact.
  - Onset of symptoms: Acute versus delayed.
  - Comorbid conditions.
    - Inquire about recent mononucleosis (EBV) infection (*increased likelihood of splenic rupture and hepatitis*).
    - Single organ (*one kidney*).
    - Recent, prolonged use of NSAID's (*increased bleeding risk*).
  - Presenting symptoms.
    - Abdominal/flank pain.
      - Diffuse versus localized.
      - Location: Right upper quadrant or superior midline tenderness—liver; left upper quadrant—splenic injury; costovertebral angle—kidney injury.
    - Dizziness.
    - Fatigue/malaise.
    - Gross hematuria.
    - Sweating.
- Physical examination.
  - General: Varied presentation, from normal vitals to obtunded athlete (*hypovolemic shock*).
  - Neck.
    - Tracheal deviation (concurrent pneumothorax).
  - Chest/pulmonary.
    - Palpate for rib fractures.
    - Tachypnea (anxiety vs. pain vs. concurrent lung injury).
    - Diminished breath sounds (concurrent pneumothorax).
  - Cardiac: Tachycardia/hypotension (pain vs. internal bleeding).
  - Abdomen.
    - Palpate each quadrant separately and ensure stability of pelvis.
    - Tenderness, guarding, rigidity (peritoneal irritation).
    - Hypoactive bowel sounds (ileus).
    - Distention (internal bleeding).
    - Ecchymosis: Grey Turner sign (flank), Cullen sign (periumbilical) are indicative of either internal bleeding or pancreatitis.
  - Genitourinary: Evaluate for blood at the urethral meatus (kidney injury complicated by gross hematuria).
  - Extremities: Decreased or absent peripheral pulses (shock).
  - Skin: Hyperhidrosis, piloerection, decreased capillary refill.
  - Additional signs (sensitivity and specificity vary).
    - Pain referred to tip of left shoulder (Kehr sign; splenic injury).
    - Increased pain during inspiration following application of posterior and superior pressure under rib cage along right midclavicular line (Murphy sign; liver injury).
    - Pain with costovertebral thump (Lloyd sign; kidney injury).

Diagnosis:

- Clinical suspicion and signs/symptoms on physical examination.
- Imaging.
  - CT with IV contrast (*gold standard*).
    - *Pros*: Rules out spleen and liver injuries that require surgery; detects small volume of fluid not ordinarily detected by ultrasonography.
    - *Cons*: Reader dependent and radiation exposure; initial images may fail to spot renal pelvis injury; contrast may need to be avoided in those with compromised renal function.
  - FAST (Focused Assessment with Sonography in Trauma; detects free fluid in abdomen).
    - If *positive*: Obtain CT.
    - If *negative*: Reasonable to perform serial abdominal examinations, repeat FAST in 6 hours, followed by CT as needed.
    - *Pros*: Decreased use of CT, fewer complications and days in hospital, and lower cost for care.
    - *Cons*: Operator dependent and unreliable in identifying solid organ injury.
  - Angiography (with embolization)—diagnostic and curative.
  - Chest a pelvis radiographs.
    - Free air under diaphragm.
    - May detect rib and/or pelvic fractures.
    - May show "*Balance Sign*"—medial displacement of gastric bubble, indicative of potential spleen injury.
- Blood tests.
  - Blood typing and screening.
  - Complete blood count.
    - Baseline and serial hematocrit (*to assess occult vs. ongoing hemorrhage*).
  - Comprehensive metabolic panel.
  - Coagulation studies.
  - Pancreatic function tests.
- Urine.
  - Gross or microscopic hematuria.
    - In patients with abdominal tenderness, 60% sensitivity and 90% specificity for intra-abdominal injury.
    - Seen in 80% to 90% of kidney injuries.
  - Pregnancy test in all athletes of childbearing age.
- Miscellaneous.
  - Diagnostic peritoneal lavage: Unstable, multisystem trauma patient, with equivocal FAST test.
  - MRI may be useful in those allergic to contrast.

Treatment:

- On-field.
  - Monitor ABC's.
  - Activate EMS and transport to nearest medical facility expeditiously.
  - Monitor vitals pending arrival of EMS.
  - If available, insert two large bore (14 or 16 gauge) peripheral intravenous catheters and commence crystalloid (normal saline) infusion.
  - Reassure athlete, teammates, parents, coaches.
- In-hospital.
  - Conservative (*if hemodynamically stable*).
    - Nonoperative management (*observation and serial blood tests/examination*).
    - Angiography with transcatheter embolization (*as needed*).
  - Operative (*if hemodynamically unstable*).
- Postsplenectomy considerations.
  - Adequate immunization and antibiotic prophylaxis are critical in the prevention of life-threatening illnesses.
  - Immunization (*initiated 14 days prior to elective surgery or 14 days postsplenectomy for emergent surgery*).
    - 23-valent pneumococcal polysaccharide vaccine; booster every 5 years.
    - Haemophilus influenza vaccine; check titers and consider booster immunization.
    - Meningococcal polysaccharide vaccine; booster every 5 years.
    - Influenza vaccine yearly; to decrease risk of secondary pneumococcal pneumonia.
  - Oral antibiotic therapy.
    - Antibiotic prophylaxis is not routinely recommended in adults.
    - Antibiotic therapy for fever is recommended followed by prompt assessment at nearest medical facility.
      - Amoxicillin/clavulanate, cefuroxime or extended spectrum fluoroquinolone (levofloxacin/moxifloxacin).
      - Ceftriaxone for suspected sepsis in outpatient setting.

Other Considerations:

- Differential diagnosis.
  - Injuries of other solid organs, including pancreas and ovaries.

- Hollow viscus perforation.
- Other genitourinary tract injuries (ureter, bladder, urethra).
- Ruptured ectopic pregnancy.
- Mesenteric vessel injuries.
- Diaphragmatic injuries.
- Pelvis or spine fractures.
- Pancreas injury.
  - Suspect with epigastric tenderness.
  - Amylase: Delayed rise, not specific or sensitive, yet rising levels should prompt further investigation.
- Hollow viscus perforations.
  - Diagnosed more effectively with CT + serial abdominal examinations.
  - Greater need for surgical intervention than solid organ injuries.
- Other genitourinary tract injuries (ureter, bladder, urethra).
  - Emergently evaluate and treat lower urinary tract injuries first.
  - Evaluate kidneys after excluding lower tract injury.
- Miscellaneous pearls.
  - 80% of those with hepatic injuries have other injuries (rib/pelvic fractures, spinal cord injuries).
  - Baseline hematocrit may be normal following hepatic injury.
  - May defer CT to rule out kidney injury in the absence of gross hematuria.
  - Vigorous hydration in the presence of gross hematuria reduces the risk of clot formation and urinary obstruction.

Return to Play Criteria:

- There are no clinical studies or specific guidelines that influence the timing for returning to activity following solid organ injury.
- Reimaging.
  - May be considered on an "individual basis" and may help guide safe return to activity.
  - At 3 months postinjury has been recommended as a reasonable option.
- Practical decisions should be made on an "individual basis" following specialist consultation based on the severity of injury, required recovery period, and the nature of the involved sport.
- It is recommended that contact sports be avoided for a longer period of time during recovery and specific protective padding to shield the flank and abdomen may be indicated.
- Recommend special attention in making decisions regarding return to play in athletes with a single kidney.
- Begin graded return to play protocol following normal clinical examination, laboratory tests, and favorable reimaging results suggestive of adequate healing.
- Return to full activity following demonstration of baseline aerobic capacity and strength.

Recommended Readings

Christmas AB, Jacobs DJ. Management of hepatic trauma in adults. *UpToDate*. Accessed March 31st, 2013.
Clinical policy: Critical issues in the evaluation of adult patients presenting to the emergency department with acute blunt abdominal trauma. *Ann Emerg Med*. 2004;43(2):278–290.
Gaines BA. Intra-abdominal solid organ injury in children: Diagnosis and treatment. *J Trauma*. 2009;67:S135.
Grinsell MM, Butz K, Gurka MJ, et al. Sport-related kidney injury among high school athletes. *Pediatrics*. 2012;130(1):40–45.
Isenhour JL, Marx J. Advances in abdominal trauma. *Emerg Med Clin North Am*. 2007;25(3):713–733.
Maung, AA, Kaplan, LJ. Management of splenic injury in the adult trauma patient. *UpToDate*. Accessed March 31st, 2013.
McCray VW, Davis JW, Lemaster D, et al. Observation for nonoperative management of the spleen: How long is long enough? *J Trauma*. 2008;65(6):1354–1358.
Melniker LA, Leibner E, McKenney MG, et al. Randomized controlled clinical trial of point-of-care, limited ultrasonography for trauma in the emergency department: The first sonography outcomes assessment program trial. *Ann Emerg Med*. 2006;48(3):227–235.
Miller KS, McAninch JW. Radiographic assessment of renal trauma: Our 15-year experience. *J Urol*.1995;154:352–355.
Pariset JM, Feldman KW, Paris C. The pace of signs and symptoms of blunt abdominal trauma to children. *Clin Pediatr (Phila)*. 2010;49:24.
Pasternack MS. Prevention of sepsis in the asplenic patient. *UpToDate*. Accessed March 31st, 2013.
Richards JR, Derlet RW. Computed tomography and blunt abdominal injury: Patient selection based on examination, haematocrit and haematuria. *Injury*. 1997;28(3):181–185.
Richardson JD. Changes in the management of injuries to the liver and spleen. *J Am Coll Surg*. 2005;200:648.
Rose JS. Ultrasound in abdominal trauma. *Emerg Med Clin North Am*. 2004;22(3):581–599.
Runyon MS. Blunt genitourinary trauma. *UpToDate*. Accessed March 31st, 2013.
Santucci RA, Wessells H, Bartsch G, et al. Evaluation and management of renal injuries: Consensus statement of the renal trauma subcommittee. *BJU Int*. 2004;93:937–954.
Scalea TM, Rodriguez A, Chiu WC, et al. Focused Assessment with Sonography for Trauma (FAST): Results from an international consensus conference. *J Trauma*. 1999;46(3):466–472.
Velmahos GC, Toutouzas K, Radin R, et al. High success with nonoperative management of blunt hepatic trauma: The liver is a sturdy organ. *Arch Surg*. 2003;138(5):475–480.

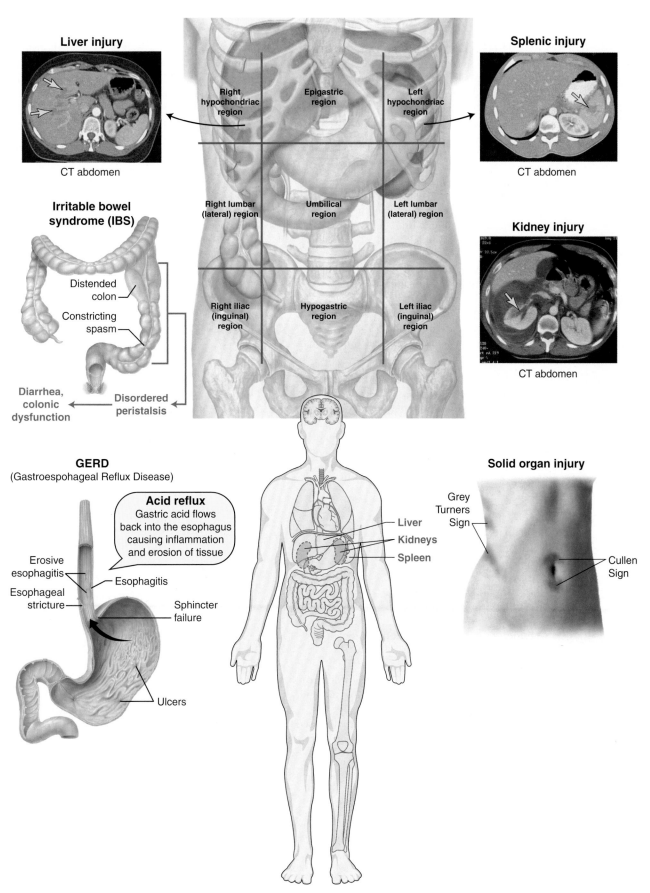

Liver injury

CT abdomen

Irritable bowel syndrome (IBS)

Distended colon

Constricting spasm

Diarrhea, colonic dysfunction

Disordered peristalsis

GERD
(Gastroespohageal Reflux Disease)

Acid reflux
Gastric acid flows back into the esophagus causing inflammation and erosion of tissue

Erosive esophagitis

Esophagitis

Esophageal stricture

Sphincter failure

Ulcers

Right hypochondriac region

Epigastric region

Left hypochondriac region

Right lumbar (lateral) region

Umbilical region

Left lumbar (lateral) region

Right iliac (inguinal) region

Hypogastric region

Left iliac (inguinal) region

Liver

Kidneys

Spleen

Splenic injury

CT abdomen

Kidney injury

CT abdomen

Solid organ injury

Grey Turners Sign

Cullen Sign

Figure 126. Abdomen

Sports Hernia

Introduction (Definitions/Classification): Also termed "Sportsman's Hernia" or "Athletic Pubalgia," is a weakness or tearing of either (and) the conjoint tendon, insertion of rectus abdominis, deep transversalis fascia, or oblique aponeurosis. This condition is typically characterized by chronic, unilateral or bilateral (less common) groin pain *without* the presence of a hernia. Imbalance, weakness, or chronic straining of the lower abdominal and groin musculature may predispose athletes to Sports Hernia.

History and Physical Examination:

- History:
  - Groin pain is the typical presenting symptom.
  - Pain worse with physical activity or Valsalva.
  - Vague, nondescript complaints: Slight bulge, sensation of weakness.
  - Onset typically insidious, although may be related to specific movements or events—cutting, pivoting, kicking, turning, torquing, twisting
- Examination:
  - *No* evidence of a true hernia.
  - Discomfort with forced hip adduction.
  - Assess area of tenderness (*related pathology*).
    - Inguinal canal (ilioinguinal nerve entrapment).
    - Pubic tubercle (osteitis pubis).
    - Adductor origin (musculotendinous strain).

Diagnosis:

- Based on clinical examination.
- Radiographic evaluation used to rule out other diagnoses (*listed below in "other considerations"*).
  - Plain XR of lumbar spine, hips, pelvis.
  - Pelvis MRI (using specific protocols to assess presence of pathology specific to athlete pubalgia).
  - CT scan.
  - Ultrasound.

Treatment:

- Conservative treatment.
  - Rest 6 to 8 weeks.
  - NSAIDs.
  - Ice, heat.
  - Massage.
  - Corticosteroid injections.
  - Stretching/strengthening exercises focusing on affected hip adductors.
- Surgery.
  - Consider for failure of conservative interventions.
  - Effective.
  - Open or laparoscopic.
    - Both approaches have >92% successful "return to play" rate.
    - Faster "return to play" for laparoscopic method.
  - "Munich repair."
    - Involves release of the isolated defect with resection of the genital nerve branch to prevent chronic pain.
    - Median time to return to sports is about 1 month versus 4 months with standard repairs.
    - Outcome studies pending.

Other Considerations:

- High prevalence.
  - Lovell review of 189 athletes with chronic groin pain; revealed sports hernias in ~50%.
- Males greater than females.
- Groin pain is often multifactorial. Consider intra-abdominal medical concerns
  - appendicitis.
  - diverticulitis.
  - testicular torsion.
  - pelvic pathology (e.g., UTI, urethritis, ovarian cyst complications, endometriosis).
- Often confused with:
  - osteitis pubis.
  - stress fractures.
  - distal rectus strain/avulsion.
  - adductor longus rupture.
  - adductor tenoperiostitis.
  - nerve entrapment syndromes.
  - referred lumbar disc or hip disease.
- Consider "*Gilmore's groin*" in soccer players.
  - Variation of a sports hernia.
  - Different pathology—torn external oblique aponeurosis or conjoint tendon, a dehiscence between conjoined tendon and inguinal ligament, a dilated superficial inguinal ring, in the setting of no palpable hernia.
  - Requires a different surgical approach.
- Consider "*hockey player's syndrome.*"
  - Elite hockey players with groin pain in the absence of a palpable hernia.
  - Involves a tear of the external oblique aponeurosis and inguinal nerve entrapment.
  - Surgical repair with mesh is the usual definitive intervention.

Return to Play:

- Trial of sports-specific movements with gradual return to full activities if pain-free.
  - Avoid "cutting-type" movements for 3 weeks following surgical repair.
  - Full return to sports typically 6 weeks post surgery.

Recommended Readings

Brooks DC. Sports-related groin pain or 'sports hernia'. *UpToDate.* Accessed October 16, 2012.
Caudill P, Nyland J, Smith C, Yerasimides J, et al. Sports hernias: A systematic literature review. *Br J Sports Med.* 2008;42:954–964.
DynaMed. Accessed October 16, 2012.
Farber A, Wilckens J. Sports hernia: diagnosis and therapeutic approach. *J Am Acad Orthop Surg.* 2007;15(8):507–514.
Gilmore J. Groin pain in the soccer athlete: Fact, fiction, and treatment. *Clin Sports Med.* 1998;17(4):787–793.
Jancin B. Munich repair hastens recovery from sports hernia. *Elsevier Global Medical News.* 2009:19.
Lovell G. The diagnosis of chronic groin pain in athletes: A review of 189 cases. *Aust J Sci Med Sport.* 1995;27(3):76–79.
Nam A, Brody F. Management and Therapy for Sports Hernia. *J Am Coll Surg.* 2008;206(1):154–164.
Omar I, Zoga A, Kavanagh E, et al. Athletic pubalgia and "sports hernia": Optimal MR imaging technique and findings. *Radiographics.* 2008;28:1415–1438.

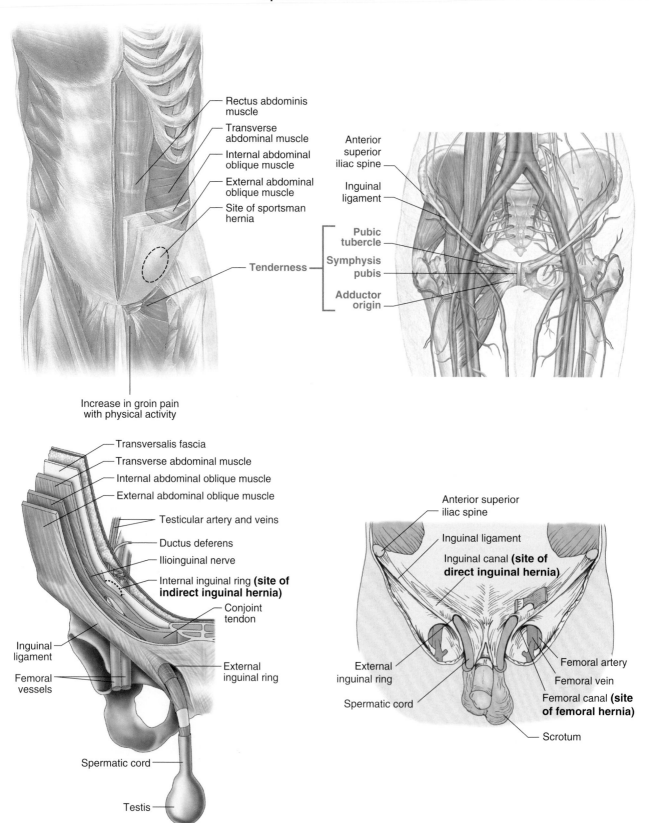

Rectus abdominis muscle

Transverse abdominal muscle

Internal abdominal oblique muscle

External abdominal oblique muscle

Site of sportsman hernia

Tenderness

Increase in groin pain with physical activity

Anterior superior iliac spine

Inguinal ligament

Pubic tubercle

Symphysis pubis

Adductor origin

Transversalis fascia

Transverse abdominal muscle

Internal abdominal oblique muscle

External abdominal oblique muscle

Testicular artery and veins

Ductus deferens

Ilioinguinal nerve

Internal inguinal ring **(site of indirect inguinal hernia)**

Conjoint tendon

Inguinal ligament

Femoral vessels

External inguinal ring

Spermatic cord

Testis

Anterior superior iliac spine

Inguinal ligament

Inguinal canal **(site of direct inguinal hernia)**

External inguinal ring

Spermatic cord

Femoral artery

Femoral vein

Femoral canal **(site of femoral hernia)**

Scrotum

Figure 127. Sportsman Hernia

Part 2: Pelvis

Urethritis

Introduction (Definitions/Classification): An inflammation of the urethra, which may be infectious or noninfectious. Common infectious etiologies include *Neisseria gonorrhoeae* and *Chlamydia trachomatis;* less frequently *Ureaplasma urealyticum, M. genitalium,* adenovirus, and HSV type 1.

History and Physical Examination: Obtain a thorough social history in addition to past medical history.

- Examine for abnormalities or lesions.
  - Perineum, rectum, and external genitalia for lymphadenopathy, lesions, or other abnormalities.
  - Collect urethral discharge by milking urethra (penile shaft for men, urethral meatus in women).
  - For women, the pelvic examination allows visualization of vaginal walls and cervix for friability, lesions, and sampling of discharge for STI testing and wet mount.

Diagnosis:

- Signs/symptoms on physical examination.
  - Discharge.
  - Dysuria.
  - Dyspareunia.
  - Urethral pruritus.
- Laboratory tests.
- Evaluation of discharge.
  - Gram stain (>5 WBCs per oil immersion field).
  - Culture.
  - Polymerase chain reaction (PCR).
  - Nucleic acid amplification test (NAAT).
- Consider CBC differential for clinical concerns of systemic spread of infection.

Treatment: Dependant on infectious etiology.

- Gonococcal—ceftriaxone or cefixime.
- Chlamydia—azithromycin or doxycycline.
- For persistent or recurrent discharge, metronidazole or tinidazole plus azithromycin.

Other Considerations:

- Recommend abstinence for 7 days after the start of therapy (following resolution of symptoms and adequate treatment of sexual partners).
- Urethritis often related to other genitourinary tract infections. Rule out cystitis, pyelonephritis, herpes genitalis, pelvic inflammatory disease in women, and proctitis/epididymitis in men.
- Consider "risk" while obtaining history. High-risk individuals include <25 years old, history of STIs, multiple sexual partners, drug users, African Americans, and homosexual population.
- With recurrent/persistent urethritis test for trichomonas—if positive, treat with metronidazole.
- If positive culture for gonorrhea or chlamydia, retest in 3 to 6 months to ensure proper resolution.

Return to Play:

- Once symptoms resolve and appropriate antimicrobial therapy has been initiated.

Recommended Readings

Bradshaw CS, Tabrizi SN, Tead TR, et al. Etiologies of nongonococcal urethritis: Bacteria, viruses, and the association with orogenital exposure. *J Infect Dis.* 2006;193:336–345.

Brunham RC, Paavonen J, Stevens CE, et al. Mucopurulent cervicitis—the ignored counterpart in women of urethritis in men. *N Engl J Med.* 1984;311:1–6.

Center for Disease Control and Prevention. (CDC 2010-08-20) www.cdc.gov.

Cook RL, Hutchison SL, Ostergaard L. Systematic review: Noninvasive testing for Chlamydia trachomatis and Neisseria gonorrhoeae. *Ann Intern Med.* 2005;142:914–925.

Swygard H, Cohen M, Sena A. Infectious causes of dysuria in adult men. *UpToDate.* Accessed October 16, 2012.

Urinary Tract Infections

Introduction (Definitions/Classification):

- Commonly known as a "UTI."
- Infection of the urethra, bladder, ureters, or kidneys.
- Prevalent medical concern particularly in sexually active adolescents and young adult women.
- Annual incidence of UTI: 12.6% for women and 3% for men.
- Classified as lower tract (acute cystitis) or upper tract (acute pyelonephritis) infections *and* uncomplicated versus complicated.
- The most common etiologic pathogens are *Escherichia coli (75% to 90%)*, *S. saprophyticus*, *Enterococci*, *Proteus*, and *Klebsiella*.

History and Physical Examination:

- Most UTIs are uncomplicated and occur in healthy individuals with normal anatomy.
- Concerns for complicated UTI:
  - History of immunosuppression.
  - Multiple UTIs.
  - Diabetes.
  - Pregnancy.
  - Infection with a resistant organism.
  - Presence of a structural or functional abnormality of the urinary tract.
  - Male patient.
- Signs and symptoms concerning for cystitis:
  - Dysuria.
  - Urinary frequency.
  - Urgency.
  - Sensation of incomplete emptying.
  - Suprapubic pressure or pain.
  - Hematuria.
- Signs and symptoms concerning for pyelonephritis:
  - Flank pain.
  - Chills and fevers.
  - Costovertebral angle tenderness (CVAT).
  - Nausea, vomiting.

Diagnosis:

- A clean-catch, mid-stream urine sample with 10 leukocytes/mcL.
- Hematuria—more common in UTI; not frequent in urethritis.
- UTI may be diagnosed on urine dipstick with either a positive leukocyte esterase or nitrite, or both.
  - A negative dipstick does not rule out UTI.
- Obtain a urinalysis and urine culture if suspicion exists for
  - failure to respond to initial treatment.
  - recurrent symptoms in <1 month after empiric therapy.
  - acute pyelonephritis.
  - UTI in a male.
  - complicated UTI.
- Men with UTI symptoms require further workup with urine culture and consideration of urologic evaluation for prostatitis.

Treatment:

- General considerations:
  - Consider local antibiotic resistance before commencing treatment.
  - A female with a history of previous UTI who presents with dysuria, frequency, hematuria, CVAT, and no vaginal discharge or irritation has a high accuracy for self-diagnosis (*can treat without diagnostic tests*).
  - If vaginal discharge is present, complete a pelvic examination and urine culture prior to treatment.
  - Moxifloxacin, an FQ, should not be used for either women or men because urine levels are insufficient and ineffective.

- Uncomplicated cystitis.
  - Trimethoprim–sulfamethoxazole (TMP-SMX) for 3 days if community resistance rates <10% to 20%.
  - Sulfa allergy—nitrofurantoin for 5 days.
  - Other options:
    - FQ for 3 days.
    - Single dose of Fosfomycin—equally effective as TMP-SMX or FQ.
    - Relief of dysuria: Phenazopyridine hydrochloride for 2 days.
- Uncomplicated pyelonephritis.
  - FQs—ciprofloxacin for 7 days, Levofloxacin for 5 to 7 days.
  - Resistance or unable to tolerate FQs—parenteral third-generation cephalosporin (ceftriaxone).
- Complicated cystitis.
  - FQs—ciprofloxacin for 7 days, levofloxacin for 5 to 7 days.
  - Resistance or unable to tolerate FQs—parenteral third-generation cephalosporin (ceftriaxone).
- Complicated pyelonephritis.
  - Consider hospitalization initially.
  - First-line broad spectrum, parenteral antibiotics.
  - Following improvement, determined by culture and sensitivity, can complete 10 to 14 days course of oral antibiotics (FQ or TMP-SMX).
- UTI in a male.
  - TMP-SMX or FQ for 7 days.
  - Limited data on Fosfomycin in men; thus avoid use.
- Recurrent UTI.
  - *Educate:*
    - Limit spermicide use.
    - Postcoital voiding.
    - Limited studies on primary prevention with cranberry juice.
  - *Medication:*
    - Prophylaxis warranted if greater than two UTIs in 6 months or greater than three UTIs in 12 months.
    - TMP-SMX or nitrofurantoin nightly for 6 months (continuous prophylaxis).
    - TMP-SMX or nitrofurantoin or FQ as a single dose (postcoital prophylaxis).

Other Considerations:

- There is no need for "test of cure" following improvement after antibiotics.
- If symptoms prolong beyond 3 days, despite treatment, check urinalysis and culture.

Return to Play:

- No debilitating symptoms such as pain, urinary frequency, or urgency.
- Proven clinical improvement of symptoms (no CVAT, suprapubic tenderness).
- Afebrile for 24 hours on appropriate treatment.
- Adequate hydration status and caloric intake.

Recommended Readings

Bent S, Nallamothu B, Simel D, Fihn S, Saint S. Does this woman have an acute uncomplicated urinary tract infection? *JAMA.* 2002;287:2701–2710.

Chapple C, Mangera A. Acknowledgements. Acute cystitis. https://online.epocrates.com/noFrame/showPage.do?method=diseases&MonographId=298&ActiveSectionId=11.

Chew LD, Fihn SD. Recurrent cystitis in nonpregnant women. *West J Med.* 1999;170:274–277.

Fihn S. Acute uncomplicated urinary tract infection in women. *N Engl J Med.* 2003;349:259–266.

Gupta K. Emerging antibiotic resistance in urinary tract pathogens. *Infect Dis Clin North Am.* 2003;17:243–259.

Hooton TM, Gupta K. Acute uncomplicated cystitis and pyelonephritis in women. *UpToDate.* Accessed November 5, 2012.

Hooton TM, Gupta K. Recurrent urinary tract infection in women. *UpToDate.* Accessed November 6, 2012.

Hooton TM. Acute uncomplicated cystitis, pyelonephritis, and asymptomatic bacteriuria in men. *UpToDate.* Accessed November 5, 2012.

Jepson R, Mihaljevic L, Craig J. Cranberries for treating urinary tract infections (Cochrane Review). The Cochrane Library 2007 Issue 1.

Krieger JN, Ross SO, Simonsen JM. Urinary tract infections in healthy university men. *J Urol.* 1993;149:1046–1048.

Milo G, Katchman E, Paul M, Christiaens T, et al. Duration of antibacterial treatment for uncomplicated urinary tract infection in women (Cochrane Review). The Cochrane Library 2007 Issue 1.

Schmiemann G, Kniehl E, Gebhardt K, Matejczyk MM, Hummers-Pradier E. The diagnosis of urinary tract infection: A systematic review. *Dtsch Arztebl Int.* 2010;107(21):361–367.

Stamm WE. Measurement of pyuria and its relation to bacteriuria. *Am J Med.* 1983;75:53–58.

Weir M, Brein A. Adolescent urinary tract infections. *Adolesc Med.* 2000;11(2):293–312.

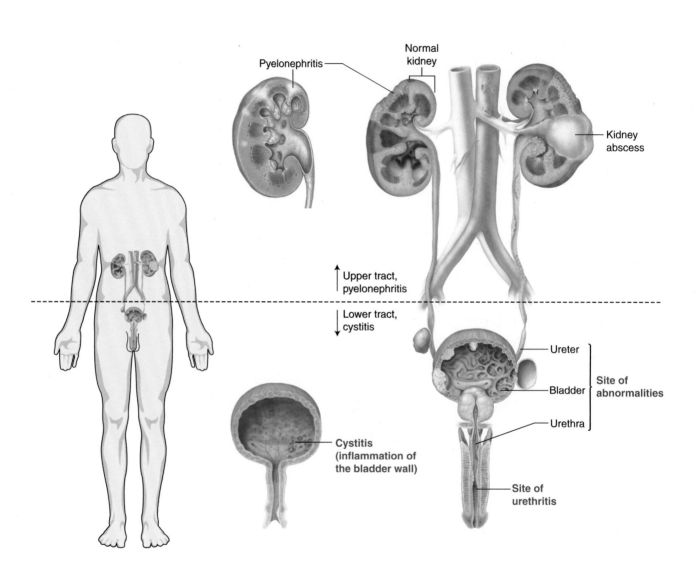

Pyelonephritis

Normal kidney

Kidney abscess

Upper tract, pyelonephritis

Lower tract, cystitis

Ureter

Bladder

Site of abnormalities

Urethra

Site of urethritis

Cystitis (inflammation of the bladder wall)

Figure 128. Pelvis

Section 7: Dermatologic

Introduction (Definitions/Classification):

- Skin diseases in athletes are very common.
- >50% of infectious diseases in sport are dermatologic.
- Athletes participating in contact sports are at high risk for transmission of skin diseases.
- Therefore, prevention, expeditious treatment, and strict adherence to return to play guidelines are critical to prevent morbidity and enhanced personal and team success in the athletic arena.
- Basic facts of dermatoses presented in this section include the following.
  - Bacterial infections.
  - Fungal infections
  - Viral infections.
  - Miscellaneous dermatoses.

History and Physical Examination:

History:
- Duration?
- Characteristics—shape, size, margins, consistency, alteration with time?
- Location and spread?
- Therapy—effectiveness or worsening with treatment?
- Associated symptoms—pruritus, pain, pus?
- Similar past personal history—recurrence or effectiveness of past treatment?
- Family history
- Inciting event(s)—stress, change in personal care products (shampoos, soaps, creams, fragrance, laundry detergent, clothing), travel, environmental exposure, insect bites, medications?
- History of allergies?
- Comorbid medical conditions?

Physical examination (general terminology/characteristics):
- **Macule:** Area of color change that is flat, nonraised, and <5 to 10 mm in size.
- **Patch:** Large macule >5 to 10 mm in size.
- **Papule:** Superficial, solid, raised lesion up to 5 to 10 mm in size.
- **Plaques:** Superficial, elevated plateaued area; diameter > depth.
- **Wheal:** Rounded or flat erythematous papule.
- **Nodule:** Deep, solid, raised area, >5 to 10 mm in width and depth.
- **Pustule:** Circumscribed, superficial, purulent elevated lesion.
- **Vesicle** (<5 mm) versus **Bullae** (>5 mm): Circumscribed, superficial, serous fluid-filled cavity.
- **Crust:** Dried serum, pus, or blood over a skin lesion.
- **Desquamation:** Scaling or peeling of skin composed of stratum corneum.
- **Ulcer:** Depression of the skin with loss of the epidermis and upper dermis.
- **Petechiae:** Small red/purple, nonblanching spots, 1 to 2 mm in size.

Diagnosis (*Dx*) and Treatment (*Rx*):

Bacterial infections:
- **Key facts:**
  - Common pathogens: *Staphylococcus aureus* (*S. aureus*) and Group A Streptococcus (*S. pyogenes*).
  - Dx.
    - Based on history and characteristics of lesions.
  - Prevention of antibiotic resistance is imperative. Therefore, whenever possible
    - incise and drain all lesions.
    - Rx of bacterial infections should be directed by culture and antibiotic sensitivity of lesions following incision and drainage of lesions.
  - Methicillin-resistant *S. aureus* (MRSA) infections are increasingly prevalent.
  - Consider empiric treatment for MRSA (sulfamethoxazole/trimethoprim [TMP/SMX], clindamycin) in geographical areas of high prevalence.

Definitions

Macule

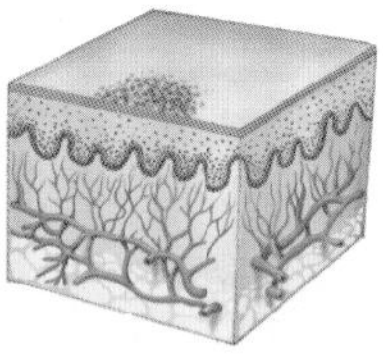

Area of color change that is flat, non-raised, and < 5-10 mm in size

Patch

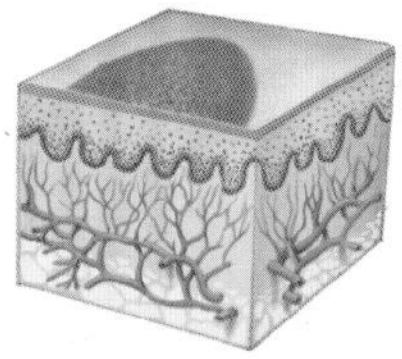

Large macule > 5-10 mm in size

Papule

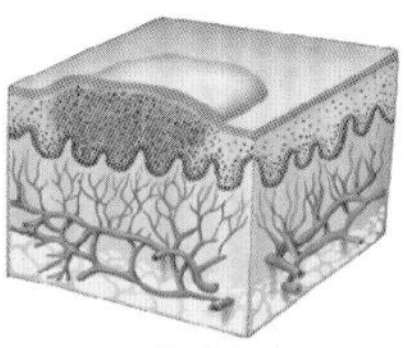

Superficial, solid, raised lesion up to 5-10 mm in size

Plaques

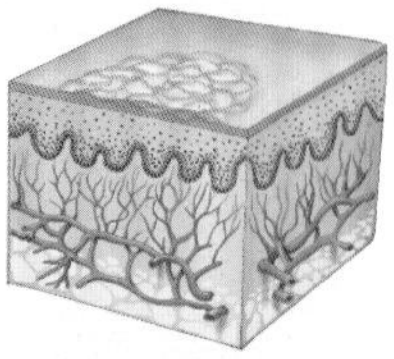

Superficial, elevated plateaued area; diameter > depth

Wheal

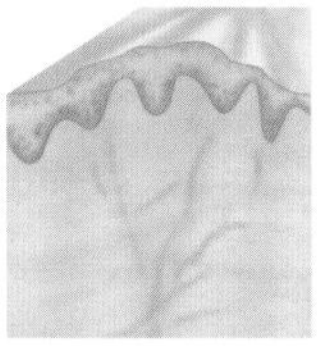

Rounded or flat erythematous papule

Nodule

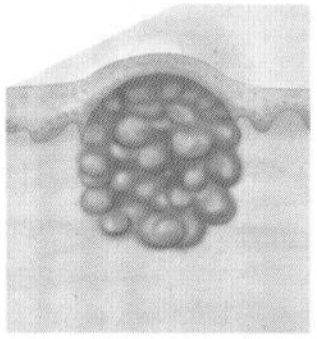

Deep, solid, raised area, > 5-10 mm in width and depth

Pustule

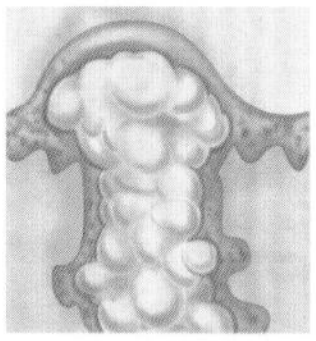

Circumscribed, superficial, purulent elevated lesion

Vesicle (< 0.5 cm) vs. Bullae (> 0.5 cm):

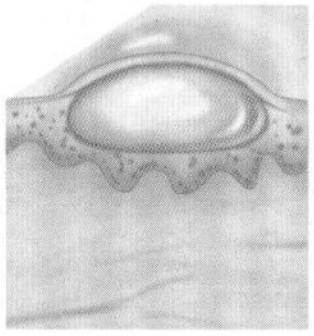

Circumscribed, superficial, serous fluid-filled cavity

Crusts

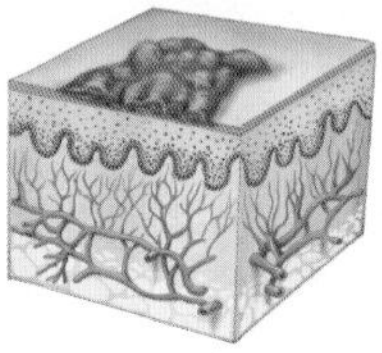

Dried serum, pus, or blood over a skin lesion

Desquamation (scaling)

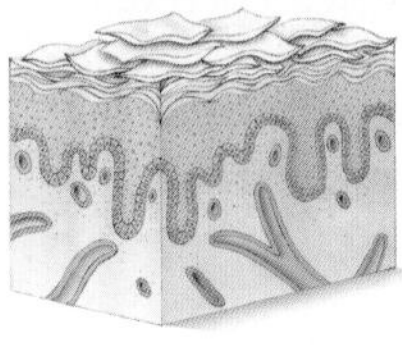

Scaling or peeling of skin comprised of stratum corneum

Ulcer

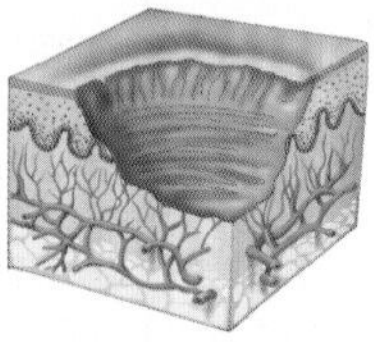

Depression of the skin with loss of the epidermis and upper dermis

Petechiae

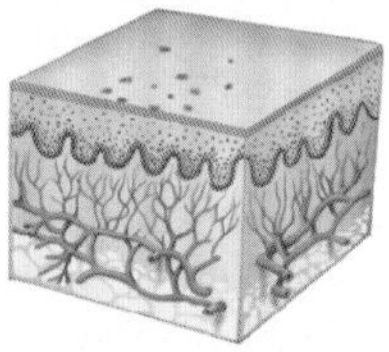

Small red/purple non-blanching spots

Figure 129. Dermatologic

- Absence of pain or pain out of proportion to appearance/clinical presentation of lesions is concerning for serious pathology (necrotizing fasciitis, myonecrosis).
- Athletes with recurrent disease.
  - Evaluate for nasal carriage of *S. aureus* (reservoir for infection).
  - Consider eradication with the following.
    - Intranasal Mupirocin 2% ointment, twice daily for 5 to 10 days.
    - Skin washing of axillae and groin daily with chlorhexidine gluconate 2% to 4% solution + dilute bleach baths (¼ cup per ¼ tub or 13 gallons of water).
    - Decolonization with oral antibiotics not routinely recommended.
- **Impetigo:**
  - *Appearance/clinical presentation.*
    - Superficial, contagious bacterial infection; red papules to vesicles which burst to form "honey-colored crust."
    - Bullous and nonbullous variants.
  - *Rx.*
    - Local wound care, wash with soap and water.
    - Topical Mupirocin three times daily for localized infection.
    - For more widespread infection, consider penicillinase-resistant antistaphylococcal antibiotics (cephalexin or dicloxacillin).
- **Cellulitis and erysipelas:**
  - *Appearance/clinical presentation.*
    - Cellulitis.
      - Infection of deeper dermis and subcutaneous fat.
      - ***"No clear demarcation"*** between involved and uninvolved tissue.
      - Overlying skin may slough and form ulcers.
      - Athletes may present with fever, chills, malaise, and/or regional lymphadenopathy.
    - Erysipelas.
      - Infection of upper dermis and superficial lymphatics.
      - ***"Clear demarcation"*** between involved and uninvolved tissues.
    - Both present with skin erythema, edema, and warmth.
  - *Rx.*
    - Empiric therapy with β-lactams, macrolides, quinolones, TMP/SMX.
    - Consider intravenous antibiotics on case-by-case basis.
- **Folliculitis, furuncles, and carbuncles:**
  - *Appearance/clinical presentation.*
    - *Folliculitis.*
      - Superficial infection (pustules) of hair follicles; multiple erythematous lesions.
    - *Furuncle.*
      - Deep, inflammatory nodules/abscess at the base of the hair follicle; may be a sequel to folliculitis.
    - *Carbuncle.*
      - Coalescence of communicating furuncles into a large abscess.
      - Athletes typically have malaise and fever.
  - *Rx.*
    - Empiric therapy with β-lactams, macrolides, quinolones, TMP/SMX.

Fungal infections:
- **Key facts:**
  - Infection is typically superficial because dermatophytes cannot penetrate dermis or affect mucous membranes.
  - Dx.
    - Based on history and characteristics of lesions.
    - Skin scrapings with KOH preparation.
  - Treatment.
    - Topical treatment is first line of management.
    - Systemic treatment reserved for refractory, widespread disease.
- **Tinea capitis** (scalp), **tinea corporis** (trunk, arms, and legs), **tinea pedis** (feet).
  - *Pathogens: Dermatophytes: Trichophyton, Microsporum, and Epidermophyton.*
  - *Appearance/clinical presentation.*
    - Typically: Pruritic (itchy), erythematous, scaling patch, or plaque with advancing border; circular or oval ring (ringworm).
    - Tinea capitis.
      - Scaly, red patches of alopecia (loss of hair).

- Tinea corporis.
  - Ring-shaped border with elevated edges.
- Tinea pedis.
  - Erythema, scaling, and maceration in toe-web spaces (fourth space common); can involve the whole foot.
- *Rx.*
  - Topical.
    - Terbinafine 1% or Ketoconazole 2% twice daily for several weeks is generally effective.
  - Systemic.
    - Fluconazole 200 mg PO weekly for 2 to 4 weeks or terbinafine 250 mg PO daily for 1 to 2 weeks.
    - Tinea capitis: Griseofulvin ultramicrosize capsules, 15 mg/kg/day in divided doses for 8 weeks.
    - Consultation with dermatologist for refractory cases despite systemic therapy.
- **Tinea versicolor.**
  - *Pathogen:* Yeast: Malassezia (Tinea versicolor).
  - *Appearance/clinical presentation.*
    - Scaly, fine, coalesced hyper- or hypopigmented macules that form irregular-shaped patches of altered skin pigmentation.
    - Scratching lesions may induce "dust-like scaling."
    - Color: Tan to brown, white to pink.
    - Location: Chest, abdomen, back neck, or proximal upper extremities and neck.
  - *Rx.*
    - Topical.
      - Ketoconazole 2% shampoo and selenium sulfide 2.5% lotion.
      - Applied for 10 minutes and rinsed, daily for at least 10 days.
      - Taper after 10 days to weekly for 1 to 2 months (prevention).
    - Systemic.
      - Anecdotal efficacy—Fluconazole 200 mg, one time dose, with acidic, caffeinated (facilitates absorption) followed by exercise (to enhance drug delivery to skin).

Viral infections:
- **Key facts:**
  - Most athletes are asymptomatic.
  - Contact sports increase risk for acquisition and transmission (asymptomatic shedding).
  - Herpes simplex.
    - Outbreaks—wrestling (*gladiatorum*), rugby (*scrumpox*).
    - Primary or recurrent.
  - Herpes zoster.
    - May present without rash and be confused as either angina, renal, or gallbladder pathology.
- **Herpes simplex:**
  - *Pathogen:* Herpes simplex: *HSV type 1.*
  - *Appearance/clinical presentation.*
    - Painful, multiple, serous fluid-filled vesicles on a red base.
    - May recur at the same site.
    - Prodromal (pre-eruptive) symptoms may include pain, burning, pruritus.
    - Fever and chills are more common in primary infection.
  - *Dx.*
    - Tzanck smear from scrapings of ulcer base.
    - Newer tests: Polymerase chain reaction (PCR) and direct fluorescent antibody (DFA) tests.
  - *Rx.*
    - Acyclovir or valacyclovir may shorten duration of lesions if commenced expeditiously.
    - Medication regimens are based on body site, and primary versus recurrent infection.
    - Consider daily suppressive therapy in athletes with recurrent disease.
    - Counsel on potential risk for nephropathy following use of acyclovir in setting of dehydration.
- **Herpes zoster (shingles):**
  - *Pathogen:* Herpes zoster: Varicella-zoster virus *(VZV).*
  - *Appearance/clinical presentation.*
    - Erythematous papules that evolve into painful, multiple, grouped vesicles.
    - Eruption typically along unilateral, thoracic, or lumbar dermatomal distribution.
    - In young, healthy athlete's lesions crust in 7 to 10 days (noninfective phase).
  - *Dx.*
    - Based on history and characteristics of lesions.

- *Tx.*
  - Either Acyclovir 800 mg, five times daily; Famciclovir 500 mg, three times daily; or Valacyclovir 1000 mg, three times daily.
  - Begin treatment within 72 hours to reduce pain and speed healing of lesions.
  - Corticosteroids do not reduce postherpetic neuralgia and may increase risk of secondary bacterial infection; thus, not recommended.
- **Molluscum contagiosum:**
  - *Pathogen:* Herpes zoster: Varicella-zoster virus *(VZV).*
  - *Appearance/clinical presentation.*
    - Dome-shaped, flesh-colored papules with soft, indented (umbilicated) centers.
  - *Dx.*
    - Based on history and characteristics of lesions.
    - Histologic examination with H&E staining may reveal keratinocytes containing eosinophilic cytoplasmic inclusion bodies (molluscum bodies).
  - *Tx.*
    - Spontaneous resolution in months to years.
    - As needed, effective treatments include liquid nitrogen cryotherapy, curettage, or the application of topical cantharidin 0.7% liquid.
    - Counsel on the avoidance of "scratching" that may extrude contagious, waxy material which can induce new lesions via autoinoculation.
- **Verruca vulgaris (wart):**
  - *Pathogen:* Human papillomavirus *(HPV)* which infects epithelial cells.
  - *Appearance/clinical presentation.*
    - Flesh-colored papules with rough, keratinized surface; papules may coalesce into plaques.
  - *Dx.*
    - Based on history and characteristics of lesions.
    - Removal of the hyperkeratotic top layer may reveal thrombosed capillaries ("seeds").
  - *Tx.*
    - Spontaneous regression can occur in up to two-thirds over 2 years.
    - Other treatments include liquid nitrogen cryotherapy, daily application of salicylic acid 40% plaster.
    - Refer refractory cases to dermatology for consideration of other treatments (immunotherapy, laser, or topical/intralesional chemotherapy).

Bacterial infections

Impetigo (staph)

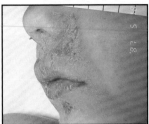

Impetigo (strep)

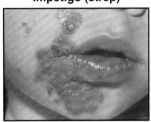

Superficial, contagious bacterial infection; red papules to vesicles which burst to form "honey colored crust"

Folliculitis

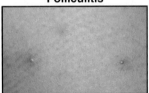

Superficial infection of hair follicles; multiple erythematous lesions

Cellulitis

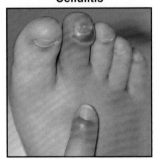

Erythema; infection of deep dermis and subcutaneous fat; **"no clear demarcation"** **between involved and uninvolved tissue**

Erysipelas

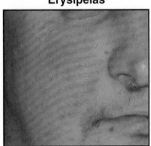

Erythema; infection of upper dermis and superficial lymphatics with **"clear demarcation"** between involved and uninvolved tissue

Fungal infections

Tinea corporis

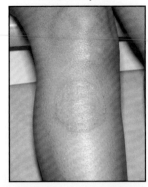

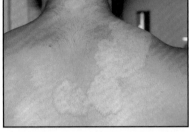

Tinea **capitis** (scalp), **corporis** (trunks, arms, legs), **pedis** (feet) - pruritic, red, scaly patch; well demarcated, advancing borders and central clearing

Tinea versicolor

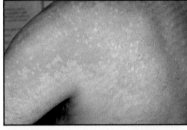

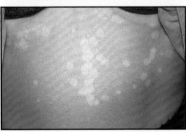

Non-contagious; change in epidermal pigmentation; light to dark macules or patches

Viral infections

Herpes simplex virus (HSV)

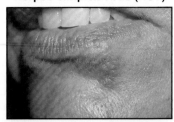

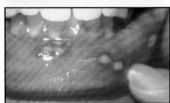

Painful, multiple serous fluid filled vesicles on a red base

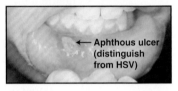

← **Aphthous ulcer** **(distinguish** **from HSV)**

Herpes zoster (shingles)

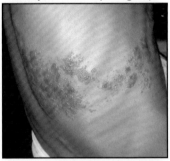

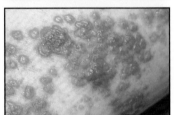

Painful, multiple serous filled vesicles on a red base; eruption along dermatome distribution

Molluscum contagiosum

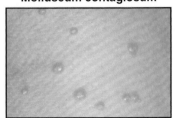

Dome shaped, flesh colored papules with soft, indented centers

Figure 130. Dermatologic

Miscellaneous dermatoses:

- **Scabies:**
  - *Pathogen: Sarcoptes scabiei* (parasitic).
  - *Appearance/clinical presentation.*
    - Exceptionally pruritic, erythematous papules, capped by hemorrhagic crusts and linear burrows.
    - Variants include "noncrusted" and "crusted."
  - *Dx.*
    - Based on history, characteristics, and location of lesions (groin, axillae, wrist, elbows, between fingers and toes).
    - Confirm with microscopic examination of skin scrapings that shows mites, eggs, or fecal pellets (scybala).
  - *Tx.*
    - Ivermectin 200 μg/kg orally.
      - "Noncrusted": One time dose, repeat in 2 weeks.
      - "Crusted": On days 1, 2, 8, 9, 15 (and days 22 and 29 if severe); use with topical scabicide.
    - Topical Permethrin cream 5%.
      - Apply ~30 g to entire body, followed by shower or bath 8 to 14 hours later.
      - "Noncrusted": One time dose, repeat in 2 weeks.
      - "Crusted": Daily for 7 days followed by 2/week until cured; use with oral Ivermectin.
    - Treat entire household and close personal contacts to prevent recurrence.
    - Contaminated clothes and linens should be washed in hot water.
- **Acne vulgaris:**
  - *Pathogen: Propionibacterium acnes.*
  - *Appearance/clinical presentation.*
    - "Noninflammatory": Open (blackheads) or closed (whitehead) comedones.
    - "Inflammatory": Erythematous papules, pustules, nodules, or cysts (with possible scarring).
    - Typically on face, upper trunk, neck, and arms.
  - *Dx.*
    - Based on history, characteristics, and location of lesions.
  - *Tx.*
    - "Noninflammatory": Topical retinoids or adapalene/benzoyl peroxide.
    - "Inflammatory":
      - Combination therapy with either erythromycin/benzoyl peroxide, clindamycin/benzoyl peroxide, or adapalene/benzoyl peroxide.
      - Azelaic acid.
      - Moderate to severe acne: Combination oral antibiotics for <6 months (tetracyclines, erythromycin, TMP-SMX, clindamycin, azithromycin) with topical benzoyl peroxide (to decrease risk of antibiotic resistance).
      - Severe, refractory acne: Oral isotretinoin, under dermatologist supervision.
- **Pityriasis rosea:**
  - *Appearance/clinical presentation.*
    - Salmon-colored, slightly pruritic, oval, maculopapular lesions and plaques along lines of skin cleavage, in a "Christmas tree distribution" on both sides of the body.
    - First, single lesion, the "Herald Patch" is round or oval, salmon colored on neck, trunk, or extremities; precedes other lesions by 4 days–2 weeks.
  - *Dx.*
    - Based on history, characteristics, and location of lesions.
  - *Tx.*
    - Self-limited with resolution in 3 to 4 weeks.
    - Refractory cases: Oral antihistamines + topical steroids for symptomatic relief of pruritus +/– oral corticosteroids (for severe cases).

Other Considerations:

- Prevention better than cure (as detailed in National Athletic Trainers' Association [NATA] Position Statement on Skin Diseases).
  - Adequate organizational support from Athletic Departments (fiscal and human resources, strict adherence to infection control policies, hygiene supplies, contract with team dermatologist).
  - Cleanliness of athletic training room, locker rooms, and athletic facilities (stadium, fields, courts, mats, pools).
  - Educate, encourage, and monitor good hygiene practices by all athletes, healthcare providers, and custodial staff include the following.
    - Regular hand washing and showering (after every practice).
    - Avoid sharing towels, hair care products (clippers, razors), water bottles.
    - Disinfection (daily laundry and equipment cleansing).
  - Educate and encourage athletes to
    - refrain from unnecessary shaving.
    - expeditiously report all skin problems.
  - Educate and encourage healthcare providers to vigilantly monitor all skin problems.

- Educate:
  - On overlapping features between different infections during the initial stages of evolution of lesions.
  - Avoid using topical or oral glucocorticoids during initial stages of skin infections (unless diagnosis of fungal infections necessitating glucocorticoid use is established).
- Be aware of NATA and National Collegiate Athletic Association (NCAA) Guidelines. Monitor websites for changes annually.
  - NATA: www.nata.org
  - NCAA: www.ncaa.org

Return to Play: (Based on guidelines adopted by the NCAA; Adopted in part from: Zinder SM, Basler RSW, Foley J, et al. National Athletic Trainers' Association Position Statement: Skin Diseases. *J Athl Train.* 2010;45(4):411–428.)

- **Bacterial infections:**
  - Appropriate antibiotic therapy for 72 hours.
  - No new skin lesions for 48 hours before competition.
  - No moist, exudative, or purulent lesions.
  - Should not cover active, purulent lesions to allow for participation.
- **Fungal infections:**
  - *Tinea corporis*—72 hours of topical therapy; lesions must be covered with a gas-permeable dressing, followed by underwrap and stretch tape.
  - *Tinea capitis*—2 weeks of oral antifungal therapy.
  - Wrestlers may be disqualified with extensive and active lesions with infection determined by KOH preparation or a review of therapeutic regimen.
- **Viral infections (herpes simplex):**
  - Primary infection.
    - Free of systemic symptoms.
    - No new vesicles in the last 72 hours.
    - No moist lesions; all lesions covered by a firm, dry, adherent crust.
    - On appropriate oral, antiviral medication for at least 120 hours before participation.
    - Not cover lesions to allow participation.
  - Recurrent infection.
    - Need to meet the last three requirements (under primary infection) before returning to event participation.
- **Molluscum contagiosum:**
  - All lesions on wrestlers must be curetted or removed before competition.
  - Single or localized, clustered lesions must be covered with a gas-permeable dressing, followed by underwrap and stretch tape.
- **Scabies:**
  - Document negative scabies test (microscopic examination of skin scrapings) at meet or tournament.
- **Warts:**
  - Warts on the face need to be treated or covered by a mask.
  - All other warts should be adequately covered.
- **Head lice:**
  - Wrestlers should be treated with an appropriate pediculicide and re-examined for healing before competition.

Recommended Readings

Albrecht MA. Clinical manifestations of varicella-zoster virus infection: Herpes zoster. *UpToDate.* Accessed March 3rd, 2013.
Albrecht MA. Treatment of herpes zoster in the immunocompetent host. *UpToDate.* Accessed March 3rd, 2013.
Dworkin MS, Shoemaker PC, Spitters C, et al. Endemic spread of herpes simplex virus type I among adolescent wrestlers and their coaches. *Pediatr Infect Dis J.* 1999;18:1108–1109.
Epocrates®, online.epocrates.com, Accessed March 2nd, 2013.
Goldstein BG, Goldstein AO. Approach to dermatologic diagnosis. *UpToDate.* Accessed March 3rd, 2013.
Graber E. Treatment of acne vulgaris. *UpToDate.* Accessed March 3rd, 2013.
He L, Zhang D, Zhou M, et al. Corticosteroids for preventing postherpetic neuralgia. *Cochrane Database Syst Rev.* 2008:CD005582.
Liu C, Bayer A, Cosgrove SE, et al. Clinical practice guidelines by the infectious diseases society of America for the treatment of methicillin-resistant Staphylococcus aureus infection in adults and children. *Clin Infect Dis.* 2011;52(3):e18–e55.
National Athletic Trainers' Association. www.nata.org, Accessed March 2nd, 2013.
2011–2012 NCAA Sports Medicine Handbook. Retrieved March 3rd, 2013, from http://www.ncaapublications.com/productdownloads/MD11.pdf.
Seidler EM, Kimball AB. Meta-analysis comparing efficacy of benzoyl peroxide, clindamycin, benzoyl peroxide with salicylic acid, and combination benzoyl peroxide/clindamycin in acne. *J Am Acad Dermatol.* 2010;63:52–62.
Zinder SM, Basler RSW, Foley J, et al. National Athletic Trainers' Association Position Statement: Skin Diseases. *J Athl Train.* 2010;45(4):411–428.

Miscellaneous

Scabies

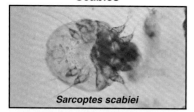

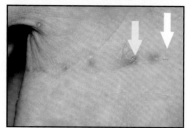

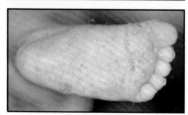

Erythematous papules capped by
hemorrhagic crusts **(yellow arrow)**;
and linear burrows **(white arrow)**

Acne vulgaris

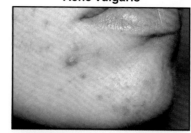

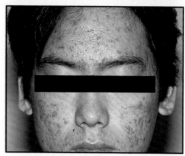

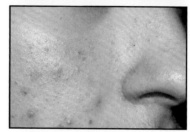

Inflamed papules, pustules, nodules,
with possible scarring

Verrucae Vulgaris (common wart)

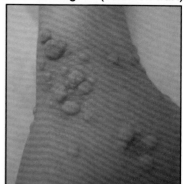

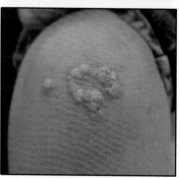

Flesh colored papules with
rough, keratinized surface

Pityriasis rosea

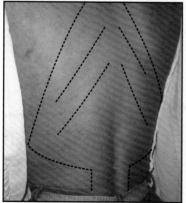

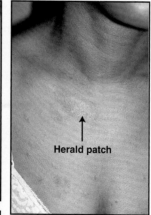

"Herald patch" precedes lesions
by 4 days – 2 weeks; single round
or oval, salmon colored lesion on
neck, trunk, or extremities

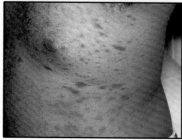

Salmon colored, papules and plaques along lines
of skin cleavage in a **"Christmas tree distribution"**
on both sides of the body

Figure 131. Dermatologic

Section 8: Neurologic

Headache

Introduction (Definitions/Classification):

- Headaches (HAs) are among the most common complaints in athletes.
- Classification:
  - *Primary* (benign, recurring, non-organic etiology) versus *secondary* (induced by underlying, organic disease process).
    - *Primary:* Migraines (with or without aura; exertional), tension, and cluster HAs.
    - *Secondary:* Posttraumatic (concussion), sinusitis, medication overuse, substance withdrawal, cranial (infection; vascular vs. nonvascular [mass]), cervical, psychiatric.
  - *Acute* versus *chronic*.
  - *Recurring* versus *nonrecurring*.
- HAs in athletes may be induced by or a sequel to
  - migraines.
  - tension HA.
  - cluster HA.
  - concussion (during acute or postconcussive phase).
  - sinusitis.
  - medication (analgesic) overuse.
  - cervical spine pathology.
  - CNS infection (e.g., meningitis; less common).

History and Physical Examination:

- History:
  - Head or neck injury, increased stress levels, recent infection and/or elevated temperature, medication overuse/withdrawal, family history of HA, change in athletes' training protocol, or cancers/tumors of the brain.
  - Inquire about
    - recent trauma (to rule out concussion).
    - age of onset.
    - onset: Abrupt versus gradual; time of day.
    - severity and duration.
    - quality (throbbing, stabbing, dull, etc.).
    - location and radiation.
    - associated symptoms.
    - number of headaches in the last month.
    - aggravating and alleviating factors.
    - past personal and family medical history.
    - recent social history changes (sleep, weight, diet, training program).
  - Red flags (that may indicate potential "*secondary headaches*").
    - New/atypical headaches in individuals <5 and >50 years of age.
    - Rapid onset of HA that reaches maximal intensity within seconds/minutes (*rule out possible subarachnoid hemorrhage*).
    - HA with concurrent fever, stiff neck, rash (*rule out meningitis*).
    - Focal neurologic symptoms or signs, including yet not limited to, seizures, confusion, or impaired consciousness (*other than typical aura of migraines*).
    - Rapid onset during intense exercise; especially posttraumatic (*rule out carotid artery dissection*).
    - HA in athletes with greater than or equal to two first-degree relatives with "*berry aneurysms.*"
    - HA in athletes with connective tissue diseases; for example, bicuspid aortic valve.
  - Physical examination (*majority of patients with HA will have a normal examination*):
    - *General:* Wearing sunglasses (*migraine*), ill appearing with fever (*intracranial infection, subarachnoid hemorrhage*).
    - *Cardiopulmonary:* Tachycardia induced by pain, murmur of mitral prolapse (*in connective tissue disorders, predisposition to subarachnoid hemorrhage*).

- *HEENT:*
  - Signs of head or cervical trauma (*blood behind the tympanic membrane or Battle sign*).
  - Injected conjunctiva, rhinorrhea, lacrimation (*suggests cluster HA if unilateral*).
  - Lymphadenopathy, bruits, dentition (*tooth abscess*).
  - Scalp tenderness (*tension headache*).
  - Funduscopic examination (*papilledema from elevated intracranial pressure*).
- *Musculoskeletal:* Tenderness/spasm of the cervical muscles (*tension HA*), nuchal rigidity (*meningitis*).
- *Neurologic:*
  - Worsening neurologic symptoms (*consider subarachnoid hemorrhage*).
  - Positive Brudzinski sign (*flexing of knees with flexion of neck*) or Kernig sign (*resistance to and painful knee extension following flexion of hips and knees*) may indicate meningitis.
- *Skin/vascular:*
  - Elevated pulse (*pain*) and BP (*hypertension as underlying etiology*).
  - Petechial rash (*meningitis*).

Diagnosis:

- Signs/symptoms on physical examination.
- "Quick check/facts" list to aid diagnosis.
  - *Migraines (with or without aura).*
    - Triggered by dietary (alcohol, caffeine, chocolate, MSG), environmental (weather changes, changes in lights, high altitude, noise), medications (OCs, cimetidine), and miscellaneous (sleep alterations, skipped meals, stress, anxiety, physical activity).
    - Auras.
      - For an hour before HA in ~30%.
      - Visual: Zig zag, scotoma.
      - Nonvisual: Sensory (paresthesias), aphasia, or dysarthria.
    - Headache: Typically unilateral, pulsatile, and severe (may progress to involve entire head).
    - Duration varies from 4 to 72 hours; ~50% last at least a day.
    - Other symptoms: Photophobia, phonophobia, nausea, blurred vision, vomiting, weakness (hemiparesis), nystagmus, vertigo, ataxia, altered hearing, diplopia, visual loss, and/or tinnitus.
    - A 3-item **ID Migraine Screener** is a validated, efficient, reliable, self or clinician-administered questionnaire.
    - Migraine variants.
      - *Hemiplegic:* Hemiparesis and nystagmus.
      - *Basilar:* Visual and nonvisual auras, diplopia, tinnitus, vertigo, altered hearing, ataxia; *no weakness.*
      - *Retinal:* Recurrent scotoma and visual loss precede headache.
  - *Tension HA.*
    - Bilateral, nonpulsatile, encircles head in a "band-like" distribution with scalp tenderness.
    - Duration: 30 minutes to 7 days.
    - No nausea, vomiting, photophobia, phonophobia, and typically not worse with exertion.
  - *Cluster HA.*
    - Deep, explosive, and excruciating unilateral presentation.
    - Males greater than females.
    - Duration: 15 minutes to 3 hours, 1 every other day up to 8 per day.
    - Associated with tearing, red eyes, nasal congestion, rhinorrhea, facial/forehead sweating, miosis, ptosis, and/or eyelid edema.
  - *Concussion (postconcussive phase).*
    - More than 80% tension HAs; less common causes include migraines, TMJ, dural shearing.
    - Symptoms: Tinnitus, dizziness, vertigo, psychological and cognitive changes.
  - *Sinusitis.*
    - Most predictive symptoms in acute viral and bacterial sinusitis include purulent rhinorrhea either *with* sinus or ear pressure/pain *and* nasal congestion.
    - Other clinical features may include **Fs—f**acial pain (unilateral tooth and maxillary tenderness; especially while leaning forward), **f**ever, **f**atigue and/or **Hs—h**eadache (worse under water), **h**alitosis, **h**yposomnia (dulled sense of smell).
    - Duration: Indefinite.
    - Multiple facial locations.

- *Medication (analgesic) overuse.*
  - Gradual onset of daily or near-daily HA with superimposed migraine attacks.
  - Associated with ergotamine, opiates, triptans, and simple/mixed analgesics.
- *Cervical spine pathology.*
  - History of neck trauma with or without radicular symptoms.
  - Consider congenital narrowing of spinal canal as potential etiology.
  - Consider Arnold–Chiari malformation in athletes with "*first*" and "*worst*" headache of life, especially after exertion.
- *CNS infection.*
  - Severe headache, flu-like symptoms, and fever.
  - Nuchal rigidity.
- Neuroimaging (CT/MRI)/other tests.
  - Postconcussion (as detailed in concussion chapter).
  - Kernig and Brudzinski sign positive, stiff neck (negative CT results require lumbar puncture with CSF analysis and pressure check).
  - CT for HA rapidly increasing in intensity/onset ("worse HA ever") or HA increasing with exertion.
  - Abnormal, focal neurologic findings.
  - New onset HAs that continue for >2 months in >40 years of age or history of cancer or HIV.
  - Physical examination findings suggest increased intracranial pressure (MRI more sensitive for tumors and recent strokes).

Treatment:

- Determine and treat underlying etiology of headaches:
  - *Migraines (with or without aura).*
    - Nonpharmacologic.
      - Migraine diary: List timing and triggers of migraines.
      - Educate: Benefits of regular exercise, sleep, and meals; limit alcohol, caffeine, chocolate, MSG, glare or flickering lights, noise, altitude.
      - Behavioral: Relaxation, CBT, biofeedback.
    - Pharmacologic.
      - Abortive (more effective when administered early in an attack).
        - Nonspecific: NSAIDs ± acetaminophen ± caffeine.
        - Prescription: Triptans, ergotamines (used less frequently, unfavorable side effects).
      - Preventive.
        - For athletes with more than four headaches per month.
        - Recommend calcium channel blockers (verapamil at low dose) in athletes.
        - Educate: May take a month for notable efficacy.
  - *Tension HA.*
    - Analgesics.
      - Mild to moderate: NSAIDs first; acetaminophen for athletes who cannot tolerate NSAIDs.
      - Severe: IM ketorolac 60 mg.
    - Combination: analgesics + caffeine.
      - For athletes who fail monotherapy with analgesics.
  - *Cluster HA.*
    - Abortive.
      - 12 L/minute for 15 minutes of oxygen.
      - Triptan: Subcutaneous or intranasal.
      - Miscellaneous: Octreotide, ergotamines.
    - Preventive.
      - 2 months: Prednisone 60 mg/day for 5 days and taper.
      - Chronic: Verapamil 240 mg/day in three divided doses.
  - *Concussion* (*as detailed in concussion chapter*).
  - *Sinusitis* (*as detailed in concussion chapter*).
  - *Medication (analgesic) overuse.*
    - Discontinue medications and counsel on alternative therapies.
  - *Cervical spine pathology.*
    - Treat underlying pathology.
  - *CNS infection.*
    - Treatment with appropriate antibiotics/antivirals based on CSF analysis.

Other Considerations:

- Evaluate "*red flags*" for *potential secondary headaches* first and refer for neurology consultation as needed.
- Recommend treatment with less-expensive drugs first, and subsequently, with more expensive drugs as needed (*step care across attacks strategy*).
- Avoid the following.
  - Triptans, ergotamine derivatives, or beta-blockers in athletes with hemiplegic migraines.
  - Triptans and ergotamine derivatives in athletes with hypertension.
- Consider prophylactic treatment for those with retinal migraines.
- "Medication-overuse headache."
  - Reduce by limiting use of analgesics in the treatment of acute migraines.
  - May be induced by triptans.
- Educate:
  - Triptans do not shorten aura or prevent an evolving headache.
  - Lack of response to one triptan does not preclude response to other triptans.
  - There are no solid data to support the preferential use of "a triptan" compared to "other triptans."

Return to Play Criteria:

- No alarm signs for secondary headaches.
- Primary headaches controlled with adequate medication regimens.
- Able to tolerate aerobic and anaerobic activities without exacerbation of symptoms.

Recommended Readings

Bajwa ZH, Sabahat A. Acute treatment of migraine in adults. *UpToDate*. Accessed March 22, 2013.

Bajwa ZH, Sabahat A. Preventive treatment of migraine in adults. *UpToDate*. Accessed March 22, 2013.

Bajwa ZH, Woottom J. Evaluation of headaches in adults. *UpToDate*. Accessed March 20, 2013.

Headache Classification Committee of the International Headache Society. The International Classification of Headache Disorders: 2nd edition. *Cephalalgia*. 2004;24(1):9–160.

Lipton RB, Dodick D, Sadovsky R, et al. A self-administered screener for migraine in primary care: The ID Migraine™ validation study. *Neurology*. 2003;61:375–382.

Lipton RB, Stewart WF, Diamond S, Diamond ML, Reed M. Prevalence and burden of migraine in the United States: Data from the American Migrine Study II. *Headache*. 2001;41:646–657.

Maizels M. The clinician's approach to the management of headache. *West J Med*. 1998;168:203–212.

May A. Cluster headache: Acute and preventive treatment. *UpToDate*. Accessed March 22, 2013.

Silberstein SD, Goadsby PJ, Lipton RB. Management of migraine: An algorithmic approach. *Neurology*. 2000;55(2):S46–S52.

Silberstein SD, for the US Headache Consortium. Practice parameter: Evidence-based guidelines for migraine headache (an evidence-based review). Report of the Quality Standards Committee of the American Academy of Neurology. *Neurology*. 2000;55:754–763.

Taylor F. Tensio-type headache in adults: Acute treatment. *UpToDate*. Accessed March 22, 2013.

Concussion

Introduction (Definitions/Classification):

- Head trauma–induced alteration in mental status (amnesia, confusion, and/or disorientation), with or without loss of consciousness (LOC).
- Rapid onset of transient neurologic function that typically resolves spontaneously.
- Clinical symptoms are induced by a functional disturbance as opposed to structural injury; neuroimaging studies are usually normal.
- Single or recurrent concussions may result in neuropathologic changes.
- 1.6 to 3.8 million/yr in USA.
- Contact sport likelihood = 20%.
- Risk in football is doubled in high school (20%) as compared to college (10%) athletes.
- The majority of concussions are frequently unobserved.
- Potential complications include the following.
  - Second impact syndrome—second concussion during symptoms of first; can be severe and life threatening.
  - Postconcussion syndrome (PCS)—headache, dizziness, vertigo, and/or psychological changes.
  - Chronic traumatic encephalopathy (CTE)—progressive degeneration of brain with increase in abnormal protein Tau due to multiple head injuries.

History and Physical Examination:

- **History:**
  - Acceleration, deceleration, or blunt trauma to the head, neck region, or impact to the body causing violent head snap (whiplash).
  - Inquire about mechanism of injury, previous concussions, past medical history, current medications (especially anticoagulants).
  - Presenting symptoms.
    - Headache (most common related symptom to concussion).
    - Confusion/disorientation.
    - Amnesia: Retrograde (memory loss before trauma) or anterograde amnesia (memory loss after trauma).
    - LOC; observed in less than 10% of concussion; inquire about the severity and duration if present.
    - Dizziness/vertigo.
    - Nausea/vomiting.
    - Diplopia (double vision), photophobia (sensitivity to light).
    - Tinnitus.
    - Numbness.
  - Subacute symptoms (observed days to weeks after concussion).
    - Aggression.
    - Depression.
    - Alteration in sleep cycle.
    - Emotional instability.
    - Irritability.
- **Physical examination:**
  - Assess A, B, C's (airway, breathing, and circulation) and exclude cervical spine injury FIRST.
  - General: Dazed/confused, vacant stare, distractable, disoriented (person, place, time), emotionally labile.
  - HEENT.
    - Ocular movements, visual acuity, pupillary asymmetry; may have diminished visual acuity, slow constriction in response to light, and bruising around eyes, scalp.
    - Nose: Possible epistaxis (nosebleed)
  - Neurologic.
    - Delayed verbal response, slurred speech.
    - Cranial nerve testing: May have some nystagmus (rapid uncontrolled eye movement) and tinnitus (ringing in the ears).
    - Cognitive dysfunction: Orientation, memory, and concentration tested using a standardized assessment tool (SAC, ImPACT, SCAT3).
    - Strength and sensation: Typically within normal limits.
    - Balance: Unable to stand in one spot with eyes closed.
    - Coordination: Rapid movement testing and tandem walking abnormal.
    - Deep tendon reflexes: Within normal limits
  - Findings that require immediate treatment.
    - Seizures.
    - Repeated vomiting.
    - Asymmetrical pupils.
    - Alteration in mental status, increased confusion, slurred speech.
    - Numbness or weakness in extremities.
    - Worsening headache.
    - CSF leak from nose or ears.

Diagnosis:

- Signs/symptoms on physical examination.
- Neuropsychological assessment tools.
  - *General Guidelines.*
    - Consider administering "Baseline" tests for all athletes (especially those in contact sports and participating on teams with a higher incidence of concussions).
  - *Standard Assessment of Concussion (SAC) Test.*
  - ***Valid, standardized, sideline assessment of cognition.***
    - Measures, in sequence, orientation, immediate memory, concentration, delayed recall, neurologic screening, and exertional maneuvers (Table 1).
    - Also includes graded, symptom checklist, a concise neurologic examination, and chronicles posttraumatic (antegrade) and retrograde amnesia (Table 2).

Table 1 Standard Assessment of Concussion SAC

Orientation (1 point each)
Month
Date
Day of week
Year
Time (within 1 hr)
Orientation score: 5

Immediate memory (1 point for each correct, total over 3 trials)			
	Trial 1	Trial 2	Trial 3
Word 1			
Word 2			
Word 3			
Word 4			
Word 5			
Immediate memory score: 15			

Concentration	
Reverse digits (Go to next string length if correct on first trial. Stop if incorrect on both trials. 1 point each for each string length.)	
3-8-2	5-1-8
2-7-9-3	2-1-6-8
5-1-8-6-9	9-4-1-7-5
6-9-7-3-5-1	4-2-8-9-3-7
Months of the year in reverse order (1 point for entire sequence correct.)	
Dec–Nov–Oct–Sep–Aug–Jul	
Jun–May–Apr–Mar–Feb–Jan	
Concentration score: 5	

Delayed recall (approximately 5 minutes after immediate memory. 1 point each)
Word 1
Word 2
Word 3
Word 4
Word 5
Delayed recall score: 5

Summary of total scores:	
Orientation	5
Immediate memory	15
Concentration	5
Delayed recall	5
Total score	30

The following may be performed between the immediate memory and delayed recall portions of this assessment when appropriate:

Neurologic screening
  Recollection of the injury
  Strength
  Coordination

Exertional maneuvers
  1 40-yard sprint
  5 sit-ups
  5 push-ups
  5 knee bends

Table 2 SAC Unscored Portion

Graded symptom checklist				
Symptom	None	Mild	Moderate	Severe
Headache	0	1	2	3
Nausea	0	1	2	3
Vomiting	0	1	2	3
Dizziness	0	1	2	3
Poor balance	0	1	2	3
Blurred/double vision	0	1	2	3
Sensitivity to light	0	1	2	3
Sensitivity to noise	0	1	2	3
Ringing in the ears	0	1	2	3
Poor concentration	0	1	2	3
Memory problems	0	1	2	3
Not feeling "sharp"	0	1	2	3
Fatigue/sluggish	0	1	2	3
Sadness/depression	0	1	2	3
Irritability	0	1	2	3
Amnesia				
Posttraumatic amnesia		Yes	No	Length
Retrograde amnesia		Yes	No	Length
Strength				
Right arm	Normal		Abnormal	
Right leg	Normal		Abnormal	
Left arm	Normal		Abnormal	
Left leg	Normal		Abnormal	
Sensation	Normal		Abnormal	
Coordination of limbs/gait	Normal		Abnormal	

The unscored portion of the Standardized Assessment of Concussion (SAC) includes a graded symptom checklist, a brief neurologic examination, and records the presence of posttraumatic and retrograde amnesia.

From: McCrea M. *J Head Trauma Rehabil.* 1998;13:27.

- Not a substitute for clinical OR neuropsychological evaluation.
- Forms A, B, and C (no change in data by using either form).
- Max score = 30 (only in 7%).
- 85% score >25 at baseline.
- No change—high school versus college OR practice versus games.
- >concussion—Score drops ~3 to 4 points
- *Immediate Postconcussion Assessment and Cognitive Testing (ImPACT).*
  - A "tool" for assessment of neurocognitive functioning.
  - Computerized test performed at baseline (for contact sport athletes) and serially after concussion.
  - Aids in making informed decisions for return to play.
- *Other (not as well validated as SAC test).*
  - Sport Concussion Assessment Tool 3 (SCAT3).
    - Endorsed by "Consensus Statement on Concussion in Sport, 2012."
    - Reviews and evaluates subjective symptoms, SAC cognitive assessment, Glasgow Coma Scale (GCS), coordination, and balance.
    - Scores 0 to 100, yet normative data and "threshold" score have not been described.
  - Modified version available for children between 5–12 years of age (Child -SCAT 3).
- Head CT.
  - Abnormality rates: 5% with GCS = 15; ≥30% with GCS = 13.
  - Evaluate need on a case-by-case basis.

- Highly recommended for worsening symptoms, LOC, seizure, amnesia >30 minutes, ≥2 episodes of vomiting, open/depressed skull fracture, bruising around both eyes or bruise behind ear (Battle sign), bleeding behind ear drum, GCS < 13, coagulapathy or use of anticoagulant medications, CSF leakage from nose or ears.
- Brain MRI.
  - Conventional brain MRI.
    - In individuals with PCS who have disabling symptoms to exclude axonal injury, contusion, petechial hemorrhage, or small extraaxial hematomas.
  - Diffusion tensor MRI (DTI).
    - Has shown abnormalities in white matter following mild traumatic brain injury (mTBI).
    - Limited data thus far, yet is more sensitive than conventional MRI in assessing slight, but clinically meaningful alterations following mTBI, and may be a valuable tool as a biomarker of recovery.
    - Thus, DTI could be helpful in diagnosis and management of concussion and to potentially prevent complications such as PCS and CTE.

Treatment:

- First—place athlete on "medical hold" from all activity.
- Provide adequate, written notification.
  - To school—stating diagnosis of concussion and mandated "medical hold" until further clearance.
  - To athlete and/or parent, guardian—information sheet detailing basic information regarding symptoms and signs of concussion, "alarm signs,, and transition back to school.
- Counsel athletes:
  - On pathophysiology of concussion and the potential for significant brain damage with a single and multiple concussions.
  - On the importance of good sleep hygiene, diet, and adequate fluid replacement, and avoidance of all alcoholic beverages.
  - On avoidance of use of any opioid analgesics. Pain management with Aleve 440 mg bid and Tylenol 1 g bid.
- Request academic accommodations as needed.
- Provide phone contact information of healthcare providers.
- Perform brain imaging as needed (as described above).
- Monitor closely with sequential, clinical assessments—CRITICAL!
- Perform neurocognitive tests in ~48 hours to assess change from baseline.
  - Helps medical providers/athletes/parents/coaches get a "sense" of how long athlete may be on "medical hold."
- Following resolution of symptoms.
  - Administer neurocognitive test and compare to "Baseline" scores.
  - If no "Baseline" test is available, consider evaluating "Postinjury" scores to normative data.
- When symptom free and following normalization of neurocognitive test scores, initiate "return to play protocol" (Table 3; as per "Consensus Statement on Concussion in Sport 3rd International Conference on Concussion in Sport Held in Zurich, November 2008").

Table 3 Return to Play Protocol

Rehabilitation Stage	Functional Exercise at Each Stage of Rehabilitation	Objective of Each Stage
1. No activity	Complete physical and cognitive rest	Recovery
2. Light aerobic exercise	Walking, swimming, or stationary cycling keeping intensity <70% MPHR; no resistance training	Increase HR
3. Sport-specific exercise	Skating drills in ice hockey, running drills in soccer; no head impact activities	Add movement
4. Noncontact training drills	Progression to more complex training drills; e.g., passing drills in football and ice hockey; may start progressive resistance training	Exercise, coordination, and cognitive load
5. Full contact practice	Following medical clearance, participate in normal training activities	Restore confidence and assess functional skills by coaching staff
6. Return to play	Normal game play	

Six-day return to play protocol. Each day the athlete makes a stepwise increase in functional activity, is evaluated for symptoms, and is allowed to progress to the next stage each successive day if asymptomatic.

Other Considerations:

- Be proactive—establish institutional "Concussion Management Protocol."
- Educate health professionals (physicians, athletic trainers, allied health professionals), athletes, parents, and coaches.
  - Need to develop a "*uniform protocol*" for diagnosis, testing, and "*safe return to play*."
  - Planning and memory have been shown to be significantly reduced following concussions.
  - Symptoms can persist beyond a week in 15% after one concussion and 30% after three or more concussions.
  - Lack of somatic symptoms (headache, nausea, vomiting) may be contrasting with objective measures of neurocognitive testing; therefore, perception of healing may provide athlete with a false sense of security.
  - Neuropsychological assessment tools (SAC, ImPACT, SCAT3) should not be used alone to make decisions regarding the "return to play" status.
- Consider the following.
  - Referral for vestibular evaluation for persistent mild or profound vertigo, ataxia, hearing difficulty, and/or nystagmus.
  - C-spine imaging (CT or MRI).
    - Neck pain and decreased range of motion.
    - Radicular symptoms in arms.
- Future trends—research and validate.
  - Use of DTI MRI to help aid diagnosis and manage concussions more thoroughly, in order to prevent PCS and CTE.
  - Use of "Baseline" and "Postinjury" neurocognitive tests for all athletes playing contact sports.
  - Use of "Postinjury" neurocognitive tests for all athletes with concussions, including those without "Baseline" tests (compare to normative data).
- Monitor websites of the NATA and National Collegiate Athletic Association (NCAA) Guidelines periodically for changes in recommendations.
  - NATA: www.nata.org
  - NCAA: www.ncaa.org

Return to Play:

- Entirely symptom free AND normal neurocognitive testing, following strict adherence and compliance with established "Concussion Management Protocol."
- Normal neurologic examination by trained health professionals following successful completion of "return to play protocol."
- As needed, normal head imaging (CT, MRI) and medical clearance by Neurologist/Neuropsychologist.

Recommended Readings

Borg J, Holm L, Cassidy JD, et al. Diagnostic procedures in mild traumatic brain injury: Results of the WHO Collaborating Centre Task Force on Mild Traumatic Brain Injury. *J Rehabil Med.* 2004;(43 suppl):61–75.

Evans RW. Concussion and mild traumatic brain injury. *UpToDate.* Accessed March 3rd, 2013.

Guskiewicz KM, McCrea M, Marshall SW, et al. Cumulative effects of recurrent concussion in collegiate football players: The NCAA Concussion Study. *JAMA.* 2003;290(19):2549–2555.

Guskiewicz KM, Weaver NL, Padua DA, et al. Epidemiology of concussion collegiate and high school football players. *Am J Sports Med.* 2000;28(5):643–650.

Marar M, McIlvain NM, Fields SK, et al. Epidemiology of concussions among United States high school athletes in 20 sports. *Am J Sports Med.* 2012;40:747.

Matser EJ, Kessels AG, Lezak MD, et al. Neuropsychological impairment in amateur soccer players. *JAMA.* 1999;282(10):971–973.

Mayer AR, Ling J, Mannell MV, et al. A prospective diffusion tensor imaging study in mild traumatic brain injury. *Neurology.* 2010;74:643.

McCrea M, Kelly JP, Randolph C. The standardized assessment of concussion (SAC): Manual for administration, scoring, and interpretation. *Clinical Instrument and Manual published and distributed by Brain Injury Association (BIA)*, Washington DC, 1997.[s7]

McCrory P, Meeuwisse W, Aubry M, et al. Consensus statement on Concussion in Sport: the 4th International Conference on Concussion in Sport held in Zurich, November 2012. *Br J Sports Med.* 2013;47(5): 250–258.

McCrory P, Meeuwisse W, Johnston K, et al. Consensus statement on Concussion in Sport 3rd International Conference on Concussion in Sport held in Zurich, November 2008. *Clin J Sport Med.* 2009;19:185.

Mittl RL, Grossman RI, Hiehle JF, et al. Prevalence of MR evidence of diffuse axonal injury in patients with mild head injury and normal head CT findings. *AJNR Am J Neuroradiol.* 1994;15:1583.

2011–2012 NCAA Sports Medicine Handbook. Retrieved March 3rd, 2013, from http://www.ncaapublications.com/productdownloads/MD11.pdf.

Practice parameter: The management of concussion in sports (summary statement). Report of the Quality Standards Subcommittee. *Neurology.* 1997;48:581.

Stiell IG, Clement CM, Rowe BH, et al. Comparison of the Canadian CT Head Rule and the New Orleans Criteria in patients with minor head injury. *JAMA.* 2005;294(12):1511–1518.

Wilde EA, McCauley SR, Hunter JV, et al. Diffusion tensor imaging of acute mild traumatic brain injury in adolescents. *Neurology.* 2008;70:948.

www.impacttest.com. Accessed March 4th, 2013.

Temporomandibular Joint Dysfunction Syndrome

Introduction (Definitions/Classification):

- Extracapsular dysfunction of the joint connecting the mandible to the temporal bone of the skull. Common causes include the following.
  - Musculoskeletal imbalance and jaw malalignment.
  - Dental malocclusion.
  - Jaw clenching and muscle fatigue.
  - Bruxism.
  - Anxiety and stress.

History and Physical Examination:

- Typically described as a dull ache of the muscles of mastication.
- Other symptoms may include the following.
  - Unilateral chronic pain.
  - Ipsilateral otalgia.
  - Headache (may be the only symptom).
  - Limited ability to open mouth.
  - Clicking, popping, grinding with opening/closing mouth.
- Physical examination:
  - Inspection.
    - Facial asymmetry.
    - Jaw deviation upon opening and closing jaw.
    - Evaluate for dental derangements (wear and tear on teeth surfaces or malalignment).
  - Palpation (for tenderness and spasm).
    - Overlying temporomandibular joint dysfunction (TMJ) (mild to severe).
    - Masseter muscle—at angle of the mandible.
    - Temporalis muscle—overlying temples, both with jaw relaxed and clenched.
    - Pterygoid muscle—posterior mouth.

Diagnosis:

- Signs/symptoms on physical examination.
- Imaging.
  - Usually not helpful.
  - In selected cases, to rule out inflammation and/or infection.
  - MRI to evaluate clinical suspicion of nonreducing, displaced disc, in athletes with restricted TMJ movement.

Treatment:

- Educate regarding etiologic factors and pathophysiology.
- Rule out, modify, and treat aggravating factors and triggers (anxiety, stress, inflammation, infection, muscle spasm, dental malocclusion).
- Acrylic bite guard while sleeping.
- Regular dental care as applicable.
- Jaw opening exercises *in conjunction with* NSAIDs.
- Consider acupuncture as an adjunct treatment. Shown to be helpful in reducing pain and improving TMJ mobility.
- Pain control: TCAs (amitriptyline) and/or muscle relaxants (cyclobenzaprine).
- For refractory cases, consider the following.
  - Joint injection with corticosteroid and local anesthetic followed by ice application for 20 minutes.
  - Botulism toxin injections directly into muscles of mastication.
- Low-level laser therapy
  - Has been shown to reduce pain and enhance TMJ mobility in limited trial.
  - Need further clinical studies.
- Surgical options include the following.
  - Arthroscopic scar tissue reduction and lavage.
  - Partial or total meniscectomy.
  - Disc repair or repositioning.
  - Total joint replacement.

Other Considerations:

- Emergent reduction under anesthesia for those with jaw locked in open or closed position.
- Consider multidisciplinary care for refractory cases including consultations with dentistry, otolaryngology, neuropsychology, neurology, and/or pain management specialist.

Return to Play:

- Consider use of mouth guard during practice and competition (even for noncontact sports).
- No debilitating pain or side effects from prescription medicines (tricyclics and/or muscle relaxants).
- Ensure that athletes are alert and oriented with normal reaction time before returning to practice and/or competition.

Recommended Readings

Alkhader M, Ohbayashi N, Tetsumura A, et al. Diagnostic performance of magnetic resonance imaging for detecting osseous abnormalities of the temporomandibular joint and its correlation with cone beam computed tomography. *Dentomaxillofac Radiol.* 2010;39:270–276.

Kulekcioglu S, Sivrioglu K, Ozcan O, Parlak M. Effectiveness of low-level laser therapy in temporomandibular disorder. *Scand J Rheumatol.* 2003;32:114–118.

Kuwahara T, Bessette RW, Maruyama T. A retrospective study on the clinical results of temporomandibular joint surgery. *Cranio.* 1994;12:179–183.

Paesani D, Westesson P, Hatala M, Tallents RH, Brooks SL. Accuracy of clinical diagnosis for TMJ internal derangement. *Oral Surg Oral Med Oral Pathol.* 1992;73(3):360–363.

Roberts C, Katzberg R, Tellents R, Espeland MA, Handelman SL. The clinical predictability of internal derangements of the temporomandibular joint. *Oral Surg Oral Med Oral Pathol.* 1991;71(4):412–414.

Sheon RP. Temporomandibular joint dysfunction syndrome. *UpToDate.* Accessed November 23, 2012.

Ta LE, Dionne RA. Treatment of painful temporomandibular joints with a cyslooxygenase-2 inhibitor: A randomized placebo-controlled comparison of celecoxib to naproxen. *Pain.* 2004;111:13–21.

The American Academy of Craniomandibular Disorders. In: McNeill C, ed. *Craniomandibular Disorders: Guidelines for Evaluation, diagnosis, and Management,* Chicago, IL: Quintessence Publishing Co; 1990.

Vicente-Barrero M, Yu-Lu SL, Zhang B, et al. The efficacy of acupuncture and decompression splints in the treatment of temporomandibular joint pain-dysfunction syndrome. *Med Oral Patol Oral Cir Bucal.* 2012;17(6):e1028–e1033.

Yuasa H, Kurita K, Treatment Group on Temporomandibular Disorders. Randomized clinical trial of primary treatment for temporomandibular joint disk displacement without reduction and without osseous changes: A combination of NSAIDs and mouth-opening exercise versus no treatment. *Oral Surg Oral Med Oral Pathol Oral Radiol Endod.* 2001;91:671–675.

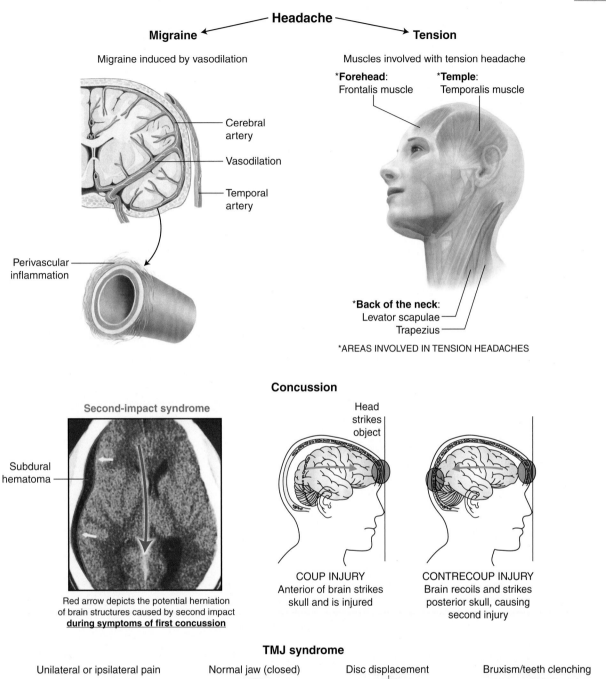

Headache

Migraine ← → **Tension**

Migraine induced by vasodilation

Cerebral artery
Vasodilation
Temporal artery

Perivascular inflammation

Muscles involved with tension headache

*Forehead: Frontalis muscle
*Temple: Temporalis muscle

*Back of the neck:
Levator scapulae
Trapezius

*AREAS INVOLVED IN TENSION HEADACHES

Concussion

Second-impact syndrome

Subdural hematoma

Red arrow depicts the potential herniation of brain structures caused by second impact **during symptoms of first concussion**

Head strikes object

COUP INJURY
Anterior of brain strikes skull and is injured

CONTRECOUP INJURY
Brain recoils and strikes posterior skull, causing second injury

TMJ syndrome

Unilateral or ipsilateral pain

Earache

Clicking, popping, grinding

Inability to open mouth

Normal jaw (closed)

Disc

Disc displacement

Musculoskeletal derangement

Bruxism/teeth clenching

Figure 132. Neurologic

Section 9: Musculoskeletal

Muscle Strain

Introduction (Definitions/Classification):

- A muscle strain is the most common musculoskeletal injury in professional and recreational athletes.
- Commonly used analogous terms include "muscle tears" or "muscle pull."
- Common feature is damage of muscle fibers.
- The severity of the injury determines the treatment and length of recovery.

History and Physical Examination:

- History:
  - Compensation from concurrent injuries.
  - Inadequate warm-up.
  - Increased training volume and fatigue predisposes athletes to injury.
  - Presence of a "pop or snap" at the time of injury.
  - Inquire about the mechanism of injury; most strains occur during the stretching or eccentric contraction phases.
  - Most frequently occurs during sudden bursts of energy or speed; can occur via both high- and low-speed stretching mechanisms.
- Physical examination:
  - Examination may be influenced by guarding in the presence of spasm, cramping, or severe pain.
  - Inspection and palpation:
    - Check skin color, tissue swelling and warmth.
    - Check for signs of neurovascular compromise.
  - Function:
    - Assess biomechanics.
    - Assess the degree of active versus passive range of motion.
    - Test strength and compare to contralateral and ipsilateral antagonist muscle groups.

Diagnosis:

- Signs/symptoms on physical examination.
- Tears classified into the following.
  - Degree I: Fascia intact, few muscle fibers ruptured, strength preserved.
  - Degree II: Fascia intact, moderate number of fibers ruptured, intramuscular hematoma, decreased strength.
  - Degree III: Torn fascia, ¼–½ of the muscle fibers torn, intramuscular hematoma, decreased strength.
  - Degree IV: Torn fascia, most or all of the muscle fibers are torn, no strength or function.
- Imaging:
  - Typically unnecessary.
  - For severe and refractory cases:
    - Ultrasound.
    - MRI.

Treatment:

- PRICE modalities: **P**rotection, **R**est, **I**ce, **C**ompression, **E**levation to decrease bleeding, swelling, and pain.
- NSAIDs.
- Graded rehabilitation:
  - Slow mobilization with gentle stretching and cautious progression to full motion.
  - Once range of motion is restored, add light strength training.
  - Stretch and strengthen antagonist muscles to prevent further injury.
- Though evidence is lacking, stretching and warm-up programs are believed to prevent strains.
- Indications for orthopedic consultation:
  - Avulsion injuries with retraction and grade IV muscle tears.

Other Considerations:

- Muscle strains are often confused with delayed onset muscle soreness (DOMS). DOMS usually presents as muscle pain and tightness following unaccustomed physical activity without acute trauma.
- Consider a more severe injury (rupture) if no improvement with therapy.
- Rehabilitate carefully. An aggressive rehabilitation program increases the risk of re-injury if the reparative scar tissue has not developed its optimum tensile strength or elasticity.
- Myositis ossificans is a possible complication of severe strains.

Return to Play:

- No general principles based on grading of muscle tears.
- To prevent recurrence, complications, increased morbidity, and prolonged loss of practice time and inability to compete effectively, return athletes to play only after they have achieved full, pain-free range of motion and strength.
- May be prolonged in athletes with stretching-type injuries opposed to high-speed running injuries.

Recommended Readings

Fields K, Copland S, Tipton J. Hamstring injuries. *UpToDate*. Accessed November 16, 2012.
Muscle strain injuries. In: *DeLee and Drez's Orthopaedic Sports Medicine*, 3rd ed. Retrieved from http://www.mdconsult.com/books. Accessed December 12, 2010.
Nelson B, Taylor D. Muscle and tendon injuries and repair. In: *Sports Medicine—Just the Facts*. McGraw Hill; 2005:55–61.

Costochondritis

Introduction (Definitions/Classification):

- A common condition induced by inflammation of the costal cartilage.
- Synonyms include "chest wall syndrome," "costosternal syndrome," and "parasternal chondrodynia" (Tietze syndrome).
- Often underdiagnosed. For patients with chest pain:
  - Costochondritis described in 30% of cases in emergency departments and 43% in primary care.
- May occur in any sport, yet more prevalent amongst volleyball and crew athletes.

History and Physical Examination:

- Patients typically present with acute chest pain, thus often require several tests to rule out cardiac etiologies.
- Has been associated with
  - Seronegative spondyloarthropathies.
  - Repetitive physical movements.
  - History of a recent illness involving prolonged coughing.
  - Recent increase in duration and intensity of exercise.
- Presenting symptoms:
  - Anterior chest pain: Dull, sharp, or pressure.
  - Tenderness usually localizes to the proximal costal cartilage of the costochondral and/or costosternal borders of ribs—two to seven.
  - *Reproducible* musculoskeletal chest pain with single-digit palpation over anterior, lateral, and posterior thoracic wall that may radiate throughout the chest wall.
  - Pain usually exacerbated by upper body movements, respiration, or exertion.
  - No associated swelling, erythema, or warmth.

Diagnosis:

- High index of suspicion based on signs/symptoms on physical examination (*following exclusion of more severe cardiopulmonary etiologies*).
- First rule out cardiac and pulmonary disease in all athletes.
- Consider specific diagnostic testing, on "individualized basis," for athletes with the following.
  - Associated palpitations, pre-syncope, syncope, and/or family history of cardiac disease or SCD less than age 50.
    - EKG, echocardiogram, Stress test, Holter and looping event monitoring (as indicated).
    - Medical clearance following cardiology consultation.
  - Either prolonged cough or eating disorders.
    - CXR (rule out concomitant pulmonary disease).
    - CT, and/or bone scan (rule out occult osseous pathology—mass/fracture).

- Fever or history of seronegative **spondyloarthropathy**.
  - CBC with differential (CBC diff).
  - ESR.

Treatment:

- No specific advantage of "one particular treatment." Best response achieved by combination therapies includes the following.
  - Rest and reassurance (following exclusion of potentially severe cardiopulmonary etiologies).
  - Discontinuation of any known triggers (e.g., increased sit-ups, weightlifting)
  - Activity modification (e.g., exercise duration and intensity).
  - Analgesics such as Tylenol and NSAIDs.
  - Educate:
    - Usually self-limited.
    - Ice reduces inflammation and heat can exaggerate inflammation.
    - Recurrence is common following poor compliance with medical recommendations.
  - Physical therapy—mobilization, manipulation, stretching.
  - Acupuncture.
- For refractory cases, consider the following.
  - Local anesthetics or steroid injections into the costochondral joints.
  - Rheumatology consultation (e.g., management of seronegative **spondyloarthropathy**).

Other Considerations:

- Additional noncardiac causes should be considered.
  - Tietze syndrome—associated swelling without erythema.
  - Inflammatory or septic arthritis—erythema or warmth.
  - Xiphodynia—pain with palpation over xiphoid thought to be secondary to inflammation.
  - Subluxations of sternoclavicular, sternocostal, or costovertebral joints.
  - SAPHO (synovitis, acne, pustulosis, hyperostosis, and osteitis) syndrome or sternoclavicular hyperostosis—a constellation of skin and osteoarticular conditions which presents with pain, swelling, and limited ranges of motion of the sternoclavicular joints.

Return to Play Criteria:

- Signs and symptoms:
  - No *reproducible* musculoskeletal chest pain with single-digit palpation over anterior, lateral, and posterior thoracic wall.
  - No radiation of pain following palpation.
  - Pain not exacerbated by upper body movements, respiration, or exertion.
- No associated swelling, erythema, or warmth.
- Other cardiopulmonary/infectious etiologies have been ruled out.
- Consider added protection for chest wall for contact sports such as football and rugby.

Recommended Readings

Disla E, Rhim H, Reddy A, Karten I, Taranta A. Costochondritis. A prospective analysis in an emergency department setting. *Arch Intern Med.* 1994;154:2466–2469.

DynaMed [Internet]. Costochondritis. Ipswich (MA): EBSCO Publishing; .Available from http://web.ebscohost.com/dynamed/detail?vid=7&hid=8&sid=2c7d02cf-250a-4c688fe99b3bbb539160%40sessionmgr11&bdata=JnNpdGU9ZHluYW1lZC1saXZlJjnNjb3BlPXNpdGU%3d#db=dme&AN=114285. Updated November 30, 2009; cited November 6, 2012; (about 24 screens).

Freeston J, Karim Z, Lindsay K, Gough A. Can early diagnosis and management of costochondritis reduce acute chest pain admissions? *J Rheumatol.* 2004;31:2269–2271.

Gregory P, Biswas A, Batt M. Musculoskeletal problems of the chest wall in athletes. *Sports Med.* 2002;32(4):235–250.

How J, Volz G, Doe S, Heycock C, Hamilton J, Kelly C. The causes of musculoskeletal chest pain in patients admitted to hospital with suspected myocardial infarction. *Eur J Intern Med.* 2005;16(6):432–436.

Proulx A, Zryd T. Costochondritis: Diagnosis and treatment. *Am Fam Physician.* 2009;80(6):617–620.

Rabey M. Costochondritis: Are the symptoms and signs due to neurogenic inflammation. Two cases that responded to manual therapy directed towards posterior spinal structures. *Man Ther.* 2008;13:82–86.

Sik E, Batt M, Heslop L. Atypical chest pain in athletes. *Curr Sports Med Rep.* 2009;8(2):52–58.

Spalding L, Reay E, Kelly C. Cause and outcome of atypical chest pain in patients admitted to hospital. *J R Soc Med.* 2003;96(3):122–125.

Stochkendahl M, Christensen H. Chest pain in focal musculoskeletal disorders. *Med Clin North Am.* 2010;92(2):259–273.

Verdon F, Herzig L, Burnand B, et al. Chest pain in daily practice: Occurrence, causes and management. *Swiss Med Wkly.* 2008;138(23–24):340–347.

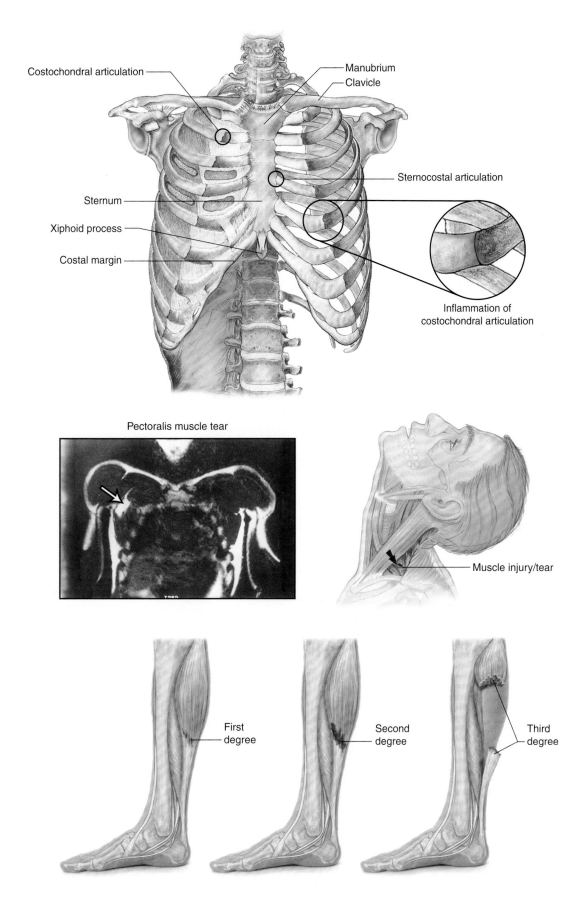

Costochondral articulation

Manubrium

Clavicle

Sternocostal articulation

Sternum

Xiphoid process

Costal margin

Inflammation of costochondral articulation

Pectoralis muscle tear

Muscle injury/tear

First degree

Second degree

Third degree

Figure 133. Musculoskeletal

Section 10: Endocrine

The Female Athlete Triad

Introduction (Definitions/Classification):

- A syndrome common among female athletes of all ability levels which results in diminished athletic performance and potentially irreversible health consequences. The three domains of "continuum" dysfunction include the following.
  - Low energy availability (energy deficits from disordered eating).
  - Menstrual dysfunction.
  - Altered bone mineral density (BMD).
- A potential fourth domain has been recently described: impaired endothelium-dependent arterial vasodilation. This may enhance cardiovascular risk.

History and Physical Examination:

- History:
  - Energy intake.
  - Attitudes toward food.
  - Dietary preferences (vegetarian, regular daily meals vs. "grazing").
  - Excessive exercise.
  - Detailed menstrual history.
  - Past history of eating disorder, secondary amenorrhea, or stress fractures.
  - Past medical history (thyroid, diabetes, psychiatric).
- Physical examination:
  - Review vitals to assess objective data—weight changes, drop in BP or pulse.
  - General—hypothermia, bradycardia, cachexia, appears fatigued.
  - HEENT—parotid gland enlargement.
  - Neck—check thyroid.
  - Skin—lanugo, skin discoloration/cold extremities, Russell sign (calluses on digits used to induce emesis).
  - Psychiatric—body image, fear of weight gain.
  - Pelvic examination—vaginal atrophic changes, if amenorrheic.
  - EKG to rule out conduction abnormalities (QT prolongation).

Diagnosis:

Signs/symptoms on physical examination, yet evaluate the following.

- Pregnancy test.
- Comprehensive metabolic panel.
- CBC with differential.
- ESR.
- Cholesterol panel.
- Thyroid function tests.
- Tests to rule out causes of primary or secondary amenorrhea (FSH, LH, prolactin).
- Densitometry evaluation for those unwilling to favorably alter energy balance or amenorrhea/oligomenorrhea >6 months, or with low impact/stress fractures.
  - Use Z-score to compare BMD to age and sex-matched controls.
  - Compared to nonathletes, athletes have 5% to 15% higher BMD.
    - Thus, investigate for BMD Z-score <−1 in athletes.
  - If BMD low, check 25 hydroxy vitamin D levels.
- Brachial ultrasound scanning (flow-mediated dilation; FMD) to evaluate for endothelial dysfunction.
  - Normal: 5% to 15% increase in brachial artery diameter after release of cuff.
  - Positive predictive value (PPV) of FMD in predicting coronary endothelial dysfunction is 95%.

Treatment:

- Multidisciplinary approach is critical to successful management.
  - Primary care physician (sports physician).
  - Sports psychologist/counselor.
  - Nutritionist/registered dietician.
  - Athletic training staff.
  - Also consider (as needed) consults with gynecologist, cardiologist, or orthopedic surgeon.
  - Family, friends, coaches.
- First goal should be to increase energy intake and reduce energy expenditure.
  - Menses may resume with this approach.
  - Helps bone formation.
- Hormonal therapy.
  - Not as effective in increasing BMD, as compared to weight gain.
  - Recommend using only as last resort.
  - Yet, monophasic, combined OCs have been shown to increase FMD.
  - Counsel on increased incidence of breast cancer and breast cancer mortality in postmenopausal women treated with OC.
- Nutritional supplementation.
  - Calcium: 1200 to 1500 mg daily.
  - Vitamin D: 400 IU daily; higher amounts with 25 hydroxy vitamin D is low.
  - Folic acid may improve endothelium-dependent vasodilation.
    - Few side effects at dose of 10 mg/day for 4 to 6 weeks.
- Weight training helps improve BMD.
- Psychological interventions for eating disorders include the following.
  - CBT may be an effective intervention, yet may not be effective in ~50%.
  - Acceptance and commitment therapy (ACT) associated with enhanced treatment outcomes.
  - Other potential interventions include dialectical behavior therapy (DBT) and enhanced CBT (CBT-E).
- Pharmacotherapy for eating disorders.
  - Selective SSRIs may be effective in combination with CBT.
  - Recommend consultation with "team psychologist" before initiating treatment.

Other Considerations:

- Prevalence of all three clinical components of triad concurrently is low. Thus, evaluate and treat presenting clinical component of triad aggressively. *Do not wait to treat until all the three components are present.*
- Be aware of athletes at increased risk.
  - Involvement in sports with weight restrictions (gymnastics, figure skating, ballet).
  - Increased pressure to win (parents, coaches, training staff).
  - Prolonged or rapid increase in training regimen.
- Early detection of endothelial dysfunction by assessment of FMD is critical for long-term health.
- Miscellaneous (including American College of Sports Medicine [ACSM] Recommendations).
  - Screen during pre-participation physical valuation or annual check-up.
  - To diagnose functional hypothalamic amenorrhea, other causes of amenorrhea must be excluded.
  - Counsel athletes practicing restrictive eating behaviors that increase in body weight.
    - May be necessary to increase BMD
    - Is more effective in increasing BMD than hormonal therapy.
  - Athletes with disordered eating and eating disorders who do not comply with treatment may need to be restricted from training and competition.
- Bisphosphonates are teratogenic and should not be used in athletes.

Return to Play Criteria:

- Attained optimal body weight.
- No metabolic or electrolyte abnormalities noted.
- EKG normal without evidence for conduction abnormalities.
- Evidence of healed acute injuries (e.g., stress fractures).
- Currently seeking treatment from multidisciplinary team and compliance with increased energy consumption and limitations of training regimen.

Recommended Readings

Anderson TJ, Uehata A, Gerhard MD, et al. Close relation of endothelial function in the human coronary and peripheral circulations. *J Am Coll Cardiol.* 1995;26(5):1235–1241.

Baer R, Fischer S, Huss D. Mindfulness and acceptance in the treatment of disordered eating. *J Ration Emot Cogn Behav Ther.* 2005;23(4):281–300.

Beals KA, Meyer NL. Female athlete triad update. *Clin Sports Med.* 2007;26(1):69–89.

Bonci CM, Bonci LJ, Granger LR, et al. National Athletic Trainers' Association position statement: Preventing, detecting, and managing disordered eating in athletes. *J Athl Train.* 2008;4380–4108.

Fredericson M, Kent K. Normalization of bone density in a previously amenorrheic runner with osteoporosis. *Med Sci Sports Exerc.* 2005;37(9):1481–1486.

Hoch AZ, Lynch SL, Jurva JW, Schimke JE, Gutterman DD. Folic acid supplementation improves vascular function in amenorrheic runners. *Clin J Sport Med.* 2010;20(3):205–210.

Mitchell JE, Agras S, Wonderlich S. Treatment of bulimia nervosa: Where are we and where are we going? *Int J Eat Disord.* 2007;40(2):95–101.

McNicholl DM, Heaney LG. The safety of bisphosphonate use in pre-menopausal women on corticosteroids. *Curr Drug Saf.* 2010;5(2):182–187.

Nattiv A, Loucks AB, Manore MM, et al. American College of Sports Medicine position stand. The female athlete triad. *Med Sci Sports Exerc.* 2007;39(10):1867–1882.

Rickenlund A, Eriksson MJ, Schenck-Gustafsson K, Hirschberg AL. Oral contraceptives improve endothelial function in amenorrheic athletes. *J Clin Endocrinol Metab.* 2005;90(6):3162–3167.

Warren MP. Amenorrhea and infertility associated with exercise. *UpToDate.* Accessed February 3, 2013.

Warren MP, Miller KK, Olson WH, Grinspoon SK, Friedman AJ. Effects of an oral contraceptive (norgestimate/ethinyl estradiol) on bone mineral density in women with hypothalamic amenorrhea and osteopenia: An open-label extension of a double-blind, placebo-controlled study. *Contraception.* 2005;72:206–211.

Warren MP, Perlroth NE. The effects of intense exercise on the female reproductive system. *J Endocrinol.* 2001;170:3–11.

Female Athlete Triad

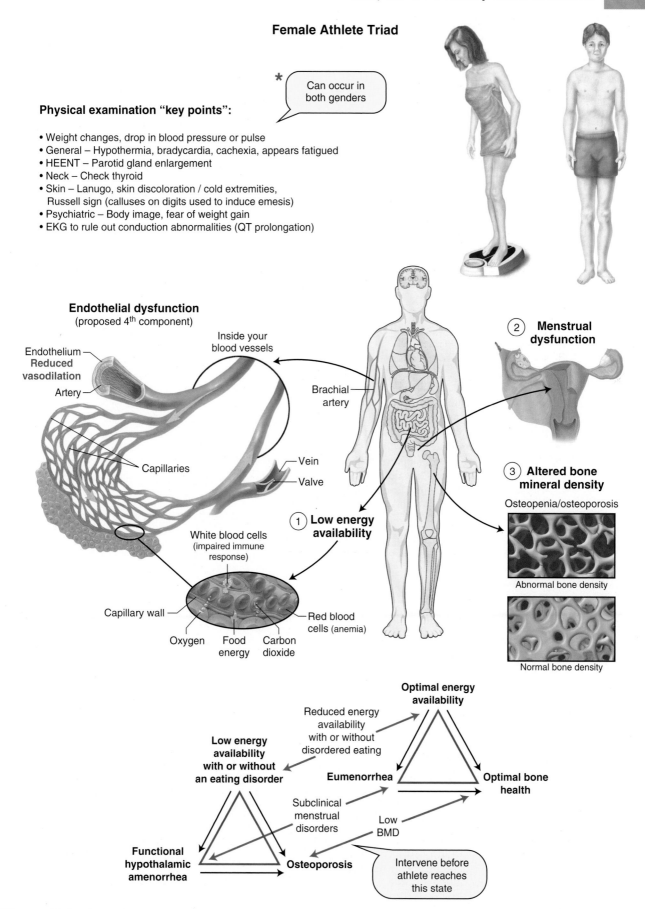

Physical examination "key points":

* Can occur in both genders

- Weight changes, drop in blood pressure or pulse
- General – Hypothermia, bradycardia, cachexia, appears fatigued
- HEENT – Parotid gland enlargement
- Neck – Check thyroid
- Skin – Lanugo, skin discoloration / cold extremities, Russell sign (calluses on digits used to induce emesis)
- Psychiatric – Body image, fear of weight gain
- EKG to rule out conduction abnormalities (QT prolongation)

Endothelial dysfunction
(proposed 4th component)

Endothelium
Reduced vasodilation

Artery

Inside your blood vessels

Brachial artery

Capillaries

Vein

Valve

White blood cells (impaired immune response)

Capillary wall

Oxygen   Food energy   Carbon dioxide

Red blood cells (anemia)

(1) **Low energy availability**

(2) **Menstrual dysfunction**

(3) **Altered bone mineral density**

Osteopenia/osteoporosis

Abnormal bone density

Normal bone density

Optimal energy availability

Reduced energy availability with or without disordered eating

Low energy availability with or without an eating disorder

Eumenorrhea

Optimal bone health

Subclinical menstrual disorders

Low BMD

Functional hypothalamic amenorrhea

Osteoporosis

Intervene before athlete reaches this state

Figure 134. Female Athlete Triad

Section 11: Hematologic

Anemia in the Athlete

Introduction (Definitions/Classification):

- This chapter discusses anemia specific to the athletic population.
- Acute exercise has nominal effects on hemoglobin and hematocrit.
- Therefore, terminologies such as "sports anemia," "athlete's anemia," "exercise-induced anemia," "swimmer's anemia," and "runner's anemia" are confounding and should not be used in the assessment and management of anemia.
- Anemia is a decrease in either hemoglobin (Hgb), hematocrit (HCT), or number of RBCs.
  - Women: Hgb < 12 g/dL, HCT < 36.
  - Men: Hgb < 13.5 g/dL, HCT < 41.
- General classification and examples of potential causes in athletes—based on the size of red blood cell (mean corpuscular volume; MCV).
  - *Microcytic:* <78 fL.
    - Iron deficiency, blood loss, sickle cell trait.
  - *Normocytic:* 78 to 100 fL.
    - Infection, drugs, and numerous other medical conditions.
  - *Macrocytic:* >100 fL.
    - Vitamin B12 and/or folate deficiency, hypothyroidism, liver disease.
- Types of anemia in athletes include the following.
  - Dilutional pseudoanemia.
  - Iron deficiency (with or without anemia).
  - Intravascular hemolysis.
  - Miscellaneous—nutritional, other medical illnesses not related to exercise.
    - Vitamin B12 and/or folate deficiency.
    - Less common and not discussed in this chapter.

History and Physical Examination/Diagnosis/Treatment/Return to Play:

(Refer Table 1 for aid with diagnosis of various types of anemia in athletes).
- *Dilutional pseudoanemia:*
  - **History:**
    - Prolonged training.
  - **Physical examination:**
    - Normal.
  - **Diagnosis:**
    - Mild anemia without consistent subjective or objective impact on physical activity or performance is not impacted.
    - Laboratory values are normal with the exception of mild decrease in Hgb: <11.5 g/dL in females, <13 g/dL in males.
  - **Treatment:**
    - None; reassurance.

Table 1 Types of Anemia in Athletes

Type of Anemia	Frequency	Hemoglobin	MCV	Ferritin	Haptoglobin
Dilutional pseudoanemia	Common	Mildly decreased	Normal	Normal	Normal
Prelatent anemia	Common	Normal	Normal	Decreased	Normal
Iron-deficiency anemia	Less common	Decreased	Decreased	Decreased	Normal
Intravascular hemolysis	Less common	Usually normal	Increased	Normal	Decreased

From Mercer K, Densmore J. Hematologic disorders in the athlete. In: Miller M, MacKnight J, eds. *Clinics in Sports Medicine—Training Room Management of Medical Conditions.* Philadelphia, PA: Elsevier Saunders; 2005;24(3):599–614, with permission.

- **Other considerations:**
  - Most common cause in athletes.
  - Induced by increase in plasma volume.
  - Transient and can resolve within 1 week of discontinuing exercise.
- **Return to play:**
  - No restrictions.
- *Iron deficiency:*
  - **History:**
    - Athletes have a higher incidence of iron-deficiency anemia, particularly those involved in endurance activities.
    - Inquire about the following.
      - Gastrointestinal (GI) or genitourinary (GU) bleeding (menstrual history in females).
      - Adequate nutrition related to level of activity.
      - Comorbid conditions: Hypothyroidism, stomach ulcer, infection with *Helicobacter pylori.*
      - Current medications—NSAIDs which can induce occult GI bleeding.
  - **Physical examination:**
    - Fatigued.
    - Pale mucus membranes; nail and/or epithelial changes.
    - Tachycardia, flow murmur (systolic) diminished capillary refill.
    - Hepatomegaly/splenomegaly.
    - Consider digital rectal or pelvic examinations.
  - **Diagnosis:**
    - Assessment of "iron stores."
      - Bone marrow biopsy (*gold standard*).
      - Ferritin assessment (*to check iron stores in most patients*).
        - <10 to 15 ng/mL = sensitivity 59%, specificity 99%.
        - <41 ng/mL = sensitivity and specificity 98%.
    - Blood tests.
      - Hgb, HCT, MCV, serum iron, total iron-binding capacity, ferritin, and transferrin saturation.
      - Assessment of iron stores.
    - On the basis of blood tests and other clinical characteristics, the following stages have been defined (Table 2).
      - Stage I: "Iron deficiency without anemia" (prelatent anemia)—more common, in 11% women/4% men.
      - Stage II: "Iron deficiency with mild anemia.
      - Stage III: "Iron-deficiency anemia—severe"—less common in ~1% to 3%.
  - **Treatment:**
    - Nonpharmacologic (Stage I).
      - Counsel on foods rich in iron (lean meats, fish, poultry, vegetables, grains).
    - Pharmacologic (Stages II and III).
      - *With:* Oral ferrous sulfate or ferrous gluconate.
      - *Key points for adequate therapy:*
        - Vitamin C supplementation during therapy may enhance iron absorption by inducing an acidic state in the gut.

Table 2 Lab Tests in Iron Deficiency

	Normal	Iron Deficiency without Anemia	Iron Deficiency with Mild Anemia	Severe Iron Deficiency with Severe Anemia
Marrow reticuloendothelial iron	2+ to 3+	None	None	None
Serum iron (SI), µg/dL	60 to 150	60 to 150	<60	<40
Total iron binding capacity (transferrin, TIBC), µg/dL	300 to 360	300 to 390	350 to 400	>410
Transferrin saturation (SI/TIBC), percent	20 to 50	30	<15	<10
Hemoglobin, g/dL	Normal	Normal	9 to 12	6 to 7
Red cell morphology	Normal	Normal	Normal or slight hypochromia	Hypochromia and microcytosis
Plasma or serum ferritin, ng/mL	40 to 200	<40	<20	<10
Erythrocyte protoporphyrin, ng/mL RBC	30 to 70	30 to 70	>100	100 to 200
Other tissue changes	None	None	None	Nail and epithelial changes

Note: Test results outlined in bold type are the ones most likely to define the various stages of iron deficiency. Thus, the presence or absence of iron stores (marrow reticuloendothelial iron) in a nonanemic patient serves to distinguish normal subjects from those with iron deficiency without anemia, respectively. (From: Schreir S. Causes and diagnosis of anemia due to iron deficiency. *UpToDate.* Accessed on April 1st, 2013, with permission.)

- Ferrous gluconate contains less elemental iron than ferrous sulfate, and is therefore better tolerated with fewer side effects.
- Iron should not be administered with foods which can reduce absorption including coffee, tea, milk, cereal, and foods rich in fiber.
- Medications that decrease absorption include calcium supplements, quinolones and tetracyclines, and antacids (proton pump inhibitors and H_2 receptor blockers).
- If athletes need antacid and iron therapy simultaneously, treat with iron 2 hours before or 4 hours after antacid therapy.
  - *How long:*
    - Recommendations vary; between 6 and 12 months is reasonable.
    - May need longer therapy; evaluate on an "individual basis."
  - *When to refer to hematologist:*
    - Refractory to oral therapy.
    - For consideration of parenteral therapy.
- **Other considerations:**
  - Iron-deficiency anemia can be induced by inadequate intake or absorption of iron; yet it is important to rule out occult blood loss to avoid misdiagnosis of a more serious underlying medical condition (GI bleeding or malignancy).
  - Important to differentiate "iron-deficiency anemia" from thalassemia and "anemia of chronic disease" (all can present with microcytosis).
  - The data on the effects of oral iron supplementation in individuals with "prelatent anemia" are inconclusive.
  - Oral iron supplementation may induce constipation, gastritis, and change composition of stool, all of which can decrease compliance to therapy.
  - There may be a role for screening athletes at "high risk" for iron-deficiency anemia; yet because of low incidence (1% to 3%), routine screening is not recommended.
  - Refer to Team Nutritionist for close monitoring.
  - Consider and manage latent eating disorders, especially if athlete presents with concomitant amenorrhea and recurrent stress fractures.
- **Return to play:**
  - No restrictions generally.
  - If athlete presents with concomitant blood abnormalities (thrombocytopenia or leukopenia), prudent to refer to a hematologist prior to medical clearance.
- **Intravascular hemolysis:**
  - **History:**
    - Painless hematuria after prolonged, intense exertion (marathons, triathlons, and long-distance swimming).
    - Athlete is generally asymptomatic because of compensatory reticulocytosis.
  - **Physical examination:**
    - Typically normal; in rare circumstances jaundice may be apparent.
  - **Diagnosis:**
    - Is a diagnosis of exclusion!
    - Obtain blood tests shortly after concluding exercise.
      - Decreased serum haptoglobin.
      - Increased lactate dehydrogenase.
      - Macrocytosis and reticulocytosis may be present.
    - Urine.
      - May show hemoglobinuria.
  - **Treatment:**
    - Activity modification.
    - Counsel on potential benefits of gait evaluation, adequate footwear, and modify training intensity (as needed).
  - **Other considerations:**
    - Current theories.
      - Possible mechanical damage during "heel strike" in runners.
      - Muscle contraction–induced compression and breakdown of RBCs in swimmers.
      - Structural changes to RBC membranes after prolonged exercise related to increased temperature and oxidative stress.
    - Rule out other causes for hemolytic anemia, especially other causes of congenital or acquired defects of RBC fragility (e.g., Vitamin E deficiency spherocytosis).

- **Return to play:**
  - No restrictions generally.
  - Yet, consider work-up for gross hematuria as indicated (e.g., GU trauma, family history of polycystic kidney disease)

Recommended Readings

Abrams SA. Iron requirements and iron deficiency in adults. *UpToDate*. Accessed on April 1st, 2013.

Brittenham G. Disorders of iron metabolism: Iron deficiency and iron overload. In: Hoffman R, Benz EJ, Shattil SS, et al., eds. *Hematology: Basic Principles and Practice*. 5th ed. Philadelphia, PA: Elsevier Churchill Livingstone; 2008, Chapter 36.

Guyatt G, Oxman A, Ali M, et al. Laboratory diagnosis of iron-deficiency anemia: An overview. *J Gen Intern Med*. 1992;7(2):145–153.

Haas J, Brownlie T. Iron deficiency and reduced work capacity: A critical review of the research to determine a causal relationship. *J Nutr*. 2001;131(2S-20):676S–88S.

Mercer K, Densmore J. Hematologic disorders in the athlete. In: Miller M, MacKnight J, eds. *Clinics in Sports Medicine – Training Room Management of Medical Conditions*. Philadelphia, PA: Elsevier Saunders; 2005;24(3):599–614.

Schreir S. Approach to adult patient with anemia. *UpToDate*. Accessed on April 1st, 2013.

Schreir S. Causes and diagnosis of anemia due to iron deficiency. *UpToDate*. Accessed on April 1st, 2013.

Schreir S, Auerbach M. Treatment of anemia due to iron deficiency. *UpToDate*. Accessed on April 1st, 2013.

Shaskey DJ, Green GA. Sports hematology. *Sports Med*. 2000;29(1):27–38.

Selby GB, Eichner ER. Endurance swimming, intravascular hemolysis, anemia, and iron depletion. New perspective on athlete's anemia. *Am J Med*. 1986;81(5):791–794.

Selby GB, Eichner ER. Hematocrit and performance: The effect of endurance training on blood volume. *Semin Hematol*. 1994;31(2):122–127.

Telford RD, Sly GJ, Hahn AG, et al. Footstrike is the major cause of hemolysis during running. *J Appl Physiol*. 2003;94(1):38–42.

Sickle Cell Trait (SCT)

Introduction/Classification:

- An autosomal recessive blood disorder that results from inheritance from one abnormal hemoglobin gene (S) coupled with a normal hemoglobin gene (A), SCT (Hb AS) is a heterozygous, benign carrier condition (not a disease).
- Individuals who are homozygous for both mutated hemoglobin genes (SS) have sickle cell diseases (Hb SS) and are highly unlikely to participate in athletics, due to severe and frequent complications. Therefore, this chapter primarily addresses SCT.
- Prevalence of SCT.
  - 8% of African Americans.
  - 0.5% of Hispanics.
  - 0.2% of Whites.
- Deaths in Division-1 football between 2000 and 2010.
  - 16 deaths during *conditioning*.
    - 15 during sprinting or high-speed agility drills and one from weightlifting.
    - 10 (63%) from exertional sickling collapse (ESC), 4 secondary to cardiac etiologies, 1 from asthma complications, and 1 from exertional heat stroke complications.
- Under specific conditions red blood cells "sickle" and block microcirculation that may induce various complications including the following.
  - ESC.
    - Typically induced by sustained, *maximal intensity* exercise.
    - Most grave complication which may cause death by inducing "explosive rhabdomyolysis."
    - Poor conditioning status + Preseason + Altitude = "Perfect storm."
  - Splenic infarction—especially at altitude.
  - Lumbar myonecrosis.
  - Compartment syndromes.
  - Gross hematuria.
  - Hyposthenuria (difficulty concentrating urine).
  - Venous thromboembolism (debated).
- Four alterations in homeostasis and that occur together are responsible for "sickling" of RBC's in microcirculation.
  - Hypoxemia.
  - Hyperosmolarity.
  - Red-cell dehydration, which concentrates hemoglobin S.
  - Lactic acidosis.

History and Physical Examination:

- **General considerations:**
  - Typically, individuals with SCT are healthy and daily activities are not impacted.
  - SCT is more common in individuals of African, Mediterranean, Middle Eastern, Caribbean, and Indian descent. However, SCT can be prevalent in all ethnicities, including Caucasians.
  - Family history.
    - If one parent is SCT carrier, athlete has 50% chance of having SCT.
    - If both parents are SCT carriers, athlete has a 50% of having SCT and 25% chance of having sickle cell disease.
- **History and physical examination concerning for ESC:**
  - **History:**
    - Recent exposure to hypoxic stimulus: Endurance athletes (football, track, basketball, cross-country, cycling, boxing, swimming), exposure to altitude, recent infection, or dehydration.
    - Ask about "concerning" symptoms.
      - Leg and low back pain.
      - Severe, diffuse musculoskeletal, abdominal, or chest pain.
      - Ascending muscle spasms.
      - Lower extremity weakness without pain; athletes may slump to the ground.
      - Immediate cessation of activity—assuming "hands on knee position."
      - Anxious.
      - Cough, dyspnea, rapid breathing.
      - Painless hematuria.
      - Lethargy.
  - **Physical examination**
    - Assess ABC's (airway, breathing, circulation).
    - During ESC, signs may include the following.
      - Rectal temperature < 39.4°C (103°F).
      - General: Anxious yet communicative.
      - Heart: Tachycardia, possible systolic murmur.
      - Lungs: Tachypnea, yet without wheezing on auscultation.
      - Abdomen: Possible hepatosplenomegaly.
      - Musculoskeletal: Weakness > pain, yet examination maybe normal.
      - Skin: Pallor.

Diagnosis:

- **SCT.**
  - Sickle solubility tests can detect Hb S; yet need hemoglobin electrophoresis or high-pressure liquid chromatography to confirm SCT and distinguish from sickle cell disease.
  - Hematology pearls.
    - Peripheral blood smear may show red cell sickling.
    - Hemoglobin, red cell indices and morphology, and reticulocyte counts can be completely normal in SCT.
- **ESC.**
  - Signs/symptoms on physical examination.
  - Urinalysis may reveal gross hematuria.

Treatment:

- **Prevention better than cure.**
  - Educate athletes, parents, and coaches.
    - That there is no "cure" for sickle cell trait or disease.
    - To have athletes acclimatize gradually to heat, humidity, altitude, and endurance.
    - To begin preseason conditioning slowly and gradually, allowing athletes to establish their "own pace."
    - To gradually increase training intensity, with "paced progressions" and longer recovery periods.
    - To avoid extreme, performance tests—particularly if not specific to their sport; "*suicide drills are a suicide.*"
    - To refrain from "maximal" exertion sustained for >2 to 3 minutes.
    - To think with the **HEAD: H**ydrate, **E**nvironmental adjustments (heat and altitude), **A**sthma control, and **D**isqualify from workouts during illnesses.
    - To be trained in CPR and use of AED.

- **ESC.**
  - Educate athlete to discontinue exercise following "initial, unjustified symptom" and treat athlete as a case of early ESC.
  - Treat any concerns for ESC as a "*medical emergency*."
    - Call 911; if unavailable, rush athlete to nearest hospital.
    - Resources permitting.
      - Administer oxygen via facemask.
      - Establish IV line.
    - Monitor vital signs frequently.
    - If indicated, cool athlete.

Other Considerations:

- NCAA guidelines.
  - All Division I and Division II athletes, regardless of race, must be tested for SCT.
  - Those who test positive, need to be
    - educated regarding exercise-induced complications of SCT.
    - monitored closely to avoid overexertion and maintain hydration.
- Caution is advised in situations known to potentiate attacks including the following.
  - Dehydration.
  - High altitude (flying, mountain climbing, living in, or visiting cities at elevation).
  - Increased pressure (scuba diving).
  - Low oxygen states (mountain climbing or extremes of exercise).
- Consider screening athletes with or without hematuria for renal medullary carcinoma ("seventh sickle cell nephropathy"; found almost exclusively in SCT).
- Educate.
  - Regarding family planning, especially if partner has SCT which increases risk for offspring having Hb SS.
  - ESC can occur without exertional heat illness.
  - ESC is often confused for cardiogenic or heat collapse, therefore make all staff aware of athlete's with SCT.
  - Hyposthenuria is typically not a major clinical concern for either high school or college aged athletes.

Return to Play:

- Sickle cell trait is not an impediment to playing sports.
- Clear athletes with SCT for sports participation after documenting education regarding adjustments to activity and detailed discussion of risks and complications.
- Return to play following episode of ESC should be individualized on the basis of nature and severity of complications.

Recommended Readings

Bonham VL, Dover GJ, Brody LC. Screening student athletes for sickle cell trait—a social and clinical experiment. *N Engle J Med.* 2010;363:997–999.

DynaMed [Internet]. Ipswich (MA): EBSCO Publishing. Sickle Cell Disease; [updated 2012 Dec 03; cited 2012 Dec 21]; Available from http://web.ebscohost.com/dynamed/detail?vid=3&hid=122&sid=37c2c93f-9d16-459b-ac90-b1a8a03c2bef%40sessionmgr113&b data= JnNpdGU9ZHluYW1lZC1 saXZlJJnNjb3BlPXNpdGU%3d#db=dme&AN=115522&anchor=References.

Eichner ER. Sickle cell trait in sports. *Cur Sports Med Rep.* 2010;9:347–351.

Eichner ER. Sickle cell considerations in athletes. *Clinics Sports Med.* 2011;30(3):537–549.

Sickle Cell Disease. Centers for Disease Control. Retrieved from http://www.cdc.gov/ncbddd/sicklecell/traits.html on January 20th, 2011.

Sickle Cell Educational Materials and Resources. National Collegiate Athletic Association. Retrieved from http://www.ncaa.org on January 20th, 2011.

Vichinsky EP. Sickle cell trait. *UpToDate.* Accessed on February 3rd, 2013.

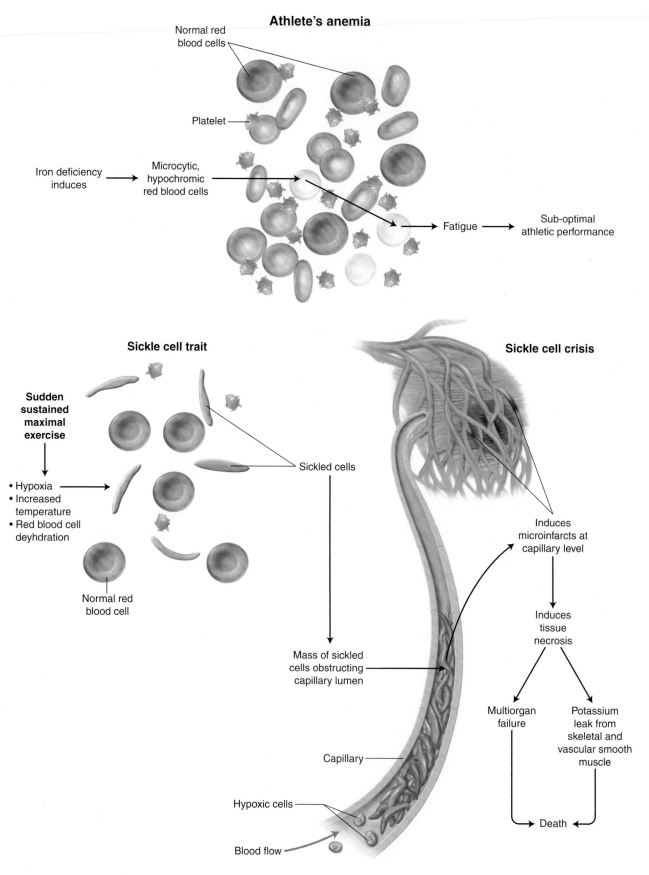

Athlete's anemia

Normal red
blood cells

Platelet

Iron deficiency
induces → Microcytic,
hypochromic
red blood cells

Fatigue → Sub-optimal
athletic performance

Sickle cell trait

**Sudden
sustained
maximal
exercise**

• Hypoxia
• Increased
temperature
• Red blood cell
deyhdration

Sickled cells

Normal red
blood cell

Mass of sickled
cells obstructing
capillary lumen

Capillary

Hypoxic cells

Blood flow

Sickle cell crisis

Induces
microinfarcts at
capillary level

Induces
tissue
necrosis

Multiorgan
failure

Potassium
leak from
skeletal and
vascular smooth
muscle

Death

Figure 135. Hematologic

Section 12: Environmental

Exertional Heat Illness

Introduction (Definitions/Classification):

- Exertional heat illness (EHI) is a leading cause of death in athletes.
- Classification in athletes.
  - Heat cramps: Exercise-associated muscle cramps (EAMC).
  - Heat syncope: Exercise-associated collapse (EAC).
  - Heat exhaustion.
  - Heat stroke: Exertional heat stroke (EHS); most severe.
- EHS is most common in football and most fatalities tend to occur during summer practices.

History and Physical Examination:

- **History (*evaluate risk factors*):**
  - **A**cclimatization—inadequate.
  - **B**ody weight—increased.
  - "**C**s."
    - **C**ongenital predisposition—sickle cell trait, malignant hyperthermia, anhidrosis.
    - **C**lothing (nonbreathable fabric).
  - "**D**s."
    - **D**ehydration: Recent illness or excessive alcohol consumption.
    - **D**rugs.
      - Anticholinergics (benadryl) and antihistamines (fexofenadine, cetirizine) for allergies.
      - Decongestants (pseudoephedrine) for common colds.
      - Stimulants: Albuterol for asthma; Amphetamines for ADHD.
      - Diuretics and beta blockers for hypertension.
      - Phenothiazines (promethazine) used to treat nausea and vomiting.
    - **D**isease: Hyperthyroidism.
    - **D**ietary supplements that contain stimulants (Ma Huang).
  - **E**xercise in detrimental environmental conditions—high temperature and high humidity.
  - **F**itness—poor shape in preseason.
- **Physical examination:**
  - **EAMC:**
    - Painful, muscle cramps of large muscle groups (legs, abdomen, and back).
    - Cardiovascular: Tachycardia.
    - Skin: Sweating.
    - CNS: Normal.
  - **EAC:**
    - Typically occurs at the end of an event following cessation of exercise.
    - Core temperature: Normal or slightly elevated.
    - Cardiovascular: Bradycardia.
    - Skin: Pallor and sweating.
    - CNS: Mental status altered, resolves in ~20 minutes with adequate treatment (distinguishing factor from EHS).
  - **Heat exhaustion:**
    - Inability to continue exercise, altered gait, nausea/vomiting, abdominal cramps.
    - Core temperature: 38.3° to 39.4°C (101° to 103°F).
    - Cardiovascular: Tachycardia and hypotension.
    - Skin: Pallor and excessive sweating.
    - CNS: Mild confusion which typically resolves with rest and cooling OR may be normal (distinguishing factor from EHS); headache, weakness.

- **EHS:**
  - Inability to continue exercise, tachypnea, altered gait, nausea/vomiting/diarrhea, dry mouth, profuse sweating, oliguria.
  - Core temperature: >40°C (104°F).
  - Cardiovascular: Tachycardia, widened pulse pressure (systolic BP—diastolic BP), arrhythmia.
  - Skin: Pallor and excessive sweating.
  - Musculoskeletal: Flaccidity.
  - CNS: Lethargic, headache, weakness, disorientation, confusion, emotionally labile, behavioral changes, seizures, altered consciousness, coma.

Diagnosis:

- Symptoms/signs on physical examination.
- Laboratory tests (as needed).
  - Complete blood count.
  - Comprehensive metabolic panel.
  - Coagulation studies.
  - Urine (ketones, protein, myoglobin).
  - Cardiac biomarkers.
- Imaging (as needed).
  - Chest radiographs.
  - Head CT.

Treatment:

- **General guidelines:**
  - Consider EHI as a continuum which can induce EHS if earlier, less severe variants are not treated expeditiously.
  - Educate medical personnel, athletes, coaches, and parents on prevention of EHI includes the following.
    - Risk factors.
    - The benefits of regular hydration (before, during, and after exercise) and frequent rest periods and altered practice during acclimatization.
    - Over hydration with excessive "free water" can induce exercise-associated hyponatremia (EAH).
    - Benefits of adequate athletic nutrition; if available, involve Team Nutritionist in educational programs.
    - Place urine color charts in bathrooms.
  - Use wet bulb globe temperature (WBGT) index to adequately modify or cancel practices in unfavorable environmental conditions.
  - Establish and diligently adhere to "emergency action plan."
  - Exercise caution in athletes with congenital disorders that predispose to EHI.
  - Communicate with and reassure athletes, coaches, parents.
- **EAMC:**
  - Hydrate.
    - First with oral fluids.
    - If ineffective, consider intravenous hydration for refractory EAMC.
  - Stretch and ice massage.
- **EAC:**
  - Monitor.
    - Airway, Breathing, Circulation (ABC's); recovery is typically spontaneous.
    - Serum sodium: EAC may be induced by EAH.
    - Core temperature: For athletes with prolonged mental status changes >20 minutes; EAC may mimic malignant hyperthermia.
    - Pulse: EAC may be induced by arrhythmias.
  - Elevate lower extremities above level of head to facilitate venous return.

- Hydrate.
  - Oral fluids when fully conscious.
  - Consider IV fluids if unable to consume oral fluids.
- Transport via EMS to nearest medical facility for
  - hyponatremia.
  - rising core temperature.
  - prolonged mental status changes >20 minutes.
  - hemodynamic instability.
- **Heat exhaustion:**
  - Stable, oriented athletes.
    - Rest in cool, shady environment.
    - Remove excessive clothing and sports equipment.
    - Initiate cooling measures: As described in EHS below.
    - Elevate lower extremities above level of head to facilitate venous return.
    - Hydration (as per guidelines above for EAMC).
  - Monitor.
    - Core temperature.
    - Mental status changes: May be normal initially.
  - Transport via EMS to nearest medical facility for
    - rising core temperature.
    - altered mental status following initial, normal assessment.
    - hemodynamic instability.
- **EHS:**
  - General guidelines.
    - "*Be aware*" that initial presentation may not be reflective of underlying severity.
    - "*Rapidly cool first and transport second*" because complications are correlated to the duration of core body temperature elevation.
    - Initiate treatment immediately and activate EMS.
  - Monitor.
    - ABC's.
    - Vitals.
      - Continuously; use rectal thermometer.
      - If possible, measure blood glucose (finger stick) and serum sodium.
  - "Cool first."
    - **How:** Follow "guidelines for cold water immersion": (Table 1)
    - **How long:** Until rectal temperature reaches 38.33° to 39°C (101° to 102°F) (*if rectal thermometer is unavailable, cool until athlete shivers or immerse athlete in cold water for 20 minutes*).
- **Observation and disposition:**
  - After close observation for 1 to 2 hours, clinical improvement and normalization of vital signs and electrolyte abnormalities, athletes may be discharged with a dependable adult.
  - Failure to improve mandates hospital admission to monitor for late development of complications related to multiorgan dysfunction (rhabdomyolysis, acute kidney injury, disseminated intravascular coagulation, liver failure, cardiac arrhythmias).

Other Considerations:

- Athletes with prior history of EHI or especially EHS are at risk for recurrence.
- **EAMC:**
  - Not necessarily induced only by heat; can also occur in cooler environments.
  - Distinguish from sickle cell trait (*as detailed in sickle cell trait chapter*).
  - The consumption of electrolyte containing sports drinks **does not** protect athletes from the development of EAH.
  - For athletes with recurrent EAMC, one-half teaspoon of table salt in sports drinks may be beneficial as a preventive measure.
  - No data exist to support the use of diazepam or magnesium sulfate.

Table 1 Cold Water Immersion Treatment of Exertional Heat Illness

Contact emergency medical services (EMS) immediately.

Assess airway, breathing, circulation, and mental status; measure vital signs before immersing the patient.

If appropriate medical staff is present on-site (e.g., team physician), equipment for aggressive cooling is readily available (e.g., cold water immersion, ice/wet towel rotation, high-flow cold water dousing), and **no other emergency medical treatment is needed** other than rapid lowering of the body temperature, follow the "cool first, transport second" guideline.

For patients to be treated with ice water immersion, prepare as follows:
    Get help.

Move patient to a shaded area.
    Half fill a tub or wading pool with water and ice. Ice should cover the surface of the water at all times.
    A whirlpool tub filled with ice water may be used if the athlete collapses near an athletic training room.

During ice water immersion treatment, assess the patient's core body temperature with a rectal thermistor continuously (a thermistor is a flexible thermometer that remains in place throughout the cooling and treatment process).

Obtain necessary assistance and cool the patient as follows:
    Place the athlete in the ice water immersion tub.
    Cover as much of the body as possible with ice water. If complete coverage is not possible, cover the torso as much as possible.
    Keep the athlete's head and neck above water. An assistant or two can do so by holding the victim under the axillae with a towel or sheet wrapped across the chest and under the arms.
    Place a towel soaked in ice water over the head and neck while the body is being cooled.
    Keep water temperature under 15°C (60°F).
    Vigorously circulate water throughout the cooling process.

Monitor vital signs approximately every 10 minutes and mental status continually during cooling.

Have several additional assistants immediately nearby in case the athlete becomes combative or must be lifted or rolled because of vomiting.

Continue cooling until the patient's rectal temperature reaches 39°C (102°F). If the rectal temperature cannot be measured and on-site ice water immersion is indicated, cool for 10 to 15 minutes and then transport to the emergency department. Cooling via ice water immersion occurs at a rate of approximately 1°C for every 5 minutes (or 1°F every 3 minutes), if the water is aggressively stirred.

Remove the patient from the immersion tub and transfer to the nearest emergency department or hospital after the rectal temperature reaches 39°C (102°F).

If ice water immersion is not feasible given the constraints of the environment, and on-site cooling is appropriate, then cool the patient using the best available means. These may include any of the following three methods:

    Fill a cooler with ice, water, and 12 towels. Place six icy wet towels all over the patient's body. Leave them in place for 2 to 3 minutes, then place those back in cooler and replace them with the six others. Continue this rotation every 2 to 3 minutes.

    Douse the patient continuously with cold water using a shower or hose.

    If ice is available but no tub, place the patient in a tarp or sheet, cover the patient with a large amount of ice, and then wrap the tarp or sheet around them. Replenish the ice as soon as a moderate degree of melting occurs.

Adapted from: The Korey Stringer Institute (ksi.uconn.edu) and Casa DJ, McDermott BM, Lee EC, et al. Cold-water immersion: The gold standard for exertional heat stroke treatment. *Exerc Sport Sci Rev.* 2007; 35:141, with permission.

- **EAC:**
  - Recommend specialist evaluation to distinguish from other causes of syncope (*as detailed in syncope chapter*) *and* other conditions that can present as EAC, including cardiac arrest, EAH, and malignant hyperthermia.
  - Consider direct measurement of serum or plasma sodium in any endurance athlete with seizures, obtundation, and coma which may reflect complications of EAH (hyponatremic encephalopathy).
  - Yet, do not assume that all "collapsed athletes" at endurance events have EAH.
- **EHS:**
  - Is a medical emergency!
  - *Profuse sweating is observed in EHS.*
  - Analgesics and antipyretics (acetaminophen, ibuprofen) can exacerbate EHS.
  - Measure sodium before administering normal saline in order to prevent worsening of occult and undiagnosed EAH.
  - Consider malignant hyperthermia or neuroleptic malignant syndrome in those with suspected EHS who have muscle rigidity.
  - Prophylactic intravenous fluids are banned by the World Anti-Doping Agency (WADA), US Anti-Doping Agency (USADA), and the National Collegiate Athletic Association (NCAA).

Return to Play:

- **EAMC:**
  - Symptom free without any concerns for worsening EHI.
  - Able to perform sports specific agility drills without recurrence.
- **EAC:**
  - Established diagnosis of EAC limited to adverse effects of heat.
  - Other potential, aforementioned causes ruled out following thorough evaluation.
- **Heat exhaustion:**
  - Symptom free without any concerns for worsening EHI.
  - Hydration and caloric status normal; attained ideal body weight (if weight loss was noted after development of heat exhaustion).
  - Demonstrated ability to complete "full practice" without symptoms.
- **EHS:**
  - No exercise for at least 1 week after discharge from medical care.
  - Follow-up with sports medicine team 1 week after discharge for targeted laboratory and imaging studies.
  - After medical clearance:
    - Commence graded, return to play protocol in a cool environment.
    - Gradually increase duration, intensity, and exposure to heat over 2 weeks.
    - Evaluate tolerance to heat exposure.
  - Resume full competition after demonstrated ability to participate fully in the heat without any adverse symptoms for 2 to 4 weeks.
  - Athletes with persistent symptoms (e.g., fatigue) after 2 to 4 weeks, should be considered for exercise-heat tolerance testing to determine if they are "heat intolerant" and are at possible increased risk for recurrent EHS.

Recommended Readings

American College of Sports Medicine, Armstrong LE, Casa DJ, et al. American College of Sports Medicine position stand. Exertional heat illness during training and competition. *Med Sci Sports Exerc.* 2007;39:556.

Asplund CA, O'Connor FG, Noakes TD. Exercise-associated collapse: An evidence-based review and primer for clinicians. *Br J Sports Med.* 2011;45:1157.

Casa DJ, Kenny GP, Taylor NA. Immersion treatment for exertional hyperthermia: Cold or temperate water? *Med Sci Sports Exerc.* 2010;42:1246.

Casa DJ, McDermott BP, Lee EC, et al. Cold water immersion: The gold standard for exertional heatstroke treatment. *Exerc Sport Sci Rev* 2007;35:141.

Centers for Disease Control and Prevention (CDC). Heat illness among high school athletes – United States, 2005–2009. *MMWR Morb Mortal Wkly Rep.* 2010;59:1009.

Dugas J. Sodium ingestion and hyponatraemia: Sports drinks do not prevent a fall in serum sodium concentration during exercise. *Br J Sports Med.* 2006;40:372.

Glazer, J. Management of heatstroke and heat exhaustion. *Am Fam Physician.* 2005 1;71(11):2133–2140.

Heled Y, Rav-Acha M, Shani Y, et al. The "golden hour" for heatstroke treatment. *Mil Med.* 2004; 169:184.

Maron BJ, Doerer JJ, Haas TS, et al. Sudden deaths in young competitive athletes: Analysis of 1866 deaths in the United States, 1980–2006. *Circulation.* 2009;119:1085.

Mueller FO, Cantu RC. Catastrophic sports injury research: Twenty-sixth annual report. University of North Carolina, Chapel Hill, 2008.

2011–2012 NCAA Sports Medicine Handbook. Retrieved March 3rd, 2013, from http://www.ncaapublications.com/productdownloads/MD11.pdf.

O'Connor FG, Casa DJ. Exertional heat illness in adolescents and adults: Epidemiology, thermoregulation, risk factors, and diagnosis. *UpToDate.* Accessed on March 30th, 2013.

O'Connor FG, Casa DJ. Exertional heat illness in adolescents and adults: Management and prevention. *UpToDate.* Accessed on March 30th, 2013.

Rosner MH, Hew-Butler T. Exercise-associated hyponatremia. *UpToDate.* Accessed on March 30th, 2013.

Sithinamsuwan P, Piyavechviratana K, Kitthaweesin T, et al. Exertional heatstroke: Early recognition and outcome with aggressive combined cooling—a 12-year experience. *Mil Med.* 2009;174:496.

Wexler R. Evaluation and treatment of heat-related illnesses. *Am Fam Physician.* 2002;65(11):2307–2315.

WHO. International Classification of Diseases, Clinical Modification (ICD-9-CM). 9th Revision, Centers for Disease Control and Prevention.

www.wada-ama.org. Accessed on March 30th, 2013.

www.usada.org. Accessed on March 30th, 2013.

Heat illness:
"Think about heat illness as a continuum"

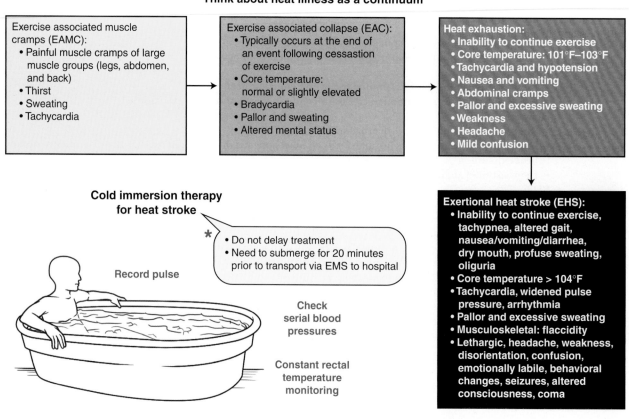

Exercise associated muscle cramps (EAMC):
- Painful muscle cramps of large muscle groups (legs, abdomen, and back)
- Thirst
- Sweating
- Tachycardia

Exercise associated collapse (EAC):
- Typically occurs at the end of an event following cessation of exercise
- Core temperature: normal or slightly elevated
- Bradycardia
- Pallor and sweating
- Altered mental status

Heat exhaustion:
- Inability to continue exercise
- Core temperature: 101°F–103°F
- Tachycardia and hypotension
- Nausea and vomiting
- Abdominal cramps
- Pallor and excessive sweating
- Weakness
- Headache
- Mild confusion

Exertional heat stroke (EHS):
- Inability to continue exercise, tachypnea, altered gait, nausea/vomiting/diarrhea, dry mouth, profuse sweating, oliguria
- Core temperature > 104°F
- Tachycardia, widened pulse pressure, arrhythmia
- Pallor and excessive sweating
- Musculoskeletal: flaccidity
- Lethargic, headache, weakness, disorientation, confusion, emotionally labile, behavioral changes, seizures, altered consciousness, coma

Cold immersion therapy for heat stroke

*
- Do not delay treatment
- Need to submerge for 20 minutes prior to transport via EMS to hospital

Record pulse

Check serial blood pressures

Constant rectal temperature monitoring

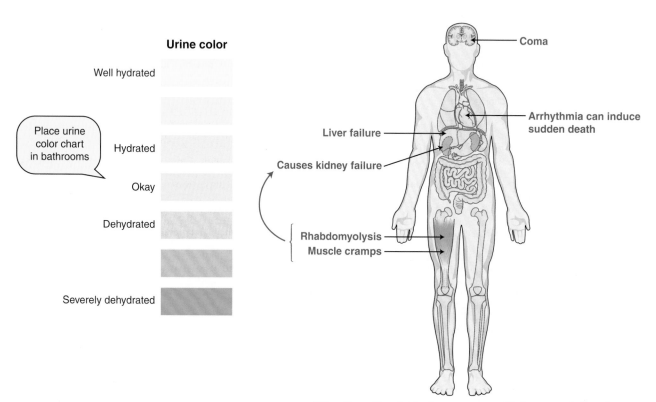

Urine color

Well hydrated

Place urine color chart in bathrooms

Hydrated

Okay

Dehydrated

Severely dehydrated

Coma

Arrhythmia can induce sudden death

Liver failure

Causes kidney failure

Rhabdomyolysis

Muscle cramps

"Exertional heat stroke causes multiple organ failure"

Figure 136. Heat Illness

Hypothermia

Introduction (Definitions/Classification):

- Hypothermia is a medical emergency and defined as a core temperature of less than 35°C (95°F).
- Hypothermia results when the body loses heat faster than generated and most commonly occurs with exposure to cold weather conditions or water; yet may result from any extended exposure to ambient temperatures colder than the body.
- Although, infants and elderly are at greatest risk, there has been an increase in incidence amongst athletes participating in cold weather sports.
- Classification (by core temperature).
  - *Mild hypothermia:* 32° to 35°C (90° to 95°F).
  - *Moderate hypothermia:* 28° to 32°C (82° to 90°F).
  - *Severe hypothermia:* <28°C (82°F).
- Mortality from moderate or severe accidental hypothermia is ~40%.

History and Physical Examination:

- **History (*evaluate risk factors*):**
  - Prolonged activity in a cold environment without appropriate warm or dry clothing.
  - Dehydration.
  - Poor nutrition: Hypoglycemia, thiamine deficiency.
  - Drugs.
    - *Impaired thermoregulation:* Opioids, anxiolytics, antipsychotics/antimanics, antidepressants.
    - *Impaired compensation to cold:* Beta-blockers, alpha-adrenergic agonists (clonidine), oral antihyperglycemics.
  - Medical illness: Anorexia nervosa, multiple sclerosis, hypothyroidism, adrenal insufficiency, psychiatric illness.
  - Sleep deprivation.
  - Intoxicants: Ethanol, carbon monoxide.
- **Physical Examination:** Nonspecific symptoms and signs classified by severity include the following.
- *Mild hypothermia:* Shivering, perioral cyanosis, dysarthria, tachycardia, hyperventilation/tachypnea, impaired memory/judgment, ataxia, "cold dieresis."
- *Moderate hypothermia:* Loss of shivering, junctional bradycardia/decreased cardiac output/atrial fibrillation/arrhythmias, hypoventilation/shallow breathing, hyporeflexia, decreased alertness/extreme fatigue, decreased renal blood flow/oliguria, paradoxical undressing.
- *Severe hypothermia:* Bradycardia/hypotension/ventricular fibrillation/asystole, pulmonary edema, absent reflexes/dilated and fixed pupils/coma, oliguria.

Diagnosis:

- Established by a combination of symptoms/signs on physical examination and history of cold exposure.
- Degree of hypothermia determined by core temperature (*as detailed above*).
- EKG.
  - Osborn or J waves.
    - Elevation of J point in V2 to V5.
    - Height of elevation is ~ proportional to degree of hypothermia.
  - Sinus bradycardia.
  - Prolonged QTc, PR, and QRS, inverted T waves.
  - Atrial fibrillation (<34°C, <93°F), ventricular fibrillation (<28°C, <82°F), and asystole (<20°C, <68°F).
  - AV block (1° < 33°C; complete <20°C, <68°F).
- Laboratory findings (in moderate and severe hypothermia) may include the following.
  - Complete blood count.
    - Elevated hematocrit due to dehydration (2% per 1° temperature drop).
    - Leukocytosis due to demargination.
    - Leukopenia and thrombocytopenia decreased due to splenic sequestration.
  - Comprehensive metabolic panel.
    - Glucose variable.
    - Inconsistent electrolyte abnormalities, thus reassess every 4 to 6 hours.
  - Pancreatic function tests.
    - Lipase elevation suggestive of hypothermia-induced pancreatitis.
  - Coagulation studies (PT/PTT).
    - Maybe reported as normal.
    - Abnormal in vivo, because coagulation cascade is inhibited.

- Blood gas.
  - Either metabolic acidosis or respiratory alkalosis, or both.
  - May not be accurate because analyzers are programmed to work at 37°C (98.6°F).
- Chest radiographs (findings consistent with either/or).
  - Pulmonary edema.
  - Vascular congestion.
  - Aspiration pneumonia.
- *Caution (miscellaneous diagnostic considerations).*
  - EKG changes.
    - J point elevation may be also noted in Brugada syndrome, hypercalcemia, or early repolarization (athlete's heart syndrome).
    - Associated with hyperkalemia are masked by hypothermia.
    - EKG machine may interpret Osborn J waves as ischemia.
  - Hyperglycemia following aggressive rewarming is suggestive of either diabetic ketoacidosis or pancreatitis because insulin function is ineffectual <30°C (86°F).
  - Toxicology screen: In individuals with mental status changes that does not match the degree of hypothermia.
  - Endocrine studies: In individuals who fail aggressive rewarming, to test for thyroid or adrenal dysfunction.

Treatment:

- Prevention by education.
  - Educate.
    - Risk factors.
    - Differential diagnosis of hypothermia.
    - Medical personnel entrusted with the care of athletes involved in winter sports should possess either low-reading glass or electronic thermometers to accurately gauge core temperature.
  - Counsel on appropriate clothing.
    - Ensure the use of loose layers of clothing, including a waterproof shell.
    - If precipitation is expected, minimize the amount of cotton clothing.
    - Carry an extra set of clothes to change into when from sweaty, wet clothes.
  - Counsel on the importance of communication.
    - Ask athletes to inform family and friends about their plans for training programs in isolated areas.
    - Keep cell phones insulated from the cold to avoid malfunction.
    - Consider training with a partner in cold temperatures in remote areas.
- General guidelines.
  - If individual is noncommunicative, stabilize the patient and immediately activate EMS.
    - Monitor airways, breathing, and circulation (ABC's).
    - Survey the entire body to assess for local areas of cold associated injury/trauma.
    - Check "central pulse" for a full minute.
    - Handle the individual gently to avoid inducing arrhythmias.
    - Minimize unnecessary movements; *do not massage*.
    - Move individuals, as needed, in a "horizontal position."
  - If alert, encourage consumption of warm, nonalcoholic, noncaffeinated beverages.
  - Monitor oxygenation by placing probe on ears or forehead.
  - Monitor core temperature during rewarming to minimize risk for iatrogenic hyperthermia.
    - Increases at ~2°C per hour with active external or active internal rewarming.
- Resuscitation.
  - Continue, regardless of duration, until core temperature is 32° to 35°C (90° to 95°F).
  - CPR as indicated, unless chest wall is frozen.
  - Cardiac defibrillation.
    - Usually ineffective until core temperature is >86°F (30°C).
  - Rehydration.
    - Insert two large bore (14 or 16 gauge) peripheral intravenous catheters.
    - Use warmed (40° to 42°C, 104° to 108°F) normal saline.
    - Avoid lactated ringers secondary to potential hypothermia-induced liver dysfunction.
- Rewarming—*goal is to reheat core temperature to 97.8°F (37°C)*:
  - *Mild hypothermia:*
    - Passive external rewarming (PER):
      - Cut away wet clothing.
      - Cover individual with dry coats or blankets covering the head, while leaving only the face exposed.

INDEX